INSTRUCTOR'S MANUAL TO ACCOMPANY

NURSING ASSISTANT

A Nursing Process Approach

10th Edition

Barbara R. Hegner, MSN, RN

(deceased)

Barbara Acello, MS, RN

Independent Nurse Consultant and Educator

Esther Caldwell, MA, PhD

Consultant in Vocational Education (CA)

THOMSON
_____
DELMAR LEARNING

Australia   Brazil   Canada   Mexico   Singapore   Spain   United Kingdom   United States

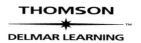

THOMSON

DELMAR LEARNING

Instructor's Manual to Accompany Nursing Assistant: A Nursing Process Approach
Tenth Edition
by Barbara R. Hegner, Barbara Acello, and Esther Caldwell

Vice President,
Health Care Business Unit:
William Brottmiller

Director of Learning Solutions:
Matthew Kane

Managing Editor:
Marah Bellegarde

Acquisitions Editor:
Matthew Seeley

Product Manager:
Jadin Babin-Kavanaugh

Editorial Assistant:
Megan Tarquinio

Marketing Director:
Jennifer McAvey

Senior Marketing Manager:
Lynn Henn

Marketing Manager:
Michele McTighe

Marketing Coordinator:
Chelsey Iaquinta

Technology Director:
Laurie Davis

Technology Product Manager:
Mary Colleen Liburdi

Technology Project Manager:
Carolyn Fox

Production Director:
Carolyn Miller

Content Project Manager:
Kenneth McGrath

Senior Art Director:
Jack Pendleton

Library of Congress Cataloging-in-
Publication Data

ISBN 10: 1-4180-6608-7
ISBN 13: 978-1-4180-6608-6

Contents

PART 1 INSTRUCTOR'S OBJECTIVES, SUGGESTED ACTIVITIES, AND ANSWERS TO UNIT REVIEWS 1

List of Procedures

List of Guidelines Included in Textbook

To the Instructor

THE NEW EDITION

The 10th edition of the *Instructor's Manual to Accompany Nursing Assistant: A Nursing Process Approach* continues to be an excellent reference for defining and clarifying instructional content for nursing assistants. The new edition of the *Instructor's Manual* contains numerous content changes. These changes were made to ensure the effectiveness and usefulness of the *Instructor's Manual* as a superior teaching tool for the instructor. To keep up with the ever-changing health care industry, the text has been updated extensively to reflect current practices, equipment, and skills. The nursing assistant of the 21st century must be a skilled paraprofessional. As the instructor, you establish the foundation and motivate the assistant to succeed. Correlated to the new edition of the text, this manual also ties the information presented to federal legislation mandated by the Omnibus Budget Reconciliation Act of 1987 (OBRA). An extensive section has been added to the student workbook on studying for and taking the state written and competency evaluation.

TEXT FORMAT

The text is organized as follows:

Student Objectives

Each lesson is preceded by a series of student behavioral objectives. These help direct the learning process by focusing student attention on the expected outcome of their work. Students should be encouraged to review these objectives before class begins and to review them once more after the lesson is completed.

The Unit

Each unit is written in simple language, well illustrated, with new words highlighted and explained. Related procedures are included where appropriate, so that students have a step-by-step guide to performance.

Vocabulary

A list of new words, medical terminology, or abbreviations is found at the beginning of each unit. Some instructors prefer to review these before the unit begins, whereas others assign students to research each new vocabulary word by looking it up in the glossary located at the back of the text.

Alert Boxes

Text alerts were added to the book in the ninth edition, and have been well received, quickly becoming a popular feature with both students and instructors. The alerts provide important information on age-appropriate care, communication, difficult patient care and important patient information, infection control, legal information pertaining to the nursing assistant, OSHA and personal injury prevention, and patient safety. New clinical information and culture alerts were added to the 10th edition. The information in the alert boxes makes the learner aware of best practices in patient care, includes practical tips based on clinical experience, and highlights critical infection control and key safety and OSHA workplace guidelines.

Guidelines

Many of the units contain guidelines, which are listed in the table of contents. These guidelines are in an easy-to-use format that highlights key points students must learn and remember for specific types of care and special situations.

Procedures

The text contains 132 procedures in an easy-to-use format. Each procedure begins with a reminder to carry out initial procedure actions and ends with a reminder to perform ending procedure actions. A list of equipment and supplies needed is included with each procedure. Notes and cautions that the nursing assistant needs to know are added to some procedures. The steps move sequentially through the procedure, all the while emphasizing patient safety, infection control, dignity, and privacy.

Unit Reviews

A variety of questions follow each unit, to allow students to assess their mastery of the subject matter. You may also use the questions as a test vehicle or as a basis for review discussion. Each unit corresponds to a section in the student workbook. Assignments in the workbook reinforce student understanding.

Glossary

A glossary of all vocabulary words is located at the back of the text.

SUPPLEMENTS PACKAGE

In addition to the newly revised and updated *Instructor's Manual*, several supplements complement the 10th edition of the text. With these supplements, *Nursing Assistant: A Nursing Process Approach* becomes a **turnkey** competency-based educational package. The supplements now available to be used with the text include:

Student Resources

- **StudyWare CD-ROM** is included in the back of the text and features quizzes, games, and case studies for each unit. Students can take the quizzes in Practice Mode to improve mastery of the material; instant feedback tells whether an answer is right or wrong, and explains why. Quiz Mode allows students to test themselves and keep a record of their scores. StudyWare games, flashcards, and image labeling exercises reinforce unit content, and the unique critical thinking case studies help synthesize and apply unit topics to real-world scenarios.

- **Student Workbook** has been updated with new content and directly correlates to the textbook. This competency-based supplement includes challenging items such as word word games, puzzles, and exercises to help students understand essential content and master defining and spelling key terms. A new section on studying for the state written and competency examination has been added to the workbook, designed to help students who will be taking a state certification exam.

- **Online Companion** features additional procedures and resources to supplement book content, plus up-to-date information on ever-changing practices and standards in nursing assisting.

- **On the Job: The Essentials of Nursing Assisting** is a handy pocket reference designed to keep critical nursing care information at the fingertrips of practicing nursing assistants. Many safety and infection control alerts, as well as suggested responses to common situations, are easily referenced using this book.

Instructor Resources

The following comprehensive tools are available to instructors:

Instructor's Manual

Contains answer keys to all text and student workbook exercises, in addition to lesson plans, student and instructor resources, quizzes and testing material, performance competency checklists for procedures, and numerous images to use as transparency masters and student handouts. The *Instructor's Manual* is available in print, and is also available electronically, both on the Electronic Classroom Manager CD-ROM and on the instructor's side of the Online Companion.

Instructor's Resource Kit

This kit provides you with in-depth resources to help simplify the planning and implementation of a nursing assisting instructional program. It integrates the use of the text, *Student Workbook*, Electronic Classroom Manager, *Instructor's Manual*, and skills videos to help you develop an efficient instructional plan. The Instructor's Resource Kit includes comprehensive teaching resources, course syllabi, unit outlines, lesson plans with supplemental materials, and English-Spanish flashcards with common terms and simple phrases.

Electronic Classroom Manager CD-ROM

This new supplement features a **Computerized Test Bank** with more than 3,000 questions in *ExamView*® *Pro* test generator software, and over 700 **PowerPoint**™ slides with illustrations from the text. Also includes electronic versions of both the Instructor's Manual and the Instructor's Resource Kit.

Online Companion

This key resource is available for the first time with the 10th edition, and includes additional procedures and skills checklists. For your convenience, the Online Companion will also include an electronic version of the *Instructor's Manual* and Instructor's Resource Kit.

Nursing Assisting: Basic Skills DVD-ROM

Finally, skills-based videos to accompany many of the procedures in the text! Each of the 76 core procedures is presented step-by-step for maximum effectiveness. These videos are great for in-class demonstration to help prepare students for exams or for clinical rotations. For your convenience, a DVD icon appears in the text on every procedure that has a corresponding video clip.

WebTutor™

This course cartridge for Blackboard and WebCT can be used to supplement on-campus course delivery or as the course management platform for an online course. WebTutor™ includes threaded discussion questions, critical thinking questions, study tips, class notes, quizzes, and Internet activities.

Yours is an exciting challenge! Good luck!

STATE AND FEDERAL REQUIREMENTS

Instructors must keep in mind that the federal rules set the core requirements for nursing assistant education, and that this program is designed exclusively for long-term care. Each state is free to modify the core program as it sees fit, and most states have done this. The only federal mandate is that the federal list of core content be presented. Some states require as little as 75 hours of education, which is the minimum federal requirement, whereas others require as much as 175. Some facilities choose to provide additional hours above the state-mandated minimums, and this is usually acceptable and encouraged. In fact, facilities should be commended for providing a thorough program that meets the needs of the nursing assistants, patients, and residents.

Considering the nature of the work nursing assistants do and the responsibilities they carry, there has been intermittent dialogue regarding the need to increase the mandatory OBRA education requirements. This suggestion is not without opposition, because of the potential expense to the employer.[1] According to the Paraprofessional Healthcare Institute (PHI), "'Raising the bar' for entrance into the field may seem counterintuitive in this time of widespread vacancies. But these recommendations are based on the observation that the most effective way of addressing vacancies is retaining more of the nursing assistants already in the field, not trying to lure a constant stream of new applicants through a revolving door—and that providing CNAs with adequate training and support is key to improving retention."[2]

At present, there is nothing related to a change in nursing assistant education on the federal legislative slate, although this is always a possibility in the future. The long-term care population has become much more fragile and unstable than it was in the past. Given the responsibilities that nursing assistants carry, most educators agree that the minimum education requirements have not kept pace with patient and resident needs. Increasing the educational requirements will better prepare nursing assistants as safe entry-level practitioners. In addition to providing better resident/patient care, increasing the educational requirements will also improve the work environment and working conditions for nursing assistants.

Some states require all nursing assistants to complete the basic nursing assistant program (which is based on the minimum OBRA requirements), including assistants who work in nursing homes, hospitals, and home health care. Others require course completion only by assistants working in long-term care and home health. Some states require completion of this course only by assistants working in long-term care. Some states require the basic 75-hour OBRA course as one part of a tiered package leading to home health care or hospital nursing assistant certification, whereas other states have separate, distinct programs for each of these positions. Some schools give certified nursing assistants advanced standing in LPN/LVN and RN programs; others do not. Some schools require successful completion of the nursing assistant program as the first rung on the ladder of the LPN/LVN or RN degree, whereas others prefer that students not be certified as nursing assistants when they enroll in the nursing class. Some nurse educators believe that current learning theory has demonstrated that it is much more difficult to change your thinking than to learn with a "clean slate." The premise is that once individuals learn to think like a CNA or LPN/LVN, it is much more difficult to learn to think like an RN. This author is unaware of any validation for this commonly held point of view, and the anecdotal information is presented only for your contemplation and consideration. You may find additional information on evaluating this type of program, or request a review of a tiered nursing program, at http://www.whatworks.ed.gov/.

Some states will not grant program approval or provider status to hospitals that wish to provide basic nursing assistant education. Because nursing assistant education is mandated only for long-term care, these states will approve only long-term care facilities and freestanding educational agencies, such as community colleges and proprietary schools. Hospitals have learned that they can usually circumvent this requirement if the facility has a skilled nursing unit which holds a separate long-term care facility license. Once the skilled unit program has been approved, the state may permit the hospital to present additional content that is specific to the acute care hospital only. For example, many hospitals teach nursing assistants to remove indwelling catheters and do fingerstick blood glucose tests. The state permits the hospital to teach this content, but may require the facility to provide all long-term care content first. This is not an unreasonable request, and many hospitals have designed their programs in this manner, to meet the needs of patients and residents throughout the facility.

---

[1] § 483.152 (c) Prohibition of charges. (1) No nurse aide who is employed by, or who has received an offer of employment from, a facility on the date on which the aide begins a nurse aide training and competency evaluation program may be charged for any portion of the program (including any fees for textbooks or other required course materials). (2) If an individual who is not employed, or does not have an offer to be employed, as a nurse aide becomes employed by, or receives an offer of employment from, a facility not later than 12 months after completing a nurse aide training and competency evaluation program, the State must provide for the reimbursement of costs incurred in completing the program on a pro rata basis during the period in which the individual is employed as a nurse aide.

[2] *Certified Nurse Aide "Model" Program* (available for download at http://www.ltccc.org/papers/cna.htm).

State-Specific Class Variations

Each state has a mandatory skills set that nursing assistants must learn. These vary widely in procedural techniques and steps, as well as procedural content. For example, some states require the federal minimum skills set. This is required "OBRA content." Other states have added to the federal skills list with additional skills, such as using the Wound V.A.C. (Vacuum Assisted Closure), caring for an artificial eye, and providing sterile eye compresses. This is state-specific content that is not required by the OBRA rules; thus, although relevant, it is not considered OBRA content. An example of procedural variations is seen in female peri care. In many states, the procedures state to clean the labia from top to bottom in this order:

- far side
- near side
- center

Many other states require this sequence:

- center
- far side
- near side

This may seem like a minor discrepancy, but in some states it is very significant. Doing the procedure out of sequence will result in failing the skill on the skills examination.

OBRA-specific content is mandated only under the federal rules. However, even the federal list is somewhat subjective. For example, consider the requirement for content on transfers. Some states consider this requirement met if the program teaches the one-person transfer and two-person transfer. However, other states believe that the content should be much more exhaustive and include procedures with and without a gait belt, transfers on and off the toilet, transfers to and from a stretcher, and transfers involving both a manual mechanical lift and an electronic lift. The mandatory OBRA content is listed in Table 1. If your state requires additional didactic content or procedures that are not generally listed here, the content is state-specific and not OBRA-required.

Each state sets its own requirements for program length. This is the total number of hours needed to successfully complete the class. (State written and skills testing hours are in addition to the class; they are not part of the class.) Each state specifies a minimum number of classroom hours, skills lab hours, and clinical hours. The most current available breakdown is listed in Table 2. This information is changed frequently, and some states do not consistently respond to surveys regarding their mandatory content requirements.

Other types of state-specific curriculum variations include:

- Number of hours required to be devoted to specific content. (For example, Illinois requires a minimum of 12 hours of content related to Alzheimer's disease and dementia. Many states require additional hours of content pertaining to HIV.)
- Minimum age at which a student may take the class. (For example, Florida and Oregon require that students be 18 years of age or older. A number of other states impose a requirement of 16 years of age or older, whereas Mississippi imposes a 17-year age limit.)
- Minimum education requirement prior to taking the class.
- Ability to speak, read, and write in English at a certain proficiency level. (For example, Illinois states that assistants "must be able to speak and understand English *or a language understood by a substantial percentage of a facility's residents.*")
- Inclusion or exclusion of home care information.
- Mandated instructor-to-student ratios, such as 1 instructor to 8 students.
- Content of state written and skills examination.
- Which examination is given first (written or skills).

Table 1   OBRA Required Nursing Assistant Program Content

(42 C.F.R. § 483.152) The nursing assistant program curriculum must include:

(1) At least a total of 16 hours of training in the following areas prior to any direct contact with a resident:

(i) Communication and interpersonal skills;

(ii) Infection control;

(iii) Safety/emergency procedures, including the Heimlich maneuver;

(iv) Promoting residents' independence; and

(v) Respecting residents' rights.

The remaining 59 hours must cover:

(2) Basic nursing skills;

(i) Taking and recording vital signs;

(ii) Measuring and recording height and weight;

(iii) Caring for the residents' environment;

(iv) Recognizing abnormal changes in body functioning and the importance of reporting such changes to a supervisor; and

(v) Caring for residents when death is imminent.

(3) Personal care skills, including, but not limited to—

(i) Bathing;

(ii) Grooming, including mouth care;

(iii) Dressing;

(iv) Toileting;

(v) Assisting with eating and hydration;

(vi) Proper feeding techniques;

(vii) Skin care; and

(viii) Transfers, positioning, and turning.

(4) Mental health and social service needs:

(i) Modifying aide's behavior in response to residents' behavior;

(ii) Awareness of developmental tasks associated with the aging process;

(iii) How to respond to resident behavior;

(iv) Allowing the resident to make personal choices, providing and reinforcing other behavior consistent with the resident's dignity; and

(v) Using the resident's family as a source of emotional support.

(5) Care of cognitively impaired residents:

(i) Techniques for addressing the unique needs and behaviors of individual with dementia (Alzheimer's and others);

(ii) Communicating with cognitively impaired residents;

(iii) Understanding the behavior of cognitively impaired residents;

(iv) Appropriate responses to the behavior of cognitively impaired residents; and

(v) Methods of reducing the effects of cognitive impairments.

(6) Basic restorative services:

(i) Training the resident in self care according to the resident's abilities;

(ii) Use of assistive devices in transferring, ambulation, eating, and dressing;

(iii) Maintenance of range of motion;

(iv) Proper turning and positioning in bed and chair;

(v) Bowel and bladder training; and

(vi) Care and use of prosthetic and orthotic devices.

(continues)

Table 1   OBRA Required Nursing Assistant Program Content (*Continued*)

(7) Residents' Rights.

    (i) Providing privacy and maintenance of confidentiality;

    (ii) Promoting the residents' right to make personal choices to accommodate their needs;

    (iii) Giving assistance in resolving grievances and disputes;

    (iv) Providing needed assistance in getting to and participating in resident and family groups and other activities;

    (v) Maintaining care and security of residents' personal possessions;

    (vi) Promoting the residents' right to be free from abuse, mistreatment, and neglect and the need to report any instances of such treatment to appropriate facility staff;

    (vii) Avoiding the need for restraints in accordance with current professional standards.

[As you can see, the OBRA-required subject matter is subjective and largely determined by each state within the parameters listed here. There is also no specific requirement for clinical time, or a mandatory number of hours specified for classroom, skills lab, or clinical. This is also left up to each individual state.]

For the specific legal citation related to the basic nursing assistant program, go to:

Code of Federal Regulations, Title 42, Volume 3, Parts 430 to End, Revised as of October 1, 1999

http://frwebgate.access.gpo.gov/cgi-bin/get-cfr.cgi?TITLE=42&PART=483&SECTION=152&YEAR=1999&TYPE=TEXT

or

http://makeashorterlink.com/?H4A423A1E

The federal rules also specify the requirements for the written and competency evaluation at 42 C.F.R § 483.154.

Table 2   Length of Nursing Assistant Program

75 hours	Alabama, Arkansas, Colorado, Iowa, Kentucky, Massachusetts, Michigan, Minnesota, Mississippi, Montana, Nebraska, Nevada, New Mexico, North Dakota, Ohio, Oklahoma, Pennsylvania, South Dakota, Tennessee, Texas, Vermont, and Wisconsin
80 hours	Georgia, Louisiana, North Carolina, South Carolina, and Utah
85 hours	Washington
90 hours	Kansas, New Jersey, and Wyoming
100 hours	Connecticut, Hawaii, Maryland, New Hampshire, Rhode Island, and New York
120 hours	Arizona, District of Columbia, Florida, Idaho, Illinois, Virginia, and West Virginia
121 hours	Indiana
140 hours	Alaska
150 hours	California, Delaware, Maine, and Oregon
175 hours	Missouri

- Whether the skills examination is given in a laboratory or facility.

- How the written and skills exam are given and proctored, including whether skills are done on manikins, student volunteers, or facility residents. (Federal testing guidelines are provided in 42 C.F.R. § 483.152.)

Additional variations include key areas in which states have augmented postcertification requirements:

- Need for criminal background checks (both initial and on renewal of certification).

- Certain character traits required for the person to work as a nursing assistant. (For example, Illinois requires that assistants be "of temperate habits and good moral character, honest, reliable and trustworthy.")

- Process for filing a complaint and conducting a hearing on abuse, neglect, or misappropriation of property.

- Method for verifying an assistant's registry status before hiring.

■ Need for enhanced and expanded curriculum for nursing assistant education.

■ Specified annual number of hours of postclass, in-service education.

■ Specified curriculum topics for in-service education (such as accident prevention, infection control, resident rights, and needs of special populations).

■ Specific requirements for annual competency checkoff. For example, the federal rules require facilities to conduct "annual competency reviews" for each nursing assistant. This is not the same as the performance evaluation that addresses appearance, dependability, attendance, and so forth. Each nursing assistant must be given an annual performance review that identifies weaknesses and is used as a basis for influencing the structure of the in-service education program. The in-service education program must also address special needs of residents to whom the assistant provides care, such as residents who are cognitively impaired.

■ Requirements and need for additional, individualized, hands-on education.

■ Specified number of hours worked biannually to renew certification; some states require as little as 7 hours, and others require as many as 64 hours. If the assistant does not work the required number of hours, he or she must repeat the class and/or state test.

The Nursing Process Approach

Nursing assistants often provide care by using either intuition or rationale. Rationale is a very important part of critical thinking for assistants who understand the nursing process. Educational programs and facilities that believe in and promote this approach usually have a structure for timely and accurate communication, and value the assistants' contribution to patient care plans. This results in nursing assistants who make good decisions and patients with better outcomes.

The nursing assistant has evolved from an unlicensed, untrained individual, to an educated, skilled paraprofessional who passes a certification examination and is listed with the state nursing assistant registry. Many are performing advanced skills that were formerly limited to nurses. Hospitals are providing ongoing education to upgrade their personnel. More is expected of the nursing assistant than ever before. Use of the nursing process is a critical element in the delivery of effective patient care, and we are committed to this method of learning and care delivery. Patient care units run more efficiently and effectively if the nursing department promotes and adheres to this model of care. Students who have learned the nursing process approach are stronger clinicians who employ the principles of critical thinking in their jobs, and this is reflected in improved performance. A breakdown of the nursing process commonly leads to negative outcomes and litigation. When making clinical judgments, nurses must base their decisions on the consideration of consequences, which prescribe and justify nursing actions.[3] The importance of the nursing assistant's contribution to the process cannot be minimized. Because of this, theory is included in the textbook when it is necessary to understand the reason for a procedure or to apply the information to other similar clinical situations. In addition to traditional nursing procedures, the text includes lists of guidelines that describe how to manage many common resident care situations.

Teaching the assistant how to contribute to the nursing process is an excellent means of ensuring high-quality nursing care. Documentation and quality of the patients' care plans are also enhanced if the plans reflect nursing assistant input. Students who have not participated in care plan decisions should be informed about how the care and services they provide improve and/or maintain the patient's condition and minimize patient decline. This information is essential to their understanding of how to employ critical thinking, use the nursing process, and recognize or identify the expected outcomes for the patient. Without knowing the reasons why they are performing particular tasks, direct care staff may not understand the relationship between the care and services they provide for a patient and the expected or actual outcomes for that patient.

Nursing Assistant: A Nursing Process Approach was written and designed to prepare the nursing assistant to work in a hospital, long-term care facility, hospital skilled unit, or subacute care center, and exceeds the core OBRA requirements

[3]American Nurses' Association (Eds.). *Code for nurses.* (2002). Washington, D.C.: American Nurses Publishing.

for nursing assistant education. Some common procedures that are considered advanced have been included for your convenience, such as performing the fingerstick blood glucose test. The text emphasizes real-world clinical practice, and provides solutions to common problems that nursing assistants encounter. Compliance with current infection control and safety practices, Joint Commission, OSHA, state and federal regulations is emphasized. Our goal is to make the instructor's job easier and make learning comprehensive, clear, and as stress-free as possible for the students. *Nursing Assistant: A Nursing Process Approach* is designed to parallel the nursing assistant curriculum, as much as possible, considering the many variables noted earlier. Although the federal requirements for nursing assistant education are standardized, as you can see, there is no universal curriculum for OBRA-approved nursing assistant education, and many instructors consider their state curriculum to be the ultimate authority on what OBRA requires. This is a common misconception. OBRA is a federal law, not a state law. We have organized your book using a modular approach and grouped material by body system. However, certain principles, such as safety, infection control, and dignity, are integrated throughout the book.

A Tiered System

A number of states have changed their laws to enable hospitals and long-term care facilities to offer a means for nursing assistant advancement. The goal of this type of program is to improve and enhance patient care and worker satisfaction, improve retention, and save money associated with staff turnover. Having a multitiered structure provides an opportunity for workers to increase their knowledge and skills, salary, and status. Increasing the pay and professionalization of jobs is very desirable for many nursing assistants. States and facilities that have implemented such programs have found them well received, and the nursing assistants are very enthusiastic about their new career opportunities. Having successful workers as mentors or role models, either formal or informal, is also an important motivator.

As a rule, employees begin on the first tier of the ladder. They have usually completed the basic nursing assistant class and are entered on the registry ("certified") to work in their state. Some facilities require assistants to be employed for a specified period of time before becoming qualified to advance to the next tier. To do so, additional education is almost always required, resulting in a higher percentage of well-trained and informed employees. Upon meeting the qualifications for this tier, the assistant usually receives an increase in pay. It is helpful for facilities to publish a booklet listing all available jobs and their requirements. Assistants can review the job description for their current job and compare it with the requirements of another position, such as attendance and length of employment, required classes, and certificates. The booklet should also list assistance available, through the facility, scholarships, or outside agencies.

Some facilities stop with two tiers, but others have three or more tiers in their program. Each level requires a specified length of employment and proficiency, with completion of another class. Sometimes the classes are offered in the facility, but some have partnered with a local community college or unions to provide the training. Successful class completion may not guarantee promotion to the next level. The nursing assistant may be required to take a test, and/or to meet certain attendance requirements or other criteria. In some facilities, a designated number of advanced positions are available, and the employee cannot advance until a position is open. In some facilities, advancing through the career ladder will provide employees with the opportunity to go to school for an LPN/LVN or RN degree.

Another consideration is that the ladder need not be linear. Some employees may wish to move laterally to obtain a broad base of education and experience, and find the area in which they derive the most job satisfaction. Examples of advanced educational classes or positions in use at present are:

- Certified Nursing Assistant (CNA) 2, 3, or 4
- Restorative Care Specialist
- Geriatric Care Specialist
- Physical and/or Rehabilitation Aide
- Feeding and Nutrition Specialist
- Dementia Care Specialist
- End-of-Life/Palliative Care Specialist

- Medication Technician

- Nursing Assistant Mentor (works with new employees)

- Advanced Skills Specialist (using skills such as dressing changes, sterile technique, ostomy care, and catheterization)

As you can see, there are many ways to implement a program of this nature. Each facility develops criteria to meet its own specific needs. When developing career ladders, facilities must also consider obstacles that prevent assistants from taking advantage of the tiered structure. For example, before making a commitment, employees must consider whether attending a class or changing positions will require trade-offs and adjustments in their personal lives. For example, parenting responsibilities, child care arrangements, costs of child care and transportation, and an overall short-age of time must be considered. The career ladder may be unusable, and advancement unattainable, without some type of financial subsidy or time off.

Career ladders are not for everyone. Some workers are satisfied in a given position and should not be made to feel that they are less desirable workers if they choose not to advance. This may be a special problem for single mothers who are struggling to manage their many responsibilities. They may choose to forego continuing education to spend time with their children. Some do not have computers or online access at home. These things are often necessary for class assignments. Although the school may have a computer lab available, the student may not have a babysitter or trans-portation enabling him or her to use the computers at the school or facility.

Although career ladders are not a panacea for improved job satisfaction and turnover reduction, they are one approach that has been used successfully to address these problems, and may be worthy of consideration in your facil-ity. A paper entitled *An Overview of Advanced or NA II Programs* provides practical suggestions for facilities that are con-sidering a program of this nature; it is available from:

Genevieve Gipson, RN, MEd, RNC

Career Nurse Assistants Programs, Inc.

National Network of Career Nursing Assistants

3577 Easton Road

Norton, OH 44203-5661

Ph 330-825 9342

Fax 330-8125 9378

E-mail: cnajeni@aol.com

Web site: http://www.cna-network.org

Another excellent, free, 161-page booklet, entitled *How Career Lattices Help Solve Nursing and Other Workforce Short-ages in Healthcare,* is available at http://www.caelhealthcare.org/pdf/healthcare_career_lattices_report.pdf.

You can easily use *Nursing Assistant: A Nursing Process Approach* for two or more tiers of a ladder program. Thomson Delmar Learning has additional books and audiovisuals available to meet facility needs for advanced skills education.

Nursing Assistant Instructor Challenges

The authors and editors of this book recognize that the job of the nursing assistant instructor is both challenging and rewarding. Finding a book that covers your state-specific content in reasonable order is a challenge in itself! As you know, we have 50 states and 50 different requirements for nursing assistant education. Satisfying the needs of programs designed by 50 states and thousands of individual facilities with a single textbook is challenging (at best) and difficult (at worst). Likewise, we understand the frustrations of the instructor who must jump from one end of the book to an-other to present the material, and have done our best to minimize this problem by grouping the material into like sec-tions. Facilities also have a say in how their curriculum is presented, and are usually free to exceed the minimum num-ber of hours required by their state. In addition to curriculum content variations, each state and facility may have a required number of hours for each unit and/or a specified order in which content must be presented. Instructors would love a textbook that flows with their program, but the task of creating one is almost impossible, for the reasons noted here. We have endeavored to meet your needs by grouping the material in logical order and providing a turnkey package of supplements to help you in your job. We welcome your suggestions and comments, and appreciate your selection and continued use of *Nursing Assistant: A Nursing Process Approach*.

TEACHING ADULT LEARNERS

There are many rewards in teaching adult learners. Students come to class with varied experiences, abilities, values, knowledge levels, and cultural backgrounds. Some of them may have been out of a classroom setting for several years—these individuals usually have high anxiety levels about their ability to succeed. You may encounter other students who have recently experienced high levels of success in the classroom but who have great difficulty in applying knowledge to the clinical situation.

Try to find the strengths of your students within the first few days of class and allow them to capitalize and build on these strengths. Assist students to strengthen their weaker areas. Here are some suggestions that may be helpful.

1. Be aware of the image you are projecting to students. It is important to:

   ■ Establish credibility. You must have confidence in your own abilities to teach and in your skills as a nurse.

   ■ Be professional, approachable, and flexible. Your appearance, posture, language, and mannerisms all send messages to students. Be sure you are sending a positive message.

   ■ Be able to say "I don't know," but be willing to work with students to find the right answer.

   ■ Reflect your enthusiasm for nursing and teaching.

   ■ Learn students' names by the end of the first class and use their names when addressing them.

2. Set and maintain standards for your students. They need to know those standards before or on the first day of class.

   ■ What criteria are used to establish pass/fail limits?

   ■ Do you have a policy for absenteeism and tardiness? (Federal law and state laws require a minimum number of hours for nursing assistant courses.) If students miss a class, how will they make it up?

   ■ What is expected of students during the time they are in your class?

   ■ Will there be breaks or mealtimes? At what point in the class do these occur, and for how long?

   ■ Is eating or drinking allowed in the classroom?

   ■ What are the regulations regarding smoking in the building?

   ■ Provide students with periodic updates throughout the course so they know how they are progressing.

3. Be consistent and fair.

   ■ Give praise and encouragement when appropriate.

   ■ Remember that the role of instructor gives you the responsibility to correct students when necessary. Do so without humiliating or embarrassing the student.

   ■ Be firm, fair, and consistent. Do not accept from one student that which you find unacceptable in another student.

4. Provide a comfortable learning environment. This includes:

   ■ Room temperature—not too hot or too cold

   ■ Elimination of noise and other distractions

   ■ Adequate nonglare lighting

   ■ Positioning of yourself, video players, screens, and blackboards so that all students can see and hear

- Physical comfort—tables and chairs are usually the most comfortable for long periods of sitting
- Adequate space so that students do not feel squeezed together
- Convenient access to bathrooms and water fountains and frequent breaks to allow students to use the facilities
- Friendly atmosphere—the tone is set by the instructor

Characteristics of Adult Learners

Adult learners have varied backgrounds. Your classes may consist of:

- College graduates who have been unable to find employment in their fields
- Recently divorced or widowed women who now find it necessary to acquire marketable work skills
- Persons who have invested several years in one job and then suddenly find they are victims of downsizing
- Persons who have "hit bottom" because of drugs or alcohol and who have been through rehabilitation and are starting over
- Individuals who are in welfare-to-work programs or other rehabilitation programs
- Single parents
- Married women whose children are now in school and who wish to return to the workforce
- Persons who are tired of their present vocations and are eager to learn a new one
- High school dropouts who have never succeeded in the world of learning
- High school graduates or students who view this class as the first step to becoming a nurse or other health care professional

It is important to understand the unique situations of your students. Empathy and compassion are prerequisites to being a successful instructor. However, your role is not that of counselor for personal problems. Express concern for their well-being, but avoid becoming enmeshed in their personal lives. Keep a list of community resources to which you can refer students if necessary.

Teaching the Experienced Worker

Even though there is a federally legislated program for the preparation of nursing assistants who are employed in long-term care, you may have students with some training and experience entering your program to achieve certification. The variance in student background and experience will offer a challenge and a source of practical application as you strive to evaluate and then improve their proficiency. Here are some suggestions:

- Have students go through the performance checklists and select those procedures that they are confident they can perform accurately and safely. Use the checklist to determine which procedures can be performed to your satisfaction and check them off for these students. This allows both you and the student to focus on the procedures that need additional practice.
- Allow experienced students to select a procedure for which they have been checked off and ask them to demonstrate for the other students. This builds self-esteem and helps motivate students to strive to reach the next goals.
- Encourage experienced students to share their own experiences that are similar to the clinical focus. If the focus is on stroke, for example, the students may relate the problems of patients they cared for and how the problems were resolved.
- Use the overhead transparencies and PowerPoint slides to review basic anatomy and physiology. Experienced students often lack knowledge in the basic sciences.
- Ask the experienced students "why." They may know "how" but have never learned "why." This limits their ability to make the adjustments necessary to meet individual patient needs.

- Ask a lot of questions to determine whether students understand the text content. An easy way to do this is to turn the behavioral objectives at the beginning of each lesson into questions.

- Help students synthesize previous and current learning by starting discussions with "Can you recall a patient or situation . . ."; "Do you remember being faced with a situation such as . . ."; "What was your response when . . ." These questions stimulate students to draw correlations between past and present experiences in a more concise way.

- Plan to spend time with vocabulary building and documentation. These are areas often deficient in the preparation of many assistants. The experienced worker with little background in these activities may feel insecure and may be resistant. Practice and patience are the keys to a positive experience.

- Work with students on developing and refining good organizational skills. The nursing assistant of the 21st century must have excellent organizational skills to be successful. Good organizational skills will make the job easier and less frustrating for the assistant.

Teaching Methods

Adults have different learning styles, so instructors must augment the traditional lecture format with other teaching methods. Your emphasis should be on student learning and retention rather than teaching. Unfortunately, the limited number of hours available in which to teach this content may stifle instructor creativity and experimentation with a variety of teaching methods. Regardless of which method(s) of teaching you use, reviewing the lesson objectives at the beginning and summarizing them at the end of the unit will help students reflect on and process the information and cement learning. This will also help you, the instructor, identify deficiencies in learning or knowledge so you can fill in the information before students are tested on the material or move on to another unit that builds on the deficient material. Use examples and clinical applications at the end of each lesson to stimulate class discussion and promote student involvement. Encourage students to build on previous lessons and draw from their previous nursing assistant experience to answer questions. Your objective is to cause them to develop and use critical thinking skills.

1. **Lecture**

   This is probably the most challenging method for the instructor. Some of the material that has to be taught is not very exciting. It is up to the instructor to capture and maintain the student's interest. Be sensitive to the facial expressions and body language of students to determine whether they are confused, bored, or tired of sitting. If so, take appropriate actions. Be prepared. No matter how often you teach the same material, most instructors need a brief outline to ensure that important material is not inadvertently omitted. However, know the subject well enough that you do not have to be constantly looking at notes. Use eye contact with everyone in the room. Avoid talking too fast and using highly technical jargon. Appropriate humor can enliven any lecture.

   Instructors sometimes make the mistake of thinking that their students need to know everything the instructors know. "Overteaching" can lead to frustration for everyone and failure for some of the students.

   The use of a blackboard, flipchart, or overhead transparencies can greatly enhance the lecture process. Most of us learn better if we can both see and hear the material simultaneously.

2. **Discussion**

   Discussion gives students an opportunity to actively participate in the learning/teaching process. The instructor remains responsible for guiding and leading the discussion. Some issues that might arise with class discussion include:

   - A timid student who never speaks out. Attempt to tactfully draw this student out without causing embarrassment.

   - A student who enjoys being center-stage. Give this student the opportunity to speak without depriving the other students of their time.

   - Keeping the discussion on track. It is all too easy to allow the discussion to wander away from the selected topic. However, sometimes learning is most successful when it is spontaneous, even though it may not be the subject that was planned for that time.

3. Demonstration

Nursing skills must be demonstrated (preferably on a live person) by the instructor if the students are to effectively learn the procedure. Before class starts, make sure you have all the equipment and supplies you will need throughout the procedure. Know the steps thoroughly so that you can give instructions while you are demonstrating. Ask a student to serve as the patient for the demonstration—be sure that all students serve in this role at some time during the course. Be tactful and sensitive to students' feelings.

Some procedures are not appropriatly demonstrated on a student. A manikin, if available, can be used for procedures such as perineal care and enemas.

4. Return Demonstrations

Students should return the demonstration soon after the instructor demonstration. Give students time to practice on each other (or the manikin) before you evaluate their competency. Use competency checklists so that you will be fair and objective. Avoid having other students as onlookers during evaluation times. Students will be self-conscious and feel awkward, and having other people around will increase their anxiety. Evaluations of this nature are time-consuming. Some procedures can be evaluated on outcome, so you need only evaluate the result. Others must be process-evaluated, and for those procedures you will have to watch the entire procedure.

5. Simulation Activities

These activities can do much to provide students with an understanding of what being old or disabled feels like. Some students may feel self-conscious at first; others will be enthusiastic and ready to perform. Guidance from the instructor is needed so that students know the purpose of the activity. Discussion should take place afterward to determine whether learning occurred.

6. Role-Playing

Role-playing can be successful with topics like communication. This activity must be well planned by the instructor before the class. Have students draw slips of paper describing their role and the topic/problem. Sensitivity is required on the part of the instructor to avoid placing students in awkward or uncomfortable positions.

7. Audio/Visuals

Videotapes, films, slides, and filmstrips are all important supplements to the teaching/learning process. They seldom take the place of the other teaching methods, but they can enhance the student's learning when used with other teaching methods. You should preview all audio/visuals before using them in class; otherwise, both you and the students may be surprised when the content proves to be different from what you expected. Use of audio/visuals always requires an introduction and a follow-up discussion.

8. Written Evaluation

Periodic written evaluations provide students with necessary feedback about their progress in the course. The quizzes or tests also help prepare them for the written competency examination required by federal law. This technique also provides you with feedback to determine the effectiveness of your instruction.

CRITERIA FOR PASSING THE COURSE

Students need to know what they must accomplish to pass the course. Several factors may be considered:

- Scores on written quizzes, tests
- Other class assignments, workbooks, worksheets, etc.
- Return demonstrations
- Attendance
- Performance during clinical assignments

Many students may perform well during clinical examinations but have problems with written tests. It is good to increase the weight of clinical performance and return demonstrations and to decrease the weight of written evaluations.

This usually gives more students the opportunity to succeed. The determination of criteria depends on the instructor, the makeup of the class, and the length of the course.

Some instructors require reading tests before the course starts. The student must be able to read and comprehend the textbook. Prior testing provides the instructor with information on the students' reading abilities. Many adults read at or below a ninth-grade level.

THE ROLE OF THE INSTRUCTOR

The instructor is the guiding force for the class. Here are several suggestions to assist you in your endeavors:

1. Be a good listener and be sensitive to the feelings and moods of students.

2. Have a sense of humor and be able to laugh at yourself (none of us is perfect). Many situations within the course can be embellished with a little appropriately used humor.

3. Be organized and know exactly what you hope to accomplish for each class. No matter how well versed you are with the course content, take time before class to go over the lesson plan. Review lecture material, assemble all the supplies and equipment that will be needed, and have the audio/visual materials ready to view. Set time frames. If you take longer for one topic and less time for another, it will all work out. Be structured but flexible.

4. Avoid interruptions. If you teach in a facility, it is especially important that the staff understand that while you are in class, the students are your first priority.

5. Facilitate students' interactions with each other. This is an important first step to building working relationships with fellow employees later on.

BASIC (MINIMUM) CLASS SKILLS LABORATORY EQUIPMENT AND SUPPLY LIST

- Alcohol hand cleaner
- Anti-embolism hose (TED hose)
- Bags, plastic
- Bath basins
- Bath blankets
- Bathing supplies (towels, washcloth, soap, etc.)
- Bed linens/pillows
- Bedpans, fracture and regular, with covers
- Briefs, disposable or reusable
- Call lights and/or tap bells (may be purchased at office supply store)
- Canes, single, quad, or tripod
- Catheter equipment with drainage bag
- Catheters, condom
- Chair, bedside
- Colostomy bag and other essential equipment for colostomy care
- Commode, bedside
- Compresses, hot and cold (commercial-type)
- Crutches/walker

- Dentures, denture cup, and oral cleaning supplies
- Eating equipment, standard (plate, cup, glass, fork, knife, spoon), nondisposable
- Emery boards
- Emesis basins
- Enemas (if taught)
- Eyewear for PPE (goggles and/or face shield)
- Forms/flow sheets used for documentation (standard)
- Gait/transfer belt
- Geri-chair
- Geri-feeder or feeding syringe (if taught)
- Gloves
- Gowns (cover gowns for PPE)
- Gowns, patient
- Graduated pitcher
- Hand cleaner, alcohol-based
- Handrolls (commercial)
- Handwashing supplies (sink, paper towels, soap)
- Heel/elbow protectors
- Height/weight measuring equipment (includes standard scales)
- Hose, anti-embolism (TED hose)
- Hospital unit, including bed with side rails, overbed table, and bedside table
- Lap board, lap buddy, devices used with wheelchairs/geri-chairs
- Lift sheets (linen pads, commercial devices such as Skil-Care TLC pad)
- Linen hampers or barrels with liners
- Lubricant, water-soluble
- Manikins (teaching)
- Masks, NIOSH-approved
- Masks, surgical
- Mouthwash
- Nail clippers
- Oral care swabs, such as Toothettes or lemon-glycerine swabs
- Orange sticks
- Oxygen cannulas, masks, signs, empty tank or concentrator for teaching
- Pillows, props, foam, and other devices for positioning
- Pitcher, graduated
- Razors, safety and electric; other shaving supplies
- Restraints (vest, pelvic, waist, and wrist)
- Scale, balance-type

- Signage as needed (biohazard, oxygen, standard precautions, isolation signs, etc.)
- Soap (for bathing)
- Specimen containers (urine, stool, and sputum, if taught)
- Sphygmomanometers
- Stethoscopes (regular and teaching)
- Straws
- Swabs for oral care, such as Toothettes or lemon-glycerine swabs
- Tape measure for measuring height and fitting anti-embolism hosiery
- Thermometer, bath
- Thermometer sheaths
- Thermometers
- Toothbrush
- Toothpaste
- Towels
- Underpads, disposable or reusable
- Urinals
- Washcloths
- Wastebaskets for bedside units
- Wheelchair

CLINICAL EXAMINATION EQUIPMENT LIST

(For facilities that present the state skills examination by using a skills laboratory)

Assemble equipment in the testing area in advance. One or more teaching manikins may be necessary for skills such as perineal care and rectal temperatures, even if you use student volunteers as simulated patients for other skills. Part of each procedure is knowing which equipment to select. When students are practicing, have them collect their own equipment, and put it away when finished. By the time they are ready for the skills exam, they should be comfortable assembling their supplies. This is a list of recommended equipment and supplies for the state skills examination. However, also consider the items on the list of minimum equipment in the preceding section. Combine them for a well-rounded skills laboratory and effective state testing.

- Aftershave
- Applicators
- Bag, appropriate for soiled linen
- Bags, isolation, for laundry & trash
- Bags, laundry
- Bandage scissors
- Basin
- Bath blanket
- Bath mat
- Bath towels (4)
- Bed with side rails
- Bedpan
- Bedspreads (2)
- Bib
- Blankets (2)
- Blood pressure cuffs
- Brush & comb
- Call light
- Cane
- Catheter, Foley (& drainage bag)
- Chair, room
- Clothing for patient

- Commode
- Container for soiled linen/laundry
- Denture cleaner
- Denture cup
- Diet cards
- Disinfectant
- Dress
- Dressing, nonsterile
- Emery board
- Emesis basin
- Enema, prepackaged
- Food tray, complete with table setting & empty milk carton
- Gait belt
- Gauze pad
- Gloves, disposable (1 box)
- Gowns
- Gowns for isolation
- Graduated cylinder
- Hand towels (2)
- I/O record
- IV setup: tubing, bottle or bag
- Linen: 2 mattress pads, 2 sheets
- Lotion
- Lubricant
- Masks
- Mattress pads (2)
- Mechanical lift
- Mouthwash
- Nail clippers
- Napkin
- Overbed table
- Paper
- Paper towels
- Pencil or nonsmearing pen
- Petroleum jelly
- Pillows (& covers if needed) (3)
- Powder
- Privacy curtain

- Razor
- Scale
- Scissors, bandage
- Shampoo
- Shaving cream
- Sheets (2)
- Shoes
- Sink
- Slippers and robe
- Soap
- Stethoscope
- Stockings
- Straw, drinking
- Swabs or Toothettes
- Swabs, antiseptic
- Tape
- Tape measure
- TED hose or elastic stockings
- Thermometer sheaths
- Thermometer, bath
- Thermometer, rectal
- Thermometer, oral (glass)
- Tissues
- Toilet paper
- Toothbrush
- Toothpaste
- Towels, paper
- Trash container (with liner)
- Tub
- Undergarments
- Urinal
- Vaseline jelly
- Walker
- Washcloths (4)
- Watch
- Water bottle & ice
- Water pitcher & glass
- Waterproof pad or Chux
- Wheelchair

CLINICAL CONTRACTUAL GUIDELINES/SUGGESTIONS[4]

Suggested Nursing Assistant Program (NAP) Guidelines

1. The NAP will be responsible for all planned learning experiences as related to program objectives, and will provide appropriate faculty for this purpose.

2. The NAP is responsible for the initiation of the contract and the renewal of same annually.

3. The NAP shall provide the clinical facility with the schedule of the clinical rotation and the names of the students and instructor(s).

4. The selection of each student's assigned patients is to be made by the primary instructor of the program in cooperation with the designated facility liaison.

5. The assignments are to be posted on the appropriate unit 24 hours in advance of student arrival and contain each student's name, as well as the names and room numbers of assigned patients.

6. The long-term care (LTC) facility is to be notified prior to each clinical rotation.

7. The LTC facility is to be notified prior to the arrival of the skills exam evaluator(s) conducting the on-site evaluation.

8. The NAP will provide one (1) instructor for every eight (8) students in the clinical area.

9. The NAP will provide RN supervision for all LPN/LVN instructors assigned to supervise students in the clinical area.

10. Orientation to the LTC facility is to be the responsibility of the NAP instructor(s) and should include introductions to the appropriate clinical facility staff and input from them regarding specific rules and regulations for the students and instructor(s).

11. All student activities and care of patients are to be with approved instructor supervision.

12. Students are not to be assigned to facility staff to provide care or to receive instruction.

13. Instructors and students will wear uniform attire as designated by the NAP and will wear name tags that designate both their status as instructors or students and the name of the NAP.

14. The NAP is responsible for any and all accidents/incidents related to student activities.

15. The NAP will provide documentation of the required immunizations/tests.

16. The NAP will abide by all policies and procedures mandated by the facility.

17. The NAP is responsible for notifying the facility of any change in schedule and for notifying the charge nurse of the need to reassign patient care in the event of a student absence.

18. The provision of patient information to students is the responsibility of the instructor(s).

19. The NAP is responsible for the selection of patient care to comply with the experiences that the students require. The selection of the unit utilized is to be made with joint approval by the NAP and the LTC facility.

Suggested Long-Term Care Facility Guidelines

1. The LTC facility will provide space for the instructor(s) and students to store personal effects before and after conferences.

2. The LTC facility will assign a liaison/contact person to assist the program coordinator/instructor in the coordination of the students' clinical rotation.

3. The LTC facility is responsible for notifying the staff of the rotation of students and the arrival of the skills exam evaluator(s).

[4]Modified from South Carolina Department of Health and Human Services guidelines.

4. The LTC facility will allow the skills exam evaluator(s) to review the patients' charts prior to the evaluation and to observe the students' performance of patient care, with the patients' approval.

5. Students are utilizing the LTC facility for a learning experience and should not be utilized or requested to render care to unassigned patients.

6. The LTC facility will specify limitations with regard to the conduct of the nursing assistant students during clinical rotation (e.g., no access to patient charts).

7. The LTC facility will designate the appropriate forms/flow sheets used for documentation by students with instructor supervision.

8. The facility must maintain survey and regulatory compliance with the mandates of various regulatory and survey agencies to qualify as a clinical training site for any state-approved NAP.

9. The LTC facility is to maintain responsibility for the overall care of patients during all clinical rotations.

10. The termination of the contractual agreement is to be initiated by either party with reasonable advance notification in order to permit the NAP to seek a contract with another LTC facility.

Resources for the Instructor

DELMAR'S FUNDAMENTAL AND ADVANCED NURSING SKILLS VIDEOS

Providing comprehensive coverage, from medication administration to hygiene and essential concepts such as drug safety principles, these videos are the perfect addition to any nursing program. Many of these procedures are covered in this text. Others, though not in the text, may be appropriate for the nursing assistants in your agency or facility. The visual materials can be used as an integral part of the curriculum in the classroom, skills laboratory, or small-group study. The procedures in the text were written for the nursing assistant who cannot assess. Although the procedures in the text are not identical to those shown in the videos, the principles and practices are essentially the same.

Basic Care

1. Physical Assessment
   Physical Assessment; Breast Examination; Male Genitalia; Hernia; Rectal Examination

2. Vital Signs
   Taking a Temperature; Taking a Pulse; Counting Respirations; Taking Blood Pressure; Weighing a Mobile Client

3. Basic Care I: Personal Care
   Oral Care; Eye Care; Hair and Scalp Care; Hand and Foot Care; Shaving a Client

4. Basic Care II: Bedmaking
   Applying Restraints; Changing Linens in an Unoccupied Bed; Changing Linens in an Occupied Bed

5. Basic Care III: Infection Control and Bathing
   Handwashing; Bathing a Patient in Bed; Perineal and Genital Care; Giving a Backrub

6. Basic Care IV: Aiding Client Movement
   Turning and Positioning a Client; Moving a Client in Bed; Preventing and Managing the Pressure Ulcer

7. Basic Care V: Aiding Client Movement
   Assisting from Bed to Stretcher; Assisting from Bed to Wheelchair, Commode, or Chair; Assisting from Bed to Walking; Administering Passive Range-of-Motion Exercises

8. Specimen Collection
   Measuring Intake and Output; Collecting a Clean-Catch, Midstream Urine Specimen; Performing a Skin Puncture; Collecting Nose, Throat, and Sputum Specimens

Intermediate Care

9. Nutrition & Elimination 1
   Inserting and Maintaining a Nasogastric Tube; Assessing Placement of a Feeding Tube; Removing a Nasogastric Tube; Feeding and Medicating via a Gastronomy Tube; Maintaining Gastrointestinal Suction Devices

10. Nutrition & Elimination II: Catheter Care
    Applying a Condom Catheter; Urinary Catheterization—Male and Female; Routine Catheter Care; Obtaining a Sterile Urine Specimen from an Indwelling Catheter; Irrigating a Urinary Catheter

11. Nutrition & Elimination III
    Administering an Enema; Digital Removal of Fecal Impaction; Inserting a Rectal Tube; Irrigating and Cleaning a Stoma; Changing a Bowel Diversion Ostomy Appliance—Pouching a Stoma

12. Wound Care
    Bandaging; General Steps for Wound Care; Procedures

13. Medication Administration I
    General Medication Guidelines; Dosage Calculation Principles; Managing Controlled Substances

14. Medication Administration II: Routes of Administration
    General Administration Guidelines; Administering Oral, Sublingual, and Buccal Medications; Administering Ear and Eye Medications; Administering Skin/Topical Medications; Administering Nasal

Medication; Administering Rectal Medications; Administering Vaginal Medications; Administering Nebulized Medications

15. Medication Administration III: Parenteral Medication
General Medication Guidelines; Administering an Intradermal Injection; Administering a Subcutaneous Injection; Administering an Intramuscular Injection; Administering Medication via Z-Track Injection; Withdrawing Medication from a Vial; Withdrawing Medication from an Ampule; Mixing Medications from Two Vials into One Syringe

16. Medication Administration IV: Intravenous Medication
General Medication Guidelines; Preparing an IV Solution; Adding Medications to an IV Solution; Administering Medications via Secondary Administration Sets (Piggyback); Administering Medications via IV Bolus or IV Push; Administering Medication via Volume-Control Sets; Administering Medication via a Cartridge System; Administering Patient-Controlled Analgesia

Advanced Care

17. Circulatory I: Venipuncture and Starting IV Therapy
General Principles of IV Therapy; Performing Venipuncture (Blood Drawing); Starting an IV; Inserting a Butterfly Needle; Preparing the IV, Bag, and Tubing

18. Circulatory II: Maintaining IV Therapy
Setting the IV Flow Rate; Assessing and Maintaining an IV Insertion Site; Changing the IV Solution; Discontinuing the IV and Changing to a Saline Lock; Discontinuing the IV

19. Circulatory III: Blood Transfusions
General Principles of Blood Transfusions; Administering a Blood Transfusion; Assessing and Responding to Transfusion Reactions

20. Oxygenation
General Principles of Oxygenation; Administering Oxygen Therapy; Assisting a Client with Controlled Coughing and Deep Breathing; Measuring Peak Expiratory Flow Rates

DELMAR'S BASIC, INTERMEDIATE, AND ADVANCED NURSING SKILLS DVD-ROMS

Each DVD-ROM contains approximately 150 minutes of step-by-step video; these are ideal for self-assessment and review of critical nursing skills. The DVD-ROMs are a perfect supplement to any course that covers nursing skills. Many of these procedures are included in this text. Others, though not in the text, may be appropriate for the nursing assistants in your agency or facility. The visual materials can be used as an integral part of the curriculum in the classroom, skills laboratory, or small-group study. The procedures in the text were written for the nursing assistant who cannot assess. Although the procedures in this text are not identical to those in the videos, the principles and practices are essentially the same.

Basic Care DVD-ROM

Physical Assessment, Vital Signs, Bedmaking, Restraints, Basic Care, Hygiene, Bathing, Ambulation/Activity

Intermediate Care DVD-ROM

Wound Care, Nutrition and Elimination, Catheter Care, Elimination, Bandaging, Medication Administration

Advanced Care DVD-ROM

IV Skills, Oxygenation, Blood Administration

DELMAR LEARNING'S BASIC CORE SKILLS FOR NURSING ASSISTANTS

Module 1   Obstructed Airway; Handwashing; Beginning and Completion Procedure Actions; Communication Skills

- Obstructed Airway, Conscious Resident
- Obstructed Airway, Unconscious Resident
- Handwashing
- Beginning and Completion Procedure Actions
  - Beginning Procedure Actions
  - Procedure Completion Actions
- Communication Skills

Module 2   Personal Protective Equipment, Standard Precautions, and Transmission-Based Precautions

- Beginning Procedure Actions
- Procedure Completion Actions
- Personal Protective Equipment
- Applying Disposable Isolation Mask, Gown and/or Gloves
- Removing Disposable Gloves, Gown and/or Mask
- Other Personal Protective Equipment Guidelines

- Isolation Procedures
  - Standard Precautions
  - Transmission-Based Precautions
    - Airborne Precautions
    - Droplet Precautions
    - Contact Precautions

Module 3   Positioning, Transfers, and Ambulation

- Beginning Procedure Actions
- Procedure Completion Actions
- General Guidelines and Precautions for Lifting and Moving
- Turning the Resident on the Side Toward You
- Moving the Resident in Bed
- Assisting the Resident to Move to the Side of the Bed
- Moving Resident to Head or Side of Bed with Assistant and Lift Sheet
- Fowler's Position
- Supine Position
- Semisupine (Tilt) Position
- Prone Position
- Semiprone Position
- Lateral Position
- Assisting the Resident to Sit Up on the Side of Bed
- Assisting the Resident to Transfer to Chair or Wheelchair
- Ambulation and Ambulation Aids
- Ambulating a Resident Using a Walker
- Ambulating a Resident Using a Cane
- Ambulation Guidelines
- Assisting a Resident during a Fall
- Assisting the Resident after a Fall
- Assisting the Resident with a Suspected Fracture

Module 4   Bedmaking and Bathing

- Beginning Procedure Actions
- Procedure Completion Actions
- Making the Unoccupied Bed
- Guidelines for Handling Clean or Soiled Linen
- Making the Occupied Bed
- Complete Bed Bath
- Partial Bath
- Tub or Shower Bath Overview

Module 5   Bladder, Bowel, and Perineal Care

- Beginning Procedure Actions
- Procedure Completion Actions
- Assisting the Resident Using a Bedpan
- Assisting the Male Resident with the Urinal
- Female Perineal Care
- Male Perineal Care
- Indwelling Catheter Care

Module 6   Personal Care

- Beginning Procedure Actions
- Procedure Completion Actions
- Backrub
- Oral Hygiene
- Special Oral Hygiene
- Denture Care
- Combing the Hair
- Shampooing the Hair
- Shaving the Resident
- Hand, Foot, and Nail Care
- AM Care
- PM Care

Module 7   Dressing, Meal Care, and Restraints

- Beginning Procedure Actions
- Procedure Completion Actions
- Assisting the Resident with Dressing/Undressing
- Preparing Residents for Meals
- Serving the Meal
- Feeding the Dependent Resident
- Measuring Intake and Output
- Restraints

Module 8   Vital Signs, Height, and Weight

- Beginning Procedure Actions
- Procedure Completion Actions
- Measuring an Oral Temperature with a Glass Thermometer
- Measuring an Oral Temperature with an Electronic Thermometer
- Measuring a Rectal Temperature with a Glass Thermometer
- Measuring Rectal Temperature Using Electronic Thermometer
- Axillary Temperature with a Glass Thermometer
- Axillary Temperature with an Electronic Thermometer
- Measuring a Tympanic Temperature
- Checking the Radial Pulse
- Counting Respiratory Rate
- Measuring Blood Pressure

- Measuring Weight and Height
  - Standing Scale
  - Chair Scale
- Weighing a Resident Using a Wheelchair Scale
- Bed Scale
- Measuring Height in a Bedfast Resident

Module 9   Observation/Reporting Guidelines and Postmortem

- Beginning Procedure Actions
- Procedure Completion Actions
- Observation and Reporting
- Postmortem Care

Module 10   Range of Motion and Mechanical Lift

- Beginning Procedure Actions
- Procedure Completion Actions
- Assisting the Resident with Range of Motion
  - Head and Neck
  - Shoulders, Arms, and Elbows
  - Wrists, Fingers, and Forearms
  - Legs, Hips, and Knees
  - Ankles, Feet, and Toes
- Mechanical Lift

EXERCISES AND ACTIVITIES TO INCREASE STUDENT LEARNING WITH AUDIOVISUAL MATERIALS

- Read each objective and ask students what part of the procedure meets each objective.
- Develop a worksheet or quiz based on the information in the video.
- Invite a guest speaker to make a presentation and answer student questions on video-related subject matter.
- Discuss the situations in the video. Question students about how they think the patient must feel and what the nursing assistant must feel.
- Give additional situations (similar to those in the video) from your personal experience and ask students what they would do in the described situation. Use their answers as a basis for group discussion.
- Discuss positive examples for the nursing assistant, such as appearance, demeanor, attitude, and skills.
- Discuss potential patient rights violations, potentially abusive actions, consequences of not reporting observations properly, and the consequences of other related actions and situations.

- Ask the group members introspective questions about what they would think or feel if they were the patient, family member, or nursing assistant.
- Develop application exercises. The objective is for students to find video-related items on their nursing units. For example, ask them to write down where the procedure manual, evacuation chart, fire extinguishers, and so on are found.
- Develop games, such as word finds, crossword puzzles, and anatomic diagrams to label based on the content of the video. Games such as "telephone" show how easily messages can be misunderstood, and emphasize the importance of providing accurate information.
- Describe the physical and emotional characteristics of a particular patient.
- Define the safety or infection control issues for a particular situation and list measures to be taken.
- Bring facility forms to class. Have students document on each patient situation shown in the videos.
- Create an imaginary family for a particular patient and define physical and emotional issues that could affect the patient's behavior and care. When discussing difficult behavior, emphasize that the key to successful behavior management is identifying and eliminating the underlying cause of the behavior. In alert patients, it is usually unmet psychosocial needs. In confused patients, it is usually unmet physical needs, too much stimulation in the environment, or boredom.
- Using videos in which safety and infection control are emphasized, have students create lists that could be used on compliance rounds. After students have completed their individual lists, develop a master list in a group discussion.
- Assign students a disability and instruct them to function as if they have the disability for the remainder of the day. Then have them report their findings in a paper or at the next class. Have students use ambulation devices, adaptive devices, or the mechanical lift.
- Bring examples of patient care equipment shown in the videos to class so that students have the opportunity to examine them and simulate use of these items.
- Role-play nursing assistant reactions to the patient or family in specific situations.
- Divide students into small groups and instruct them to role-play responses to physical, emotional, social, or spiritual needs. Emphasize the needs of confused patients. Write various patient needs and situations on index cards and give one to each member of the group. Each person in the group will express his or her need, based on the

information on the card. Each member of the group should offer suggestions on how the nursing assistant can help meet the need.

■ Have a discussion on students' first experiences with death, sickness, hospitalization, chronic disease, long-term care, and the like.

■ Respond to an interaction or procedure and relate this to specific incidents in the nursing assistant's interaction with the patient. Would students do anything differently? Why?

■ Develop simulated care plans for patients in the videos. Ask students to contribute to and discuss the care plans and respond to the goals and approaches.

■ Provide copies of the facility's daily assignment sheet and have students practice documenting the care given to a particular patient.

■ Define and review facility policies, such as reporting, safety, incident reports, and infection control requirements, in the context of specific patient care situations.

■ Develop a panel of experienced nursing assistants. Hold panel discussions and allow students to ask questions on situations similar to those depicted in the videos.

■ Prepare worksheets or questionnaires based on the information in the videos. Use these as homework assignments, or allow independent study time to complete the worksheets. Offer assistance as needed. Allow students to work alone or in small groups, according to individual learning styles.

■ Incorporate ideas, concepts, and principles from the videos into classroom quizzes.

■ Ask nurses from various units to view the videos with the students. After the viewing, ask the guests to speak to the students about guidelines, training, and qualities that are important to them in nursing assistants who care for patients similar to those depicted in the videos.

■ Identify, define, and discuss regulations and public policy issues. Nursing assistants do not deliberately break the law, but someone must tell them what the law requires.

■ Show a video at the end of class, then ask students to use the information as a basis for a research paper or other homework assignment.

■ Develop exercises and games that focus on team-building skills and working together.

■ Introduce information and ideas that will benefit the student as an individual and as a paraprofessional, such as how to cope with stress, negative behavior, and other problems similar to those experienced in clinical practice.

■ Cover an area of the wall with flipchart paper. At the end of the video (or unit), ask students to write comments in each of the following categories: (1) How I feel about the subject matter; (2) Best idea I got from this material; (3) One way I will use this information right away. Discuss each comment with the group.

■ Prepare the skills lab area with unacceptable conditions before students arrive. For example, place a bottle of chemicals on the table. Make the mock unit look untidy, with linen on the floor. Place a urinal on the overbed table and food on the shelf with the bedpan in the bedside stand. Create as many realistic, unfavorable conditions as possible. Tell students the number of incorrect conditions. Have them tour the area, writing down as many problems as possible. Discuss the problems and identify them as a group, then relate the scenario to nursing assistant responsibilities in the context of the job description and state regulations.

■ Have each student draw a slip of paper listing a subject studied in this unit or used in the video. Each student should prepare a five-minute presentation describing how the information is used, and the nursing assistant responsibilities regarding this subject, to present at the next class session.

■ Have students create a commercial or advertisement describing the video. List important information and highlights.

OTHER CLASSROOM ACTIVITY SUGGESTIONS

■ Review vocabulary terms.

■ Gather various pain rating scales and review how each is scored.

■ List items that interfere with comfort, rest, and sleep (such as the following) on separate pieces of paper:

> pain, hunger, thirst, need to eliminate, illness, exercise, noise, temperature, ventilation, light intensity, physical discomfort, nausea, some medications, caffeine intake, alcohol, drugs, some foods and beverages, lifestyle changes, anxiety, stress, fear, emotional problems, worry, changes in the environment, unfamiliar environment, treatments and therapies, staff providing routine care.

Have each student draw one item and explain how it interferes with comfort, rest, and sleep, and describe nursing assistant actions to assist the patient.

■ With a student volunteer acting as the patient, create a lab situation in which the student is poorly positioned and in pain. Have each student throw a die. The student must demonstrate the number of nursing comfort measures he or she rolled on the die to make the patient more comfortable.

■ Have students stand up. Do an aerobic quiz using true or false questions, such as, "A patient who is smiling cannot be having pain." If the answer to the question is true, students touch their chairs as if to sit down, and then stand back up. If the answer is false, students remain standing. Make sure students are directly over their chairs so they do not fall. A variation is to have students sit down if they answer correctly and remain standing if their answer is incorrect. Continue until all students are seated.

■ Give each student blank index cards. Throughout the lecture or video, pause momentarily and ask each student to create a flashcard of important information. Collect the cards at the end of the lecture. File them in an accessible area where students can use them to study.

■ Have students design adaptive equipment for mock patients, such as wrapping adhesive tape or a sponge around a toothbrush to make it easier to grip, or fastening it to the hand with wide rubber bands.

■ Have a career day in which students read various want ads, job descriptions, or other related information. Assign each student a subject to present to the class to introduce nursing assistant responsibilities for this area.

■ Develop trivia questions about nursing history or hospital information for students to answer. Keep score. Give the winning student a prize, such as a pass to skip a homework assignment or increase the grade on a paper of the student's choice one level.

■ List members of the interdisciplinary and/or restorative team on pieces of paper. Have each student draw one slip of paper. Each student must write a paper or give a verbal overview of the role and responsibilities of the team member selected. Identify key points of the history of your profession, important principles or standards of the profession, how members of the profession are educated, practice environments in which practitioners work, and key responsibilities of the professional practice.

■ Develop a case study. Have students list team members' positions (RN, nursing assistant, OT, etc.) within circles. If team members' responsibilities overlap, have students overlap or interlock those circles. Have students answer questions, such as how to resolve situations in which responsibilities overlap, what are team members' priorities, and so forth.

■ As a group, have students identify and list key leadership behaviors.

■ As a group, have students identify and list key responsibilities of team members.

■ Create a bulletin board of a specific subject with photos, drawings, or pictures that students clip from magazines.

■ Assign an essay contest. Ask students to complete a sentence, such as "Responsible employee behavior is important because . . ." and then write an essay explaining and supporting the completed sentence.

■ Have a "Survivors Challenge," using the format of the popular television series. The object is for each student to survive an obstacle course of biohazards, infections, and other potential accidents. Set up stations on tables, then give students a list of questions to answer about each table. Then stage real scenarios and potential accidents around the room. Include subtle hazards, such as an unlit EXIT sign, a blocked fire exit, and an extension cord plugged into a multiplug outlet. Instruct students to list the problems and describe how these problems could potentially cause accident or injury.

■ Create other activities based on popular games, such as "Safety Bingo" or "Infection Control Jeopardy."

■ *Team building activity 1.* Have students form a circle, holding hands. Place a hula hoop between two students. The students must move the hula hoop around the circle without dropping their hands. If anyone drops the hoop or lets go of the other students' hands, start over at the beginning. After the group accomplishes this, add a second hula hoop, moving it in the opposite direction.

■ *Team building activity 2.* Form a circle. Give one student a softball. Time how long it takes to pass the ball to each student in the circle. Now add two more softballs. See how long it takes to pass three balls. Each student must touch each ball. The game is finished when the balls are returned to the person who started with them.

By using these suggestions, students are exposed to the material to be learned in many different ways. This encourages a competency-based format with active student participation and instructor intervention. Use of these methods ensures that students see, hear, touch, and feel, which optimizes the learning experience.

STAFF DEVELOPMENT RESOURCES

In 2003, Thomson Delmar Learning purchased Frontline Publishing Corporation. Frontline Publishing Corporation was established to help today's health care providers educate, develop, and keep their quality frontline caregivers. Its educational model was to build self-esteem and professionalism as the prerequisites for providing excellent service. Thomson Delmar Learning continues to support this model. We believe that the future of the U.S. economy depends, in large measure, on the skills and dedication of frontline workers. As a result of the shift from a manufacturing economy to a service economy, demand for frontline service workers is at an unprecedented high, and is expected to soar even higher. Worker shortages already plague the industry, and the pool of available workers is shrinking. For those people who do frontline work, there is a terrible gap between the education they get, the respect they are accorded, and the increasingly complex requirements of consumers. Thomson Delmar Learning's goal is to produce and market ongoing educational programs to close that gap.

Many frontline health care workers enter their jobs with a genuine desire to help people. However, their self-esteem and enthusiasm often diminish within one year; these workers then describe their jobs as stressful and report feelings of burnout and lower concern for customers. The fallout from this situation hurts both quality and profitability. Companies lose the confidence of their customers; frontline workers perform below their potential and below expectations; managers have to cope with chronic service problems and staff turnover. Together, these factors contribute to a vicious cycle that becomes more difficult to break the longer it continues.

Outstanding service is the key to many of the nation's best-publicized corporate success stories. These companies all understand that employee commitment is indispensable.

They know that staff who receive the ongoing training and recognition they need are also motivated to align themselves with their company's long-term mission and goals. They know that those goals are most often undermined by staff who feel unappreciated, resentful, and unequipped to deal with the demands of the job.

Thomson Delmar Learning has recognized that while teaching discrete skills is highly effective in the manufacturing environment, it is not enough in service industries, where a feel for the "big picture" and the capacity to manage interpersonal relationships take on greater importance. Only comprehensive, ongoing professional development programs can resolve the demographic and economic crisis that confronts the service sector. What's more, in areas such as health care, elder care, and child care, more than profitability is at stake. The education provided to those who care for society's most vulnerable members must not be left to ill-conceived, haphazard, and inadequate models.

Thomson Delmar Learning offers a variety of products, including subscription-based staff development programs, practical guides for caregivers, professional development books, and family resource books. See http://www.delmarhealthcare.com or call 1-800-347-7707.

Contact us to learn more about our newsletters:

- *The Long-Term Care Nurses Companion*
- *Nursing Assistant Monthly*
- *The Resident Assistant*

Course Syllabus for 75–90 Hour Nursing Assistant Program

PART I: CLASSROOM INSTRUCTION

INTRODUCTION AND ORIENTATION

Community Health Care	Section 1, Unit 1
Role of the Nursing Assistant	Section 1, Unit 2
Infection Control	Section 4, Units 12, 13
Environmental and Nursing Assistant Safety	Section 5, Unit 14
Patient Safety and Positioning	Section 5, Unit 15
Consumer Rights and Responsibilities in Health Care	Section 1, Unit 3
Ethical and Legal Issues	Section 1, Unit 4
	12 hours

PART II: CLASSROOM INSTRUCTION

BASIC HUMAN NEEDS AND COMMUNICATION

Communication Skills	Section 3, Unit 7
Meeting Basic Human Needs	Section 3, Unit 9
Developing Cultural Sensitivity	Section 3, Unit 11
Principles of Observation, Reporting, and Documentation	Section 3, Unit 8
Comfort, Pain, Rest, and Sleep	Section 3, Unit 10
	8 hours

PART III: CLASSROOM INSTRUCTION

SAFETY AND MOBILITY

Patient Mobility: Transfer Skills	Section 5, Unit 16
Patient Mobility: Ambulation	Section 5, Unit 17
	6 hours

PART IV: CLASSROOM INSTRUCTION

PERSONAL CARE SKILLS

Bedmaking	Section 7, Unit 23
Patient Bathing	Section 7, Unit 24
General Comfort Measures	Section 7, Unit 25
	8 hours

PART V: CLASSROOM INSTRUCTION

BASIC NURSING SKILLS

BODY SYSTEMS, COMMON DISORDERS, AND RELATED CARE PROCEDURES

Body Temperature	Section 6, Unit 18
Pulse and Respiration	Section 6, Unit 19
Blood Pressure	Section 6, Unit 20
Measuring Height and Weight	Section 6, Unit 21
Admission, Transfer, and Discharge	Section 7, Unit 22
Nutritional Needs and Diet Modifications	Section 8, Unit 26
Integumentary System	Section 11, Unit 38
Respiratory System	Section 11, Unit 39
Circulatory (Cardiovascular) System	Section 11, Unit 40
Musculoskeletal System	Section 11, Unit 41
Endocrine System	Section 11, Unit 42
Nervous System	Section 11, Unit 43
Gastrointestinal System	Section 11, Unit 44
Urinary System	Section 11, Unit 45
Reproductive System	Section 11, Unit 46
Caring for the Patient with Cancer	Section 11, Unit 47
	16 hours

PART VI: CLASSROOM INSTRUCTION

SPECIAL CARE

Caring for the Emotionally Stressed Patient	Section 9, Unit 30
Caring for the Bariatric Patient	Section 9, Unit 31
Death and Dying	Section 9, Unit 32
Basic Emergencies	Section 13, Unit 52
Employment Opportunities	Section 14, Unit 53
	5 hours
Total Classroom Hours	55 hours
Total Clinical Hours	20 hours
Total Program Length	75 hours

NOTE: The minimum federal requirement for nursing assistants in long-term care is 75 hours. About half the states mandate the 75-hour course. The remaining 50% require courses of varying length, ranging from 80 hours to 175 hours.

Instructor Information

Instructors who have used *Nursing Assistant: A Nursing Process Approach* in the past are probably aware that instructor input, comments, suggestions, and complaints drive and largely dictate the content for each revision of the book. Reviewer suggestions and instructor surveys also provide information for each revision. We also consider trends in regulatory and accreditation agencies, current litigation, and new infection control information. If you have provided suggestions and information in the past, please accept our sincere thanks for helping to ensure that this book remains a comprehensive source of the most current information available for health care in general, and nursing assistants and patient care technicians (PCTs) in particular. Some of the changes in this edition and some of the concerns conveyed to us follow a pattern, and an explanation of some recurring issues follows. If nothing else, this may provide an insight into the thought process behind adding, removing, or modifying information in the book. We take all user comments seriously and research them when necessary. We hope that this information clarifies instructor concerns regarding these issues, and gives insight into the decision-making process.

USE OF 1:100 SODIUM HYPOCHLORITE SOLUTION FOR DISINFECTION

With each revision, we receive a number of concerns regarding the recommendation for using 1:100 sodium hypochlorite (bleach) solution for disinfection. Many of the comments suggest that this is an error, either in typography or content. This is not an error for most patient care situations, although a large blood or body fluid spill may require a heavier concentration. If bleach is used to decontaminate a spill in the laboratory, a 1:10 concentration is definitely required. The Centers for Disease Control and Prevention (CDC) states:[5]

> D. An EPA-registered sodium hypochlorite product is preferred, but if such products are not available, generic sodium hypochlorite solutions (e.g., household chlorine bleach) may be used.
>
> 1. Use a 1:100 dilution (500–615 ppm available chlorine) to decontaminate nonporous surfaces after cleaning a spill of either blood or body fluids in patient-care settings (*301,304*). Category IB
>
> 2. If a spill involves large amounts of blood or body fluids, or if a blood or culture spill occurs in the laboratory, use a 1:10 dilution (5,000–6,150 ppm available chlorine) for the first application of germicide before cleaning (*279,301*). Category IB

UC Davis also addresses this issue, noting that

> [m]any active chlorine compounds are available at various strengths; however, the most widely used for chemical disinfection is sodium hypochlorite. Household or laundry bleach is a solution of 5.25% or 52,500 ppm of sodium hypochlorite. Note that a 10% or 1:10 dilution of bleach will result in a 0.525% or 5,250 ppm solution of chlorine. The Center for Disease Control (CDC) recommends 500 ppm (1:100 dilution of household bleach) to 5,000 ppm (1:10 dilution of bleach), depending on the amount of organic material present, to inactivate Human Immunodeficiency Virus. The strength of chlorine to be used for disinfection must be

---

[5]Centers for Disease Control and Prevention. (Eds.). (2003). Guidelines for environmental infection control in health care facilities: Recommendations of CDC and Healthcare Infection Control Practices Advisory Committee (HICPAC). *Morbidity and Mortality Weekly Report, 52* (No. RR-10), 1–44; Rutala, W. A. (1996). APIC guideline for selection and use of disinfectants. *American Journal of Infection Control, 24,* 313–342.

clearly indicated when described in the Biological Agent Use Authorization and/or training documentation such as standard operating procedures.[6]

The CDC Web site also addresses the dilution issue: "Extraordinary attempts to disinfect walls, floors, or other environmental surfaces are not necessary. However, cleaning and removal of soil should be done routinely. An inexpensive environmental surface germicide effective against HIV is a solution of sodium hypochlorite (1 part household bleach to 99 parts water or 1/4 cup bleach to 1 gallon of water) prepared daily. Bleach, however, is corrosive to metals (especially aluminum) and should not be used to decontaminate medical instruments with metallic parts."[7]

As you can see, the use of 1:100 sodium hypochlorite solution is recommended in most situations. In the laboratory or operating room, a large spill of blood or body fluid may require a stronger concentration. Please adjust your lesson plans to reflect the concentrations listed here, or follow facility policies if they differ from CDC recommendations.

HANDWASHING

In previous editions of this book, we have always instructed the student to turn the faucet on by using a paper towel. Although not required, this is a sound infection control practice. We have received a surprising number of complaints about this procedure, probably because this step is not required in most state tests. We have removed the paper towel from the "turning the faucet on" step at the beginning of the handwashing procedure. The portion of the procedure involving turning the faucet off is unchanged from previous editions and instructs students to use a paper towel for turning the faucet off.

FEMALE CATHETER CARE/PERINEAL CARE

This is another procedural step about which we have received a number of complaints. Formerly, the procedures instructed the student to wash the far side of the labia, then the near side, then the center. Over the year, this procedure has evolved and become quite technical for the student. Instructions have been added to turn the washcloth with each step of the procedure. The sequence for washing the perineum reflects another change that a number of states have adopted. Many states now require the student to wash the center of the perineum first, then one side, then the other. This is a skill on which there are a surprisingly high number of failures in state skills examinations, but variations from one state to the next continue to be problematic. We have modified the procedure in the textbook to correspond with this sequence: center of labia, far side, near side. The procedure also instructs the student to turn the washcloth and use a clean section for each downward stroke.

TRENDELENBURG POSITION

Over the years, we have had a number of instructors voice their concerns about the Trendelenburg position pictured in Unit 28 (Assisting with the Physical Examination). This is because the feet are down in the photo. The instructors called our attention to the fact that the feet should be elevated when this position is used. This is true *if* the position is being used for the treatment of shock or hypotension. There are several accepted variations of the Trendelenburg position, including the modification in the photo we have used in this book for many years. The "foot down" position would not be acceptable in an emergency, but it is not provided for use in that context. We have added a drawing of the "other" Trendelenburg position that is used in emergencies, with the exception of head injuries.

However, instructors may wish to consider additional information from the literature. Research has shown that using the Trendelenburg position in emergencies may be a "sacred cow." Current recommendations state that the position should not be used as a treatment for shock or hypovolemia.[8] This is a subject on which additional research is

[6]University of California–Davis. (2003). SafetyNet #68—Use of Chlorine Compounds as Disinfectants. Retrieved November 1, 2006, from http://ehs.ucdavis.edu/ftpd/sftynet/sn_68.pdf

[7]Centers for Disease Control and Prevention. Retrieved November 1, 2006, from http://www.cdc.gov/ncidod/dhqp/bp_hepatitisb_prevent.html

[8]Johnson, S., & Henderson, S. (2003). Myth: The Trendelenburg position improves circulation in cases of shock. *Canadian Journal of Emergency Medicine, 6*(1), 48–49. Retrieved August 20, 2006, from http://www.caep.ca/template.asp?id=DF61785B363D4460835A593243E70058

probably needed. Because of this, we have also added an online reference to this information in the "Exploring the Web" section of Unit 28. An online search will readily bring up additional peer-reviewed articles related to this subject.

ERGONOMICS

Over the past decade, there has been a movement underway to reduce the incidence of back injuries in health care workers and others. At the time of this writing, the following states have passed safe patient handling legislation:

- Hawaii
- New York
- Ohio
- Rhode Island
- Texas
- Washington

These states have introduced safe patient handling legislation:

- California (the governor vetoed this bill three times in three years; another died in committee)
- Florida (died in committee)
- Illinois
- Massachusetts
- New Jersey

The Nurse and Patient Safety and Protection Act was introduced in the federal House of Representatives in 2006 and is pending. The American Nurses' Association, OSHA, and a number of unions are supporting efforts and legislation to reduce the incidence of back injuries. Studies of back-related workers' compensation claims reveal that nursing personnel have the highest claim rates of any occupation or industry.[9]

No nursing-assistant studies are available related to back injury data. However, a literature review reveals that the licensed nurse workforce in the United States is aging, and there is a severe shortage of nursing personnel. The estimated increase in demand is approximately 40% annually. However, the number of available nurses has increased by only about 6 percent.[10] Patients and residents are getting larger, and obesity has become an issue in hospitals and long-term care facilities. Bariatric care units are becoming common. Combine the increased patient size with the loss of agility associated with aging and the effects of a nursing shortage. This makes it clear that the industry must consider methods of preventing back and other musculoskeletal injuries in the nursing workforce. Research regarding the impact of musculoskeletal injuries on nurses reveals:

- 52% of nurses complain of chronic back pain.[11]
- 12% of nurses report that they have left nursing "for good" because of back injuries and/or back pain.[12]
- 20% of RNs requested a transfer to a different unit, position, or employment because of low back pain, with 12% considering leaving the profession.[13]
- 38% of RNs have suffered occupation-related back pain severe enough to require taking leave from work.[14]
- 6%, 8%, and 11% of RNs reported changing jobs because of neck, shoulder, and back problems, respectively.[15]

Addressing back injuries is largely a facility-specific and/or state-specific subject. We have added content on sliding-board transfers, introduced and described a number of new types of equipment, and added a chapter on

[9]American Nurses Association. (2004). *Handle with care*. Washington, DC. American Nurses Publishing. Retrieved January 20, 2006, from http://www.NursingWorld.org/handlewithcare

[10]Id.

[11]Nelson, A. (2003, March 3). State of the science in patient care ergonomics: Lessons learned and gaps in knowledge. Presented at the Third Annual Safe Patient Handling and Movement Conference, Clearwater Beach, FL.

[12]Stubbs, D. A., Buckle, P. W., Hudson, M. P., Rivers, P. M., & Baty, D. (1986). Backing out: Nurse wastage associated with back pain. *International Journal of Nursing Studies, 23*(4), 325–336.

[13]Owen, B. D. (1989). The magnitude of low-back problem in nursing. *Western Journal of Nursing Research, 11*(2), 234–242.

[14]Owen, B. D. (2000). Preventing injuries using an ergonomic approach. *AORN Journal, 72*(6), 1031–1036.

[15]Trinkoff, A. M., Lipscomb, J. A., Geiger-Brown, J., Storr, C. L., & Brady, B. A. (2003). Perceived physical demands and reported musculoskeletal problems in registered nurses. *American Journal of Preventive Medicine, 24*(3), 270–275.

bariatric patients. We have also strengthened the existing information on lifting and moving patients. We will monitor this subject carefully and revisit it again in the next edition to ensure that the information in your book reflects current practice and legislation. For additional information on back-injured nurses and state legislation, refer to http://wingusa.org/.

TYMPANIC TEMPERATURES

We have received a number of instructor comments regarding the use of tympanic thermometers. These fall largely into two categories:

- Tympanic temperatures are not accurate.

- Rectal temperatures are the "gold standard" in infants and small children and the tympanic thermometer should not be used for children under the age of 5.

Donna Wong, PhD, RN, PNP, FAAN, maintains a Web page for her renowned book on pediatrics. Dr. Wong has a number of position papers and other writings on her Web site. She states, "The ear drum's anatomic location is superior to the rectal site, and a poor correlation between the two sites may actually indicate more accurate, not less accurate, temperature values from ear thermometry. Perhaps aural temperatures should be considered the 'gold standard,' and studies showing a poor correlation between ear and rectal temperatures should be used to discourage use of the rectal route."[16]

Regarding inaccurate tympanic temperatures, Dr. Wong writes,

Also, technique must be considered. For the sensor to detect heat from the drum, not from the cooler canals, the ear canal must be straightened as when using an otoscope—the pinna pulled down and back for children under 3 years and up and back for children above 3 years. With the ear tugged correctly and the probe tip pointing at the midpoint between the eyebrow and sideburn on the opposite side of the face, higher temperature readings are obtained. A review of 19 studies concluded that aural thermometers are best used with a standardized ear tug in children older than three months. The agreement between tympanic and referent temperature (oral, rectal, axillary, pulmonary artery, and bladder) was consistently lower, suggesting a difference in site of temperature measurement. Pontious and others (1994) have found that accuracy and reliability of temperature measurement from the rectum, mouth, and axilla were significantly improved when experienced nurses received moderate to intensive education. The researchers poignantly conclude, *the single most important implication for nursing is that no procedure performed on patients is routine.*[17]

Although Dr. Wong's missive was written specifically for pediatrics, it applies to use of the tympanic thermometer in other patients as well. Many facilities have returned to electronic thermometers because of inaccurate tympanic readings. Thus brings up Dr. Wong's point that "no procedure is routine." For the most part, tympanic thermometers are accurate. User technique is usually the cause of the problem. The tympanic thermometer is similar to a camera. It takes a picture (the temperature) of whatever the lens is aimed at, which in this case is the tympanic membrane. For accurate values, the lens cover must be flat against the tympanic membrane. If it is tipped even slightly to the side, the value will not be accurate. Part of the solution involves using the ear tug that Dr. Wong noted, and part of it involves rotating the thermometer after it has been inserted in the ear canal. It should be positioned so the handle looks like a telephone receiver, with the patient talking into the end.

A list of guidelines to improve accuracy in using the tympanic thermometer was added to the ninth edition of your book. The guidelines were further strengthened with the 10th edition revision. The URLs in the "Exploring the Web" section also provide guidance on using the tympanic thermometer. Instructors may also find the information in the paper, *Ear and oral temperatures under usual practice conditions,* useful.[18]

---

[16]Wong on Web Paper. Sites of temperature measurement in children. Retrieved April 27, 2007, from http://www3.us.elsevierhealth.com/WOW/op019.html
[17]Id.
[18]Ear and oral temperatures under usual practice conditions. (1999, June). *Research for Nursing Practice, 1*(1). Retrieved April 27, 2007, from http://www.graduateresearch.com/lee.htm

GLASS THERMOMETERS

We have also received complaints about retaining the glass thermometer procedures in the eighth edition of the book. Some of these note that the procedures are outdated, and others note that "mercury is illegal." Although mercury has proven toxic and should be eliminated, it is not universally illegal throughout the United States. Some state laws have banned mercury in thermometers, but others have not addressed this issue legislatively.

We removed all references to "mercury" thermometers in the ninth edition revision and provided an explanation and several cautions regarding problems associated with mercury. We have advocated the use of galinstan and other mercury alternatives since then. Simply put, a 2006 survey revealed that *34 states continue to include the glass thermometer procedure in either classroom or clinical curricula.* Some ask students to define the mercury thermometer, whereas others require using and reading a glass, non-mercury thermometer as part of the state skills examination. Inability to read the value on the glass thermometer results in the student failing the skill. We recognize that these are dated procedures, but do not feel that we can responsibly eliminate them as long as they continue to be part of the curriculum and skills examination in a majority of states. Although not a solution to the problem, we have retained one glass thermometer procedure in print and moved the others to the Online Companion so that the material can remain available to programs that need it.

Instructors may find the "Mad as a Hatter" materials at http://orf.od.nih.gov/Environmental+Protection/ Mercury+Free/useful. In *Alice in Wonderland* (1865), Lewis Carroll selected a hat maker as the demented host for the tea party. Hatters of the time commonly exhibited signs of dementia because of their exposure to high levels of mercuric nitrate during the hatmaking process. Carroll and others were, of course, unaware that the problem was associated with mercury toxicity. Instructors may wish to use this interesting example in teaching. Many other resources are also available through this Web site.

Instructors have also called our attention to the variables in the length of time the glass thermometer must remain in place for the oral, rectal, and axillary temperatures. We can find no consistent standard for oral and rectal thermometers. Recommendations we have reviewed vary from leaving the thermometer in place from 2 to 8 minutes. We have opted to use the 3-minute standard for oral and rectal temperatures and 10 minutes for axillary values. These are the most universal time frames found in our review of state curricula and current literature. If your state guidelines differ from these values, by all means use them! We have added the following notation to the glass thermometer procedures: "The guidelines for this procedure vary slightly from state to state, and from one facility to the next. Your instructor will inform you if the sequence in your state or facility differs from the procedure listed here. Know and follow the required sequence for your facility and state."

PATIENT ROOM TEMPERATURE

The textbook has always listed 70°F as a comfortable patient room temperature. One reader of the ninth edition informed us that "the regulations require" a temperature range of 71°F to 81°F. There is nothing in the *State Operations Manual* (federal rules) for hospitals addressing room temperature. We found the 71°F to 81°F temperature in the *State Operations Manual* for long-term care facilities.[19] We have changed the value in the textbook to match this range, which is reasonable in patient care units. Please make the necessary adjustment if your facility maintains a different temperature range.

USE OF THE WHEELCHAIR

Several readers objected to instructions advising the nursing assistant to lock the wheelchair brakes when the chair is not in motion. This is the standard of care in the literature. Although a chair may be stopped or parked, tipping is possible if the patient bends down to pick up an item on the floor, or adjusts a shoe or sock while the feet are on the footrests. Locking the brakes protects patient safety.

[19]Centers for Medicare and Medicaid Services. (2005). *State operations manual—Appendix PP—Guidance to surveyors for long-term care facilities.* F257, §483.15(h)(6).

Another concern is the instruction to position the small front wheels of the wheelchair with the large part facing forward during transfers and when the chair is parked. (The brakes must also be locked.) This is not so much a complaint as it is a lack of understanding. This instruction on front-wheel position is not commonly known by nurses, although we have been promoting this safety feature for quite some time. Positioning the large part of the small front wheel facing forward and locking the brakes stabilizes the chair and prevents tipping by changing the center of gravity. This method is safer for the patient.

RESTRAINT STRAP POSITION

Several instructors commented that the directions to tie a restraint to the *movable* part of the bed frame is incorrect. These individuals contend that the straps must be tied to the *stationary* part of the bed frame. This is not safe. Elevating the head of the bed with the strap tied to the stationary frame increases the risk of injury, including choking and strangulation.

Another concern is that when the patient is in bed, the restraint strap must be tied to the inner bed spring, not the frame. Tying it in a bow to the frame provides a great temptation for a patient to reach down and untie the strap. We have also strengthened this information and provided a line drawing showing how to tie straps to the inner bed springs. If the bed has a solid lower surface, contact the manufacturer of the restraints used by your facility. Although this is not well known, they will supply rings that attach to the lower deck of the bed to fasten and secure the restraint on the inner surface, where the patient cannot reach the knot.

Another concern is the position of the straps for a vest or belt restraint when the patient is up in the wheelchair. Always follow the manufacturer's instructions for the restraint you are using. The information in the textbook does not support threading the straps *through the armrests* and tying the restraint behind the patient's back. There are several reasons for this:

- Tying the straps in this manner does not keep the hips down. Some patients can stand up with the restraint intact when this type of strap placement is used. Depending on the patient's size and strength, the wheelchair may end up on his or her back.

- The patient can often reach behind the chair and untie the slip knot.

The book recommends threading the straps *between* the seat and armrests, then crossing the straps over each other in back, then using a slip knot to fasten them to the kick spurs. This is in keeping with the restraint manufacturers' recommendations for vests, belts, and other commonly used devices.

OTHER CHANGES

Please review the front matter of the textbook for a listing of other changes. The most notable change is the addition of a chapter on caring for bariatric patients. We announced our plans as part of a survey and approximately 50% of the respondents stated that they were not familiar with the term "bariatrics." *Bariatrics* is a newer field of medicine that focuses on the study of obesity, including its causes, prevention, and treatment. We believe this is a timely and useful change due to a recent shift in patient populations, an increase in weight loss surgery, and the emphasis on ergonomics and back injury prevention.

The author and publishing staff welcome your suggestions and comments. Please feel free to e-mail the author at bacello@spamcop.net or contact Thomson Delmar Learning via their Web site at www.delmarhealthcare.com.

PART 1   Instructor's Objectives, Suggested Activities, and Answers to Unit Reviews

SECTION 1 INTRODUCTION TO NURSING ASSISTING

UNIT 1 Community Health Care

Instructor Objectives

When using this unit, you will be able to teach students to:
- Spell and define terms.
- List the five basic functions of health care facilities.
- Describe four changes that have taken place in health care in the past few years.
- Describe the differences between acute care and long-term care.
- Name the departments within a hospital.
- Describe the functions of the departments within a hospital.
- Explain three ways by which health care costs are paid.
- State the purpose of health care facility surveys.

Suggested Activities

1. Review the vocabulary terms.
2. Arrange a visit to the local health department. Discuss the range of health-oriented activities conducted by the department.
3. Discuss employment opportunities for nursing assistants in the community.
4. Discuss the community's responsibility for the health of its citizens.
5. Discuss how information gathered in the community about health problems can be of value to people throughout the world.
6. Ask the director of nursing of a hospital or skilled care facility to speak to the class about the way their facilities operate.
7. Take students on a field trip to a hospital or skilled care facility.

Unit Review Answers

A. True/False

1. T	2. T	3. T	4. F	5. T
6. F	7. F	8. T	9. T	10. F

B. Multiple Choice

11. c	12. b	13. c	14. b	15. a
16. b	17. b	18. c	19. b	20. c
21. c	22. a	23. b		

C. Word Choice

24. skilled care facility
25. Hospitals
26. Patient-focused care
27. Prenatal

28. residents
29. surgicenter
30. Pathology
31. Occupational therapy
32. Physical therapy
33. Medicare

D. Nursing Assistant Challenge

34. Mrs. Hernandez will need to receive prenatal care throughout her pregnancy so she and the baby will remain healthy and so that if complications occur they can be detected and treated early.
35. Prenatal care may be given in the physician's office, prenatal clinics, public health clinics, or hospitals.
36. Many communities have programs on the labor and delivery experience, Lamaze classes, new baby care, and breast feeding. They may also have classes for other children in the family and for new grandparents.
37. Mrs. Hernandez will receive the services of the obstetrical department, newborn nursery, laboratory for routine tests, from the surgical department if she needs a cesarean section, from environmental services, and dietary. She may also receive social services.
38. The baby will need to be seen at regular, frequent intervals during the first year by the pediatrician or a pediatric nurse practitioner. Some hospitals provide nurses who go to the home during the first few weeks to check the baby's progress.

UNIT 2 Role of the Nursing Assistant

Instructor Objectives

When using this unit, you will be able to teach students to:
- Spell and define terms.
- Identify the members of the interdisciplinary health care team.
- Identify the members of the nursing team.
- List the job responsibilities of the nursing assistant.
- Make a chart showing your facility's lines of authority.
- Describe the legal importance of working within the established scope of nursing assistant practice.
- Discuss the potential for career growth and advancement, and identify opportunities for expanding the scope of nursing assistant practice.
- Describe the importance of good human relationships and list ways of building productive relationships with patients, families, and staff.
- List the rules of personal hygiene and explain the importance of a healthy mental attitude.
- Describe the appropriate dress for the job.

Suggested Activities

1. Review vocabulary terms.
2. Invite a nursing assistant to talk to the class about nursing assistant activities and the scope of nursing assistant practice.
3. Begin a discussion of good grooming with introductory questions.
4. Have students pair up. Instruct the pairs to interview each other to find out why they chose to become a nursing assistant, what expectations they have about the class, and what they know about the responsibilities and role of the nursing assistant. Each pair will then introduce one another to the rest of the class and share each other's responses.
5. Encourage students to discuss how attitude and stress affect working relationships and steps that can be taken to defuse stressful situations.

Unit Review Answers

A. True/False

1. T	2. T	3. F	4. T	5. T
6. T	7. T	8. F	9. T	10. T
11. T	12. F	13. T	14. T	15. F
16. T	17. T	18. T	19. F	20. T

B. Multiple Choice

| 21. c | 22. b | 23. b | 24. c | 25. d |

C. Matching

| 26. b | 27. e | 28. c | 29. a | 30. d |

D. Completion

31. The nursing assistant is not legally qualified to do this.
32. a. Give the nursing assistant recognition.
    b. Help define the scope of nursing assistant practice.
    c. Assure better uniformity of care provided by nursing assistants.
    d. Promote educational standards for nursing assistants.

E. Nursing Assistant Challenge

33. a. his charge nurse.   b. Yes.   c. No.
34. a. Yes.
    b. Three opportunities to pass the state test.
    c. At least 12 hours per year.
35. No jewelry or nail polish.
    Maintain uniforms in good repair, mending when necessary.
    Clean shoes daily.

UNIT 3 Consumer Rights and Responsibilities in Health Care

Instructor Objectives

When using this unit, you will be able to teach students to:
- Spell and define terms.
- Explain the purpose of health care consumer rights.
- Describe six items that are common to Residents' Rights, the Patients' Bill of Rights, and the Clients' Rights in Home Care.
- List three specific rights from each of the three documents.
- Describe eight responsibilities of health care consumers.

Suggested Activities

1. Review vocabulary terms.
2. Ask an administrator or director of nursing from a hospital, skilled care facility, or home care agency to describe situations in which there was a conflict between the rights of the patient, resident, or client and the welfare of that person and how the conflict was resolved.
3. Lead a discussion in which students think about which of the rights would be most important to them as individuals.
4. Discuss the ways in which nursing assistants participate in the consumer's rights.
5. Discuss the responsibilities of the consumer.

Unit Review Answers

A. True/False

1. F	2. T	3. T	4. F	5. T

B. Multiple Choice

| 6. b | 7. a | 8. a | 9. d |

C. Completion

10. informed consent	11. grievance
12. advance directive	13. involuntary seclusion
14. privacy	15. respect

D. Nursing Assistant Challenge

16. #11—to expect reasonable continuity of care and to be informed of all the options he has for continuing care.
17. #1—to participate in the planning of his care; #5—accommodation of needs and to be assisted to maintain independence as much as possible; #8—to participate in social, religious, and community activities.
18. #1, 2, and 10.

UNIT 4 Ethical and Legal Issues Affecting the Nursing Assistant

Instructor Objectives

When using this unit, you will be able to teach students to:
- Spell and define terms.
- Discuss ethical and legal situations in health care.
- Describe the legal and ethical responsibilities of the nursing assistant concerning patient information.
- Describe tactful ways to refuse a tip offered by a patient.
- Describe the legal responsibilities of a nursing assistant.
- Describe how to protect the patient's right to privacy.
- Define sexual harassment and give examples of activities that may be perceived as being sexually harassing.

Suggested Activities

1. Review vocabulary terms.
2. Initiate a discussion with the class about why the basic rule of medical ethics is the preservation of life.
3. Discuss students' feelings about a "no code" order.
4. Have students role-play these situations:
   - The patient offers a tip.
   - You observe someone taking drugs.
   - A patient asks you to reveal personal information about another patient.

- You are reporting the fact that you have observed another person stealing from a patient.
5. Divide the class in half and have them debate the values and ethics of a current issue, such as heroic measures for a terminally ill patient or maintaining life to preserve organs for transplant.

Unit Review Answers

A. Multiple Choice
1. d   2. d   3. c   4. b   5. a
6. d   7. d   8. b   9. a   10. c

B. True/False
11. F   12. T   13. F   14. F   15. T
16. T   17. T   18. T   19. T   20. T
21. T   22. F   23. T   24. F   25. T
26. T   27. F   28. F   29. T

C. Nursing Assistant Challenge
30. To assist Mrs. Harvey to be as physically and mentally comfortable as possible. She needs frequent attention for mouth care, sips of water if she can take it, position changes, back care, and general personal cleanliness. She may be incontinent and need linen changes. For mental comfort, she needs to know that people care, that her loved ones can be with her at any time, and that her needs will be met.
31. She should be allowed to say her prayers and then be given her breakfast.
32. Refer her question to the nurse.

SECTION 2 SCIENTIFIC PRINCIPLES
UNIT 5 Medical Terminology and Body Organization

Instructor Objectives
When using this unit, you will be able to teach students to:
- Spell and define terms.
- Recognize the meanings of common prefixes, suffixes, and root words.
- Build medical terms from word parts.
- Write the abbreviations commonly used in health care facilities.
- Describe the organization of the body, from simple to complex.
- Name four types of tissues and their characteristics.
- Name and locate major organs as parts of body systems, using proper anatomic terms.

Suggested Activities
1. Review vocabulary terms.
2. Select a prefix. Combine it with several suffixes and ask students to define the resulting words.
3. Select a suffix. Combine it with several prefixes and ask students to define the resulting words.
4. Have a "spelling bee" in which students have to correctly spell and/or define medical terms.
5. Use care plans and medical records and have students interpret the abbreviations and medical words.

6. Provide a skeleton/torso/chart for students to examine.
7. Divide students into small groups. Have them try to determine the general location of major muscle groups and basic movements such as abduction, adduction, flexion, and extension.

Unit Review Answers

A. Matching
1. d   2. i   3. e   4. b   5. f
6. j   7. c   8. l   9. k   10. h

B. Matching
11. j   12. i   13. a   14. l   15. g
16. b   17. d   18. c   19. e   20. f

C. Define
21. Difficult urination   dys
22. Absence of breathing   a
23. Surgical opening into skull   crani
24. High blood pressure   hyper
25. Rapid pulse or heartbeat   tachy

D. Define
26. Pain in a nerve   algia
27. Lack of breathing   pnea
28. Surgical removal of appendix   ectomy
29. Study of blood   ology
30. Tumor of fibrous or connective tissue   oma

E. Short Answer
31. nephrolithiasis   32. proctoscopy
33. thoracotomy   34. gastritis
35. leukocyte

F. Identification
36. Prefix: an, suffix: emia   37. Prefix: neur, suffix: itis
38. Prefix: pharyng, suffix: itis   39. Prefix: pan, suffix: emic
40. Prefix: trache, suffix: otomy

G. Measurements
41. mL   42. kg   43. lb   44. F   45. in

H. Print the Roman numerals
46. II   47. V   48. VI   49. IX   50. X

I. Multiple Choice
51. c   52. b   53. a   54. c   55. b
56. b   57. d   58. a   59. b   60. d

J. True/False
61. F   62. T   63. T   64. T

K. Nursing Assistant Challenge
(see care plan)

UNIT 6 Classification of Disease

Instructor Objectives
When using this unit, you will be able to teach students to:
- Spell and define terms.
- Define disease and list some possible causes.
- Distinguish between signs and symptoms.
- List six major health problems.
- Identify disease-related terms.

- List ways in which a diagnosis is made.
- Describe malignant and benign tumors.

Suggested Activities

1. Review vocabulary terms.
2. Ask students who have been ill themselves or who have had illness in their family to describe signs and symptoms they have observed.
3. Make a list of signs and symptoms. Let students select one and identify it as a sign or a symptom.
4. Select a common disease and discuss possible types of therapy.
5. If students are in a clinical area, let each select a patient for whom they have cared. Have each present: diagnosis, signs and symptoms, type of therapy, nursing care.

Unit Review Answers

A. Matching

1. g	2. h	3. d	4. b	5. i
6. a	7. j	8. c	9. e	10. f

B. Fill-In

11. sign	12. symptom	13. symptom
14. sign	15. sign	

C. Matching

16. d	17. g	18. h	19. a or h	20. c
21. f	22. g	23. d	24. b	25. b

D. True/False

26. F	27. T	28. F	29. T	30. T
31. T	32. F	33. F	34. T	35. T

E. Completion

36. Change in bowel or bladder habits.
37. A sore that does not heal.
38. Unusual bleeding or discharge.
39. Thickening or lump in breast or elsewhere.
40. Indigestion or difficulty in swallowing.
41. Obvious change in wart or mole.
42. Nagging cough or hoarseness.

F. Nursing Assistant Challenge

43. a. Age and nutritional status.   b. More difficult.
    c. Infection.
44. a. A genetic condition, because it was inherited.
    b. This is a predisposing factor for fractures.
    c. Yes.
45. a. Overweight.
       Lack of exercise.
    b. Heart problems.
       Stroke.
    c. Condition of heart regulation.

SECTION 3 BASIC HUMAN NEEDS AND COMMUNICATION
UNIT 7 Communication Skills

Instructor Objectives

When using this unit, you will be able to teach students to:
- Spell and define terms.
- Explain the types of verbal and nonverbal communication.

- Describe and demonstrate how to answer the telephone while on duty.
- Describe four tools of communication for staff members.
- Describe the guidelines for communicating with patients with impaired hearing, impaired vision, aphasia, and disorientation.
- State the guidelines for working with interpreters.

Suggested Activities

1. Review vocabulary terms.
2. Role-play answering the phone, taking a message, and properly writing out the message.
3. Ask a speech language pathologist to talk to the class about communicating with patients who have hearing impairments and patients who have aphasia.
4. If you have access to these manuals, have students skim through them and discuss the types of information contained within each manual: employee's personnel handbook, disaster manual, procedure manual, nursing policy manual. If your class is facility-based or in clinical, give each student a list of items to locate on a scavenger hunt. You may include other important items for which students must know the location, such as the fire extinguishers and evacuation map. Have students locate each item and bring it to the classroom or write down the location of the items on the list.
5. Obtain a copy of an organizational chart from the facility in which students have clinical experience. Discuss the person you would go to for specific types of situations.

Unit Review Answers

A. Multiple Choice

1. d	2. a	3. b	4. a	5. d
6. c	7. a	8. d	9. a	10. b
11. a	12. b	13. d	14. b	15. d
16. a	17. d	18. d	19. c	20. c

B. Completion

21. aphasia	22. disorientation
23. shift report	24. medical chart
25. memo	26. body language
27. care plan	28. nonverbal communication
29. verbal communication	30. braille
31. interpreter	

C. Nursing Assistant Challenge

32. Arrange the food in clock fashion—for example, with potatoes at 12:00, meat at 3:00, vegetable at 6:00, etc. This should be on the care plan so that each staff member does it the same way.
33. Get everything out that she will need and then tell her where everything is—the soap, washcloth, towel, and any other items.
34. Get everything out that she will need and then tell her where everything is. These actions (and those for her bath) should also be on the care plan so all staff members do it the same way. For grooming procedures, give her feedback—let her know in a tactful manner, for example, if her hair needs to be recombed.

35. Other helpful actions include offering to read her mail to her and assisting her to learn how to use the telephone, the television, and the radio. Find out if talking books are available.

UNIT 8 Observation, Reporting, and Documentation

Instructor Objectives

When using this unit, you will be able to teach students to:
- Spell and define terms.
- List the components of the nursing process.
- Explain the responsibilities of the nursing assistant for each component of the nursing process.
- Describe two observations to make for each body system.
- Describe the purpose of the care plan.
- List three times when oral reports are given.
- Describe the information given when reporting.
- Describe the purpose of the patient's medical record.
- Explain the rules for documentation.
- State the purpose of the HIPAA laws.
- List at least 10 guidelines for computerized documentation.

Suggested Activities

1. Review vocabulary terms.
2. Using the assessment tool in the student text, explain and discuss the types of information required.
3. Obtain a care plan and discuss the types of nursing diagnoses listed and the approaches specified in it. Discuss which ones a nursing assistant would be responsible for.
4. Role-play a shift report. Have students take notes for specific patients they would be assigned to.
5. Give students examples of various situations and have them document the situations appropriately.

Unit Review Answers

A. True/False
1. F   2. F   3. T   4. F   5. T
6. T   7. T   8. F   9. T   10. T

B. Multiple Choice
11. b   12. d   13. d   14. a   15. c
16. c   17. a   18. b   19. b   20. b
21. d   22. a   23. c   24. b

C. Nursing Assistant Challenge
- Walked to bathroom with assistance. Difficulty walking and almost fell.
- Refused to eat breakfast.
- Threw washcloth across room when assisted with bath.
- B/P 146/88
- Smiled, hugged wife.
- Passive range of motion done on all joints without difficulty.
- Reddened area noted on coccyx.
  Examples of verbal communication: refusing breakfast (could also be nonverbal)
  Examples of nonverbal communication: almost falling, throwing washcloth, smiling and hugging wife.

Rights as a patient: refusing breakfast, having wife visit, walking and range-of-motion exercises to prevent complications and increase his independence, receiving prompt attention for the reddened coccyx to prevent skin breakdown.

UNIT 9 Meeting Basic Human Needs

Instructor Objectives

When using this unit, you will be able to teach students to:
- Spell and define terms.
- Describe the stages of human growth and development.
- List five physical needs of patients.
- Define self-esteem.
- Describe how the nursing assistant can meet the patient's emotional needs.
- List nursing assistant actions to ensure that patients have the opportunity for intimacy.
- Discuss methods of dealing with the fearful patient.
- List the guidelines to assist patients in meeting their spiritual needs.

Suggested Activities

1. Review vocabulary terms.
2. Role-play situations in which patients show fear, anger, frustration. Show how the nursing assistant should respond to these situations.
3. Initiate a discussion of ways the nursing assistant can help patients protect their self-esteem.
4. Have students describe a learning experience that made them feel good about themselves and motivated them to continue to want to learn.
5. Take an example of a situation in which a person went through a crisis—either a patient in the health care facility or an example from a newspaper. Discuss the hierarchy of needs and how they might fluctuate during such a crisis.
6. Discuss people in different age groups and how serious illness would affect those individuals.

Unit Review Answers

A. True/False
1. T   2. T   3. T   4. T   5. T
6. F   7. F   8. T   9. F   10. T
11. T   12. F   13. T   14. T   15. T
16. T   17. T   18. F   19. T   20. T
21. F

B. Matching
22. e   23. b   24. a   25. c   26. d

C. Multiple Choice
27. d   28. a   29. a   30. a

D. Nursing Assistant Challenge
31. Difficulty with rest and sleep because of pain, inability to meet need for food because of lack of appetite.
  Nursing staff can determine which foods she would like to try and present them to her when she feels she can eat, not necessarily just at mealtime. Her family may be able

to bring food from home or from a restaurant if that sounds better to her.

Do everything possible to ease pain. Report promptly to nurse so medication can be given, reposition, and do range-of-motion exercises if it helps.

32. She may have trouble meeting security needs because she feels fear and anxiety about the pain and about dying.

33. She may be fearful that her physical appearance will affect her family. She may be worried about the things she cannot do for them because of her illness.

34. The loss of a breast, hair, and weight will probably affect her sexuality.

35. Her physical needs may be uppermost when she is in pain or when she cannot eat. If her physical comfort needs are met, she may be concerned about her appearance.

UNIT 10 Comfort, Pain, Rest, and Sleep

Instructor Objectives

When using this unit, you will be able to teach students to:

- Spell and define terms.
- Explain how loud noise affects patients and hospital staff.
- Explain why nursing comfort measures are important to patients' well-being.
- List six observations to make and report for patients having pain.
- State the purpose of the pain rating scale and briefly describe how a pain scale is used.
- Describe nursing assistant measures to increase comfort and relieve pain.
- List nursing comfort measures that promote rest.
- Describe the phases of the sleep cycle and the importance of each.
- List nursing measures to promote sleep.

Suggested Activities

1. Review vocabulary terms.
2. Gather various pain rating scales and review how each is scored.
3. List items that interfere with comfort, rest, and sleep, such as the following, on separate pieces of paper.

    Pain, hunger, thirst, need to eliminate, illness, exercise, noise, temperature, ventilation, light intensity, physical discomfort, nausea, some medications, caffeine intake, alcohol, drugs, some foods and beverages, lifestyle changes, anxiety, stress, fear, emotional problems, worry, changes in the environment, unfamiliar environment, treatments and therapies, staff providing routine care.

    Have each student draw one item, explain how it interferes with comfort, rest, and sleep, and describe nursing assistant actions to assist the patient.

4. Invite a respiratory therapist or individual who specializes in diagnosis or care of patients with sleep disorders to speak with the class about sleep problems, observations to make, and ways of assisting patients.

5. With a student volunteer acting as the patient, create a lab situation in which the student is poorly positioned and in pain. Have each student throw a die. The student must demonstrate the number of nursing comfort measures he or she rolled on the die to make the "patient" more comfortable.

6. Have students stand up. Do an aerobic quiz using true or false questions, such as "A patient who is smiling cannot be having pain." If the answer to the question is true, students should touch the chair as if to sit down, then stand back up. If the answer is false, students should remain standing. Make sure students are directly over their chairs so they do not fall. A variation is to have students sit down if they answer correctly and remain standing if the answer is incorrect. Continue until all students are seated.

Unit Review Answers

A. True/False

1. F	2. T	3. T	4. F	5. T	6. F
7. F	8. F	9. T	10. T	11. F	12. T

B. Matching

13. e	14. d	15. f	16. c	17. h	18. b
19. a	20. g				

C. Completion

21. REM	22. Comfort	23. hypersomnia
24. narcolepsy	25. sleep apnea	26. somnambulism

D. Multiple Choice

27. b	28. d	29. a	30. b	31. c	32. c
33. a	34. c	35. d	36. c	37. a	38. a

E. Nursing Assistant Challenge

39. Yes.   40. pillows or props
41. Yes.   42. Yes.
43. Assist him into a comfortable position, using pillows or props as necessary. Provide extra pillows or blankets. Adjust the environmental temperature for comfort. Straighten the bed linen. Give a backrub. Offer to help wash the face and hands or provide a cool cloth for his forehead. Play soft music for distraction. Let the patient talk and listen to his concerns. Provide emotional support. Provide a quiet, dark environment.

UNIT 11 Developing Cultural Sensitivity

Instructor Objectives

When using this unit, you will be able to teach students to:
- Spell and define terms.
- Name six major cultural groups in the United States.
- Describe ways the major cultures differ in their family organization, communication, need for personal space, health practices, religion, and traditions.
- List ways nursing assistants can develop sensitivity about cultures other than their own.
- List ways the nursing assistant can help patients in practicing rituals appropriate to their cultures.
- State ways the nursing assistant can demonstrate appreciation of and sensitivity to other cultures.

Suggested Activities

1. Review vocabulary terms.
2. Ask students to think about their lifestyles and their families and to discuss the rituals, traditions, and customs that are important to them.
3. Discuss stereotypes students may have had about a person of another race or culture and how their ideas may have changed after they got to know the person better.
4. Discuss ways in which people can overcome stereotypes and prejudices.
5. Discuss opportunities available in the community that can provide information on various cultures and races.

Unit Review Answers

A. Matching
1. b   2. e   3. d   4. a   5. c

B. Completion
6. stereotypes   7. race   8. culture
9. beliefs   10. rituals

C. Multiple Choice
11. c   12. a   13. d   14. b   15. b
16. a   17. b   18. d   19. b   20. c

D. Short Answer
21. a. Treat a rosary, Bible, or crucifix with respect.
    b. Allow privacy for prayer.
    c. Assist her to attend religious services if possible.
    d. Relay to the nurse her requests to have a priest visit.
22. [Variable depending on students.]
23. Learn about the patient's culture; respect the patient's cultural beliefs and practices.

E. Nursing Assistant Challenge
24. F   25. F   26. F   27. T   28. F

SECTION 4 INFECTION AND INFECTION CONTROL
UNIT 12 Infection

Instructor Objectives

When using this unit, you will be able to teach students to:
- Spell and define terms.
- Identify the most common microbes and describe some of their characteristics.
- List the steps in the chain of infection.
- List the ways that infectious diseases are spread.
- Name and briefly describe five serious infectious diseases.
- Identify the causes of several important infectious diseases.
- Define spores and explain how spores differ from other pathogens.
- Describe common treatments for infectious disease.
- List natural body defenses against infections.
- Explain why patients are at risk for infections.

Suggested Activities

1. Review vocabulary terms.

2. Explain how each of these measures helps to prevent the spread of disease:
   - Washing dishes with hot water and detergent and rinsing well
   - Covering the mouth and nose when sneezing or coughing
   - Handwashing after using the bathroom
   - Handwashing before eating
3. Have students think of things in a typical patient unit on which microorganisms can grow.
4. If laboratory resources are available, obtain some culture plates and inoculate each plate with micro organisms from various sources: a student's fingers, a student's hair, swab from a bedpan or urinal, swab from a faucet, and other sources. Incubate the plates so that colonies grow. If possible, have the lab identify the types of microorganisms and discuss the findings with students.
5. You may wish to explore the Internet for games and activities related to infection control. These may be useful:
   - Chain of Infection Matching Game—flashcards, study tools for chain of infection http://www.studystack.com/ matching-1670
   - Chain of Infection—Learning Activity http://www.wisc-online.com/ objects/index_tj.asp?objid=NUR1603
   - GloGerm™—numerous infection control activities; explore the entire site http://www.glogerm.com/
   - Microbiology Experiments http://www.microbeworld.org/ resources/experiment.aspx
   - Resources for Educators http://www.microbeworld.org/ resources/educate.aspx
   - Merlot (go to Science, Health, Learning Materials) http://www.merlot.org/merlot/
   - HealthFinder Games (consider Amazing Microbe Hunters) http://www.healthfinder.gov/ scripts/kids_games.asp
   - Just for Fun http://4faculty.org/public/ just4fun.htm

Unit Review Answers

A. Matching
1. g   2. f   3. c   4. e   5. a

B. Word Choice
6. a. susceptible host   b. method of transmission
   c. portal of exit   d. reservoir
7. sexual contact   8. sneezing
9. water   10. insects

C. True/False
11. F   12. T   13. T   14. T   15. F
16. T   17. T   18. T   19. F   20. T

D. Multiple Choice
21. b   22. a   23. c   24. d   25. a
26. b   27. c   28. a   29. b   30. d
31. a   32. c   33. d

E. **Nursing Assistant Challenge**
34. a. Virus.   b. No.   c. By droplets.
35. a. Bacteria.   b. Round.
    c. By direct contact from a visitor or caregiver.

UNIT 13 Infection Control

Instructor Objectives

When using this unit, you will be able to teach students to:
*   Spell and define terms.
*   Explain the principles of medical asepsis.
*   Explain the components of standard precautions.
*   List the types of personal protective equipment.
*   Describe nursing assistant actions related to standard precautions.
*   Describe airborne precautions
*   Describe droplet precautions.
*   Describe contact precautions.
*   Demonstrate the procedures in the text.

Suggested Activities

1. Review vocabulary terms.
2. Demonstrate and have students return demonstrations on these procedures:
    #1—Handwashing
    #2—Putting on a mask
    #3—Putting on a gown
    #4—Putting on gloves
    #5—Removing contaminated gloves
    #6—Removing contaminated gloves, mask, gown
    #7—Serving a meal in an isolation unit
    #8—Measuring vital signs in an isolation unit
    #9—Transferring nondisposable equipment outside of the isolation unit
    #10—Specimen collection from patient in an isolation unit
    #11—Caring for linens in an isolation unit
    #12—Transporting patient to and from the isolation unit
    #13—Opening a sterile package
3. Wash your hands. Wash and dry an apple, then cut it in half. Rub half the apple on your clean hands. Place it in a jar with a lid in a warm, dark place. Write your name on the jar. Rub the other half of the apple on the hands of a student who has not washed his or her hands recently. Place it in a second jar with a lid in a warm, dark place. Write the student's name on the jar. Remove the apples at the next class session and compare the difference in appearance. Then return them to the cupboard for a week. Remove and compare the apples before discarding them.
4. Fill a shallow cake pan with one inch of water. Sprinkle pepper (to represent germs) liberally on the surface of the water. Put a tiny drop of liquid soap in the corner of the pan. Discuss the outcome with students. The objective is to show why germs do not like soap, and why using soap and water to wash hands is better than using water alone.
5. Obtain GloGerm™ cream (see http://www.glogerm.com). Have students apply gloves, then apply cream to the

hands of the gloves, all the way to the cuffs. The cream represents contaminants picked up during patient care. Have students remove the gloves. Use an ultraviolet light to show that the contamination may end up on the hands even if gloves were worn during contact with the patient. Use this activity to show why handwashing is important when gloves are removed.

6. At the beginning of the day, apply GloGerm liberally to your own hands and let it dry. Stand outside the open classroom door. Shake hands with each student as he or she enters the room. (If you wish, you may prepare the class in advance by discussing how a firm handshake projects a positive image.) After all students have taken their seats, have them get up and wash their hands. Do not tell them there is GloGerm on their hands yet. When there is one student left at the sink, tell the students about the GloGerm and shine the light on the last student before he or she washes the hands. Then use the black light to see how many "germs" are left over on their hands immediately after handwashing. Because students do not know they have GloGerm on their hands, they may not be as careful with handwashing. This interesting surprise makes a point about unseen pathogens on the hands that are not removed with inadequate handwashing. Hand lotion with food coloring or washable paint may also be used for a modified version of this activity if GloGerm is not available, but it ruins the element of surprise and tends to be messier. You can blindfold students as they wash their hands, which helps make the same point about unseen pathogens. When the blindfold is removed, the students are usually surprised at how much of the colored product is still on their hands.

Unit Review Answers

A. True/False
1. F   2. F   3. F   4. T   5. F
6. T   7. T   8. F   9. F   10. F
11. F   12. T   13. F

B. Completion
14. washing hands
15. exposure incident
16. personal protective equipment
17. 1:100 dilution of bleach
18. sharps container (puncture-resistant container)

C. Complete the Chart
19. Contact   20. Airborne   21. Droplet
22. Contact   23. Droplet

D. Multiple Choice
24. b   25. b   26. c   27. a
28. b   29. d   30. a   31. b

E. Nursing Assistant Challenge
32. a. Gowns, masks, gloves, goggles or face shields, plastic bags marked for biohazardous waste, color-coded biohazard plastic bags for soiled linen—these items are placed in a cart outside the isolation room. Place wastebasket in room with plastic, labeled bag. Place laundry hamper in room, lined with color-coded

biohazard laundry bag. Put paper towels and soap in wall dispenser or foot-operated dispenser by sink in room.

b. She may feel alone and afraid of passing disease to other people; may be fearful of staff entering room wearing personal protective equipment.

c. Spend extra time with patient and provide more emotional support.

d. Visitors may be fearful of catching the disease; they may not like to wear the personal protective equipment.

33. a. Before handling food trays.

b. After straightening overbed tables.

c. After changing an incontinent patient.

d. After using facial tissue.

e. After using the restroom.

f. Before and after making the bed.

SECTION 5 SAFETY AND MOBILITY

UNIT 14 Environmental and Nursing Assistant Safety

Instructor Objectives

When using this unit, you will be able to teach students to:

• Spell and define terms.
• Describe the health care facility environment.
• Identify measures to promote environmental safety.
• List situations when equipment must be repaired.
• Describe the elements required for fire.
• List five measures to prevent fire.
• Describe the procedure to follow if fire occurs.
• Demonstrate the use of a fire extinguisher.
• List at least 10 guidelines for dealing with a violent individual.
• List techniques for using ergonomics on the job.
• Demonstrate appropriate body mechanics.
• Describe the types of information contained in Material Safety Data Sheets (MSDS).

Suggested Activities

1. Review vocabulary terms.
2. Demonstrate the operation of different types of hospital beds and have students work with beds.
3. Take students to a patient unit and point out:
   • Bedside table and the equipment
   • Overbed table and how to use it
   • Call light—how it works and how it is turned off
   • Privacy curtains
   • Glove dispensers
   • Bathrooms
     Take students through other areas of the patient floor: utility rooms, nurses' station, linen and supply cupboards.
4. Tour the clinical facilities and point out the location of fire alarms, fire extinguishers, fire exits, and the evacuation plan.
5. Ask a member of the local fire department to demonstrate the use of fire extinguishers and have students use them.

6. Have students participate in a drill if possible.
7. Demonstrate and have students return demonstrations for body mechanics:
   • Picking up an item from the floor
   • Carrying a moderately heavy item
   • Moving a patient up in bed
   • Hold an "exercise session" with the exercises illustrated in the text
   • Discuss other ergonomic issues that may pertain to the facility, such as the use of back supports, wrist supports, and so on.
8. Set up a number of tables or stations in a room. Each table should have a display to review and one or more questions to answer. Give each student a paper with the questions on it, with room to write the answers. For example, one station might have chemical bottles with no labels, or those that have been improperly repackaged with the product name crossed out and another name written in marker on the label. Questions for this station apply to repackaging chemicals and adhering to labeling requirements. Another question may pertain to the MSDS. You may instruct students to compare the labels with the MSDS. Another station may ask staff questions, such as, "How would you get the box from the floor to the table?" (The question refers to a large, heavy box on the floor.) You may want to have stations representing items such as the chemical spill kit and ask questions about what is missing from the kit. Another good activity is to place colored water in a plastic gallon milk jug. Write the name of the product on a piece of paper and tape or rubber-band it to the bottle. Put some MSDSs on the table. Ask the students what information is missing from the label. This can be enlightening, because students may not realize that chemicals should never be transferred to a container used for food. Create stations to illustrate safety factors that students have discussed in class. You also may place a number of hazards (about 25 to 30) around the room and have students identify them on the paper for the station. These may be subtle or simple, such as an electrical cord across the floor in the center of the room, an overloaded outlet, an unlit exit sign, or soiled linen on the floor. Place other items in the room that are not safety hazards so students have to think critically to identify the problems.

Unit Review Answers

A. Multiple Choice

1. d	2. c	3. c	4. a	5. b	6. a
7. c	8. a	9. c	10. c	11. b	12. c

B. Completion

13. body mechanics	14. hips and knees
15. incident	16. ergonomics
17. mechanical lift	18. call light
19. Material Safety Data Sheets (MSDS)	20. OSHA
21. RACE	

C. True/False

22. T	23. T	24. T	25. T	26. T
27. T	28. F	29. T	30. F	31. F

D. Nursing Assistant Challenge

32. She needs to know facility policies for smoking and use of oxygen. She needs to know the fire procedure, where fire alarms are located, where extinguishers are located and how to use them, and the evacuation route.
33. Thermometers, blood pressure equipment, wheelchairs, stretchers, mechanical lifts.
34. Use good body mechanics, follow principles of ergonomics, know information on MSDS.
35. Soaps, possibly alcohol, hydrogen peroxide, cleaners, disinfectants.

UNIT 15 Patient Safety and Positioning

Instructor Objectives

When using this unit, you will be able to teach students to:
- Spell and define terms.
- Identify patients who are at risk for having incidents.
- List alternatives to the use of physical restraints.
- Describe the guidelines for the use of restraints.
- Demonstrate the correct application of restraints.
- Describe two measures for preventing accidental poisoning, thermal injuries, skin injuries, and choking.
- List the elements that are common to all procedures.
- Describe correct body alignment for the patient.
- List the purposes of repositioning patients.
- Demonstrate the procedures included in the text.

Suggested Activities

1. Review vocabulary terms.
2. Obtain an assortment of supportive devices and explain their uses to students.
3. Obtain an assortment of restraints and explain how they are used.
4. Demonstrate application of commonly used restraints.
5. Demonstrate and have students return demonstrations:
   #14—Turning the patient toward you
   #15—Turning the patient away from you
   #16—Moving a patient to the head of the bed
   #17—Logrolling the patient
6. Demonstrate and have students practice:
   - Supine and semisupine positions
   - Prone and semiprone positions
   - Lateral position
   - Fowler's position
   - Orthopneic position

Unit Review Answers

A. Multiple Choice

1. d	2. d	3. a	4. a	5. a
6. c	7. c	8. a	9. c	10. b
11. a	12. a	13. d	14. a	15. a

B. True/False

16. F	17. T	18. F	19. T	20. T
21. F	22. T	23. F	24. T	25. T

C. Matching

26. f	27. g	28. e	29. a
30. d	31. b	32. c	33. h

D. Nursing Assistant Challenge

34. She is at risk for falling because of her shuffling walk and disorientation.
    Disorientation may cause swallowing problems.
    She may cause other patients to strike out by walking into their rooms.
    She may drop things because of the tremor and fall when trying to retrieve them.
35. Her right to remain as independent as possible. Her right not to be restrained.
36. Take to bathroom regularly, promptly. Provide adequate foods and fluids. Observe for complications such as urinary infections, constipation. Observe and report pain and discomfort.
    These will all lower her risk of falling.
37. Help her do active range-of-motion exercises. Allow her to walk, with assistance if necessary.
38. She may enjoy homemaker types of activities, such as cooking, folding clean laundry, dusting. Other activities include musical activities, pets.
39. Meet physical needs promptly, provide appropriate activities and exercise.

UNIT 16 The Patient's Mobility: Transfer Skills

Instructor Objectives

When using this unit, you will be able to teach students to:
- Spell and define terms.
- List at least seven factors to consider, before lifting or moving a patient, to determine whether additional equipment or assistance is necessary.
- Apply the principles of good body mechanics and ergonomics to moving and transferring patients.
- List the guidelines for safe transfers.
- Describe the difference between a standing transfer and a sitting transfer.
- Demonstrate correct application of a transfer belt.
- Demonstrate the procedures in the text.

Suggested Activities

1. Review vocabulary terms.
2. Demonstrate and have students return demonstrations for:
   #18—Applying a transfer belt
   #19—Transferring the patient from bed to chair, one assistant
   #20—Transferring the patient from bed to chair, two assistants
   #21—Sliding-board transfer from bed to wheelchair
   #22—Transferring the patient from chair to bed, one assistant
   #23—Transferring the patient from chair to bed, two assistants

#24—Independent transfer, standby assist
#25—Transferring the patient from bed to stretcher
#26—Transferring the patient from stretcher to bed
#27—Transferring the patient with a mechanical lift
#28—Transferring the patient onto and off the toilet

Unit Review Answers

A. Multiple Choice
1. c   2. b   3. b   4. c   5. a

B. True/False
6. F   7. T   8. T   9. F   10. T
11. T   12. T   13. F   14. T   15. T

C. Nursing Assistant Challenge
16. Tell her where she is going and then tell her what she can do to help with the transfer.
17. Make sure the bed is ready for her return. Raise the bed to the same height as the stretcher, make sure the bed wheels are locked, and be sure there are enough people to help with the transfer.

UNIT 17 The Patient's Mobility: Ambulation

Instructor Objectives

When using this unit, you will be able to teach students to:
- Spell and define terms.
- Describe the purpose of assistive devices used in ambulation.
- List safety measures for using assistive devices.
- Describe safety measures for using a wheelchair.
- Describe nursing assistant actions for
  - Ambulating a patient using a gait belt
  - Propelling a patient in a wheelchair
  - Positioning a patient in a wheelchair
  - Transporting a patient on a stretcher
- Demonstrate the procedures in the text.

Suggested Activities

1. Review vocabulary terms.
2. Gather several different assistive devices and explain their uses to students. Have students examine and use the devices.
3. Invite a physical therapist to speak to students about the role of the physical therapist in the health care of patients.
4. Demonstrate all procedures and have students return demonstrations for:
   #29—Assisting the patient to walk with a cane and three-point gait
   #30—Assisting the patient to walk with a walker and three-point gait
   #31—Assisting the falling patient

Unit Review Answers

A. Multiple Choice
1. b   2. b   3. b   4. b   5. c
6. c   7. c   8. a   9. a   10. c

B. True/False
11. T   12. F   13. T   14. F   15. F
16. F   17. T   18. F   19. F   20. T

C. Nursing Assistant Challenge
Mr. Santozi is using the walker to raise himself out of the bed, which he should not do. Keep the walker out of his reach until he is standing upright.

He is putting the walker down by the front legs first and then the back legs—instruct him to set all four legs down at the same time.

He is using a two-point gait and is putting his strong leg first—instruct him to place the walker ahead, then his weak leg, then his strong leg.

SECTION 6 MEASURING AND RECORDING VITAL SIGNS, HEIGHT, AND WEIGHT

UNIT 18 Body Temperature

Instructor Objectives

When using this unit, you will be able to teach students to:
- Spell and define terms.
- Name and identify the three types of clinical thermometers and tell their uses.
- Read a thermometer.
- Identify the range of normal values.
- Demonstrate the following procedures:
  #32—Measuring temperature using a sheath-covered thermometer
  #33—Measuring an oral temperature with an electronic thermometer
  #34—Measuring a rectal temperature with an electronic thermometer
  #35—Measuring an axillary temperature with an electronic thermometer
  #36—Measuring a tympanic temperature

Suggested Activities

1. Review vocabulary terms.
2. Set out several glass thermometers with varied readings and have students read and record the temperatures. (Use warm water to obtain different readings.)
3. Demonstrate all procedures and have students return demonstrations. Use a manikin to allow students to practice rectal and groin temperatures.

Unit Review Answers

A. True/False
1. T   2. F   3. T   4. T   5. F
6. F   7. F   8. F   9. F   10. F
11. F   12. F   13. T   14. F   15. F
16. F   17. T   18. T   19. T   20. F
21. T   22. T   23. F   24. T   25. F

B. Completion
26. temperature, pulse   27. Fahrenheit   28. tympanic
29. higher   30. less

C. Nursing Assistant Challenge
31. d   32. d   33. a

UNIT 19 Pulse and Respiration

Instructor Objectives

When using this unit, you will be able to teach students to:
- Spell and define terms.
- Define pulse.
- Explain the importance of monitoring a pulse rate.
- Locate the pulse sites.
- Identify the range of normal pulse and respiratory rates.
- Measure the pulse at different locations.
- List the characteristics of the pulse and respiration.
- List eight guidelines for using the stethoscope.
- Demonstrate the following procedures:
  #37—Counting the radial pulse
  #38—Counting the apical-radial pulse
  #39—Counting respirations

Suggested Activities

1. Review vocabulary terms.
2. Have students find the pulse in every pulse site on their own bodies.
3. Demonstrate all procedures.
4. Encourage students to use stethoscopes to find apical pulses on several other students.
5. Have students return all demonstrations.

Unit Review Answers

A. True/False
1. T   2. T   3. F   4. F   5. T
6. T   7. F   8. T   9. T   10. F

B. Matching
11. h   12. d   13. g   14. b   15. e
16. i   17. a   18. k   19. f   20. c

C. Nursing Assistant Challenge
21. a. tachycardia   b. dyspnea   c. rales
    d. tachypnea   e. apical   f. radial
22. a. For an irregular pulse.
    b. For a patient receiving heart medication.

UNIT 20 Blood Pressure

Instructor Objectives

When using this unit, you will be able to teach students to:
- Spell and define terms.
- Describe the factors that influence blood pressure.
- Identify the range of normal blood pressure values.
- Identify the causes of inaccurate blood pressure readings.
- Select the proper size blood pressure cuff.
- List precautions associated with use of the sphygmomanometer.
- Demonstrate the following procedures:
  #40—Taking blood pressure
  #41—Taking blood pressure with an electronic blood pressure apparatus

Suggested Activities

1. Review vocabulary terms.
2. Allow students time to manipulate sphygmomanometers and stethoscopes before attempting to take blood pressures.
3. Demonstrate the procedure for taking blood pressure.
4. Have students return the demonstrations on several other students.

Unit Review Answers

A. True/False
1. T   2. F   3. T   4. F   5. T
6. F   7. F   8. T   9. T   10. T

B. Matching
11. g   12. b   13. h   14. a   15. e

C. Completion
16. systolic   17. hypertension   18. lost
19. exercise   20. forward

D. Nursing Assistant Challenge
21. Will need to use a very large cuff.
22. Right.
23. Yes.
24. Because the blood pressure was elevated at the last reading. The nurse needs to know whether it is still elevated.

UNIT 21 Measuring Height and Weight

Instructor Objectives

When using this unit, you will be able to teach students to:
- Spell and define terms.
- Explain why having an accurate height and weight for each patient is important.
- Describe and demonstrate how to weigh the patient on a standing balance scale, chair scale, wheelchair scale, digital scale, and bed scale.
- Describe and demonstrate how to measure a patient's height using a standing balance scale.
- Describe and demonstrate how to measure a patient using a tape measure and explain when this type of measurement is necessary.
- Demonstrate the following procedures:
  #42—Weighing and measuring the patient using an upright scale
  #43—Weighing the patient on a chair scale
  #44—Measuring weight with an electronic wheelchair scale
  #45—Measuring and weighing the patient in bed

Suggested Activities

1. Review vocabulary terms.
2. Demonstrate the procedures in the text.
3. Have students return all demonstrations.

Unit Review Answers

A. True/False
1. F   2. T   3. T   4. T
5. F   6. T   7. F

B. **Short Answer**
  8. pounds, kilograms   9. inches, centimeters
  10. ambulatory   11. kilograms
  12. away

C. **Nursing Assistant Challenge**
  13. b   14. b   15. a   16. c

SECTION 7 PATIENT CARE AND COMFORT MEASURES
UNIT 22 Admission, Transfer, and Discharge

Instructor Objectives

When using this unit, you will be able to teach students to:
- Spell and define terms.
- List the ways the nursing assistant can help in the processes of admission, transfer, and discharge.
- Describe family dynamics and emotions that occur when a loved one is admitted to the hospital.
- List ways in which the nursing assistant can develop positive relationships with a patient's family members.
- Demonstrate the following procedures:
  #46—Admitting the patient
  #47—Transferring the patient
  #48—Discharging the patient

Suggested Activities

1. Review vocabulary terms.
2. Demonstrate the procedures in the text.
3. Have students return demonstrations with another student as the patient.
4. Have students record their activities.

Unit Review Answers

A. **True/False**
  1. F   2. T   3. F   4. F   5. T
  6. T   7. F   8. T   9. T   10. T

B. **Multiple Choice**
  11. c   12. a   13. d   14. b   15. a

C. **Nursing Assistant Challenge**
  16. No.   17. Yes.   18. No.   19. Yes.   20. Yes   21. No.

UNIT 23 Bedmaking

Instructor Objectives

When using this unit, you will be able to teach students to:
- Spell and define terms.
- List the different types of beds and their uses.
- Operate each type of bed.
- Properly handle clean and soiled linens.
- Demonstrate the following procedures:
  #49—Making a closed bed
  #50—Opening the closed bed
  #51—Making an occupied bed
  #52—Making the surgical bed

Suggested Activities

1. Review vocabulary terms.
2. Demonstrate the operation of all types of available beds, if this has not been done previously.
3. Display the various types of linens used in health care facilities so that students can learn the difference between bath blankets, bedspreads, and so on.
4. Demonstrate bedmaking.
5. Have students return demonstrations.

Unit Review Answers

A. **True/False**
  1. F   2. T   3. T   4. T   5. F
  6. T   7. T   8. T   9. T   10. T

B. **Multiple Choice**
  11. d   12. c   13. a   14. c   15. b
  16. d   17. c   18. a   19. c   20. b

C. **Nursing Assistant Challenge**
  21. Pillowcases, 2 large sheets, drawsheet, waterproof sheet, or pillowcase, 1 flat sheet, 1 fitted sheet, optional draw sheet, optional underpad(s), according to patient need and facility policy

Unit 24 Patient Bathing

Instructor Objectives

When using this unit, you will be able to teach students to:
- Spell and define terms.
- Describe the safety precautions for patient bathing.
- List the purposes of bathing patients.
- State the value of whirlpool baths.
- Demonstrate the following procedures:
  #53—Assisting with the tub bath or shower
  #54—Bed bath
  #55—Changing the patient's gown
  #56—Waterless bed bath
  #57—Partial bath
  #58—Female perineal care
  #59—Male perineal care
  #60—Hand and fingernail care
  #61—Bed shampoo
  #62—Dressing and undressing the patient

Suggested Activities

1. Review vocabulary terms.
2. Discuss safety issues and the routines/procedures at the facility where students' clinical practice is being completed.
3. Demonstrate procedures on a student; have the student wear a swimsuit or shorts and a tank top and avoid embarrassing the student. Provide privacy.
4. Have students return demonstrations on other students.
5. Discuss with students their feelings about being bathed. Discuss any issues they may have about bathing patients of the opposite sex.

Unit Review Answers

A. True/False
1. T   2. F   3. F   4. F   5. T
6. T   7. F   8. F   9. T   10. T

B. Matching
11. c   12. d   13. a

C. Multiple Choice
14. c   15. a   16. a   17. d   18. a

D. Nursing Assistant Challenge
19. nursing assistant
20. should
21. transporting him by wheelchair
22. off
23. wrap him in a bath blanket

UNIT 25 General Comfort Measures

Instructor Objectives

When using this unit, you will be able to teach students to:
- Spell and define terms.
- Discuss the reasons for early morning and bedtime care.
- Identify patients who require frequent oral hygiene.
- List the purposes of oral hygiene.
- Explain nursing assistant responsibilities for a patient's dentures.
- State the purpose of backrubs.
- Describe safety precautions when shaving a patient.
- Describe the importance of hair care.
- Explain the use of comfort devices.
- Demonstrate the following procedures:
  #63—Assisting with routine oral hygiene
  #64—Assisting with special oral hygiene
  #65—Assisting the patient to floss and brush teeth
  #66—Caring for dentures
  #67—Backrub
  #68—Shaving a male patient
  #69—Daily hair care
  #70—Giving and receiving the bedpan
  #71—Giving and receiving the urinal
  #72—Assisting with use of the bedside commode

Suggested Activities

1. Review vocabulary terms.
2. Invite a dental hygienist to visit the class and discuss the importance of and procedure for routine oral examination and dental care.
3. Demonstrate all procedures.
4. Have students return demonstrations.
5. Review the following material online:
   - PowerPoint presentation and other materials— http://www.oda.org/gendeninfo/Smiles.cfm
   - Review the classroom activities—http://www.ada.org/

Unit Review Answers

A. True/False
1. F   2. T   3. T   4. F   5. T
6. F   7. T   8. T   9. T   10. F

B. Matching
11. e   12. a   13. b   14. d   15. c

C. Completion
16. down   17. PM care   18. hand, name
19. surgery   20. breakfast

D. Multiple Choice
21. d   22. b   23. d   24. a   25. a

E. Nursing Assistant Challenge
26. a. heavy smoker   b. mouth breather
27. In a denture cup.   28. Wet.   29. Yes.   30. Cool.

SECTION 8 PRINCIPLES OF NUTRITION AND FLUID BALANCE

UNIT 26 Nutritional Needs and Diet Modifications

Instructor Objectives

When using this unit, you will be able to teach students to:
- Spell and define terms.
- Define normal nutrition.
- List the essential nutrients.
- Name the food groups and list the foods included in each group.
- State the liquids/foods allowed on the basic facility diets.
- Describe the purposes of the following diets:
  - clear liquid
  - full liquid
  - soft
  - mechanically altered
- State the purpose of calorie counts and food intake studies.
- Define dysphagia and explain the risks of this condition.
- Describe general care for the patient with dysphagia and swallowing problems.
- State the purposes of therapeutic diets.
- List types of alternative nutrition.
- Describe the nursing assistant actions when patients are unable to drink fluids independently.
- Demonstrate the following procedures:
  #73—Assisting the patient who can feed self
  #74—Feeding the dependent patient

Suggested Activities

1. Review vocabulary terms.
2. Invite a dietitian to speak with the class.
3. Ask students to keep a diary of their food/fluid intake for three days and then analyze the results.
4. Have students pair up. On day one of this activity, student A will spoon-feed student B, who must wear a blindfold throughout the meal. Halfway through the meal, have students set up the tray in a clock formation, and instruct the blindfolded students to finish the meal by themselves. On day two of the activity, student B will spoon-feed student A, who must also wear a blindfold. Have a discussion about how it felt to be fed food that students could not see, what it was like to eat and drink food they could not see, and what they learned about feeding a person who is blind. Ask each student to list a tip they

would give a new nursing assistant about feeding a blind person. Write the tips on a paper and post it on the bulletin board.

5. Obtain sample trays of the various facility diets, including clear liquid, low sodium, mechanical soft, and pureed. Have students sample each of the diets. Discuss what they liked and disliked about the food preparation, and how they can use this information to benefit patients.

6. Obtain samples of various types of supplements, both pudding and liquid. Have students sample each flavor. Make sure some of the supplement is not refrigerated. Discuss students' feelings about the supplements and their taste/texture, and how they can use this information to benefit patients. Ask students if they noticed a difference between the warm and cold supplements.

7. Use food thickener to mix various thickened liquids that are nectar, honey, and pudding consistencies. Have students sample each. Next, ask students to mix solutions comparable to their perceptions of nectar, honey, and pudding consistencies. Determine if they were able to reliably mix their relative perceptions of each consistency. Discuss how the thickener tasted. Did it alter the taste? Did the liquid taste milder or stronger than usual? Is there a difference between liquids (such as coffee) that are normally served warm, compared with liquids (such as juice) that are normally served cold? Did the liquid continue to thicken if it sat unused for a while? Discuss how students can use this information to benefit patients.

8. Demonstrate all procedures.

9. Have students return demonstrations.

Unit Review Answers

A. True/False
1. T	2. F	3. T	4. F	5. T
6. T	7. F	8. T	9. T	

B. Matching
10. c	11. e	12. d	13. g	14. a	15. b

C. Multiple Choice
16. c	17. a	18. c	19. b	20. c
21. a	22. d	23. a	24. c	

D. Nursing Assistant Challenge
25. Choking (aspiration) because of trouble swallowing.
26. There should be no conflict. Coffee, tea, alcohol are not permitted on Seventh Day Adventist diets, but do not need to be served to a person on a diabetic diet. Pork is not allowed and the dietitian would need to be sure not to include pork or pork products on her menu.
27. She may have problems feeding herself because of the tremors. However, people with Parkinson's usually have "resting" tremors, so this may not present a problem. She needs to be monitored during eating to see if she needs help.
28. The diabetic diet is a part of the treatment for diabetes. Perhaps the dietitian or nurse could talk with her about her food intake. The family and friends may need to be

informed about the restrictions on her diet. Depending on the severity of her disease, the dietitian may be able to plan her food intake so that she can have some treats and still maintain a reasonably good diet.

SECTION 9 SPECIAL CARE PROCEDURES
UNIT 27 Warm and Cold Applications

Instructor Objectives

When using this unit, you will be able to teach students to:
- Spell and define terms.
- List the physical conditions requiring the use of heat and cold.
- Name types of heat and cold applications.
- Describe the effects of local cold applications.
- Describe the effects of local heat applications.
- List safety concerns related to application of heat and cold.
- Demonstrate the following procedures:
  #75—Applying an ice bag
  #76—Applying a disposable cold pack
  #77—Applying an Aquamatic K-Pad
  #78—Giving a sitz bath
  #79—Assisting with application of a hypothermia blanket

Suggested Activities

1. Review the vocabulary terms.
2. Obtain as many different items as possible that are used for heat and cold treatments, both disposable and reusable.
3. Demonstrate all procedures and have students return demonstrations.

Unit Review Answers

A. True/False
1. T	2. T	3. F	4. F	5. T
6. F	7. F	8. T	9. F	

B. Multiple Choice
10. b	11. b	12. c	13. a
14. d	15. d	16. c	

C. Matching
17. e	18. c	19. a	20. b	21. d

D. Nursing Assistant Challenge
22. Reduces pain; reduces swelling.
23. Half-full.
24. To remove sharp edges.
25. Not directly on patient.
26. Before ice is melted.
27. With tape or gauze.
28. Discoloration, numbness.

UNIT 28 Assisting with the Physical Examination

Instructor Objectives

When using this unit, you will be able to teach students to:
- Spell and define terms.
- Describe the responsibilities of the nursing assistant during the physical examination.

- Name the various positions for physical examinations.
- Drape patient for the various positions.
- Name the basic instruments necessary for physical examinations.

Suggested Activities

1. Review the vocabulary terms.
2. Obtain various pieces of equipment used in physical examinations. Encourage students to handle the equipment and to become familiar with it.
3. Display all pieces of equipment and instruct students to name each piece.

Unit Review Answers

A. True/False

1. F	2. T	3. F	4. F	5. F
6. T	7. F	8. T	9. T	10. F

B. Multiple Choice

11. b	12. b	13. c	14. a

C. Matching

15. c	16. d	17. a	18. b

D. Nursing Assistant Challenge

19. reassure	20. on, off	21. drape
22. anticipate	23. dorsal recumbent	

UNIT 29 The Surgical Patient

Instructor Objectives

When using this unit, you will be able to teach students to:

- Spell and define terms.
- Describe the concerns of patients who are about to have surgery.
- List the various types of anesthesia.
- Shave the area to be operated on.
- Prepare the patient's unit for the patient's return from the operating room.
- Give routine postoperative care when the patient returns to the room.
- Assist the patient with deep breathing and coughing.
- Apply elasticized stockings or bandages and pneumatic hosiery.
- Demonstrate the following procedures:
  #80—Assisting the patient to deep breathe and cough
  #81—Performing postoperative leg exercises
  #82—Applying elasticized stockings
  #83—Applying elastic bandage
  #84—Applying pneumatic compression hosiery
  #85—Assisting the patient to dangle

Suggested Activities

1. Review vocabulary terms.
2. If any students have had surgery, ask them if they would share their experiences and their feelings during this time.
3. Invite a surgical technician or surgical nurse to speak to the class.
4. Demonstrate procedures.
5. Have students return demonstrations.

Unit Review Answers

A. True/False

1. F	2. T	3. F	4. T	5. T
6. F	7. T	8. T	9. F	10. T

B. Matching

11. l	12. h	13. g	14. c	15. b
16. a	17. f	18. k	19. j	20. d

C. Multiple Choice

21. b	22. a	23. c	24. c	25. b

D. Nursing Assistant Challenge

26. Every 15 minutes for 4x.
    Pulse, respiration, blood pressure (temperature not taken each time).
    Pulse: 60-100; respirations: 16-20; blood pressure: systolic 140-100; diastolic 98-60.
    Changes noted with shock, hemorrhage
27. Observe amount, color, clarity, presence of foreign material such as blood.
    Foley is inserted to keep bladder empty, to avoid incontinence during surgery, to avoid accidental nicking of a full bladder if surgery is in abdomen, and to ensure that urine output is adequate after surgery.
28. Observe drip rate and insertion site for swelling, redness, leaking. IV is started to avoid dehydration and to provide a route for medication.
29. Coughing and deep breathing help clear the lungs of anesthetic and prevent pneumonia. Splinting the incision helps minimize discomfort.
30. Elastic stockings are used to reduce the risk of thrombophlebitis. They are taken off and reapplied at least every 8 hours. In some cases they may be removed for the night. Remember to put them on before the patient gets out of bed. Make sure they fit and are not too tight. They must be wrinkle-free. Observe toes for circulation after stockings are put on.
31. Report complaints of pain by indicating: where pain is occurring (left upper quadrant, lower right quadrant, etc.), how long pain has occurred, type of pain (sharp, ache, etc.).
32. Check dressing frequently. Note whether blood is seeping out through or under the dressing.

UNIT 30 Caring for the Emotionally Stressed Patient

Instructor Objectives

When using this unit, you will be able to teach students to:

- Spell and define terms.
- Define mental health.
- Define anxiety disorder, affective disorder, eating disorder, and substance abuse and give examples of each.
- Explain the interrelatedness of physical and mental health.
- Understand mental health as a process of adaptations.
- Identify commonly used defense mechanisms.
- Describe ways to help patients cope with stressful situations.
- Identify signs and symptoms of maladaptive behaviors that should be documented and reported.

- List nursing assistant measures in providing care for patients with adaptive and maladaptive reactions.
- Identify professional boundaries in relationships with patients and families.

Suggested Activities

1. Review vocabulary terms.
2. Role-play caring for patients who are:
   - disoriented
   - depressed
   - agitated
   - demanding
   - manipulative
3. Invite a psychiatric nurse to speak with the class.
4. Discuss stress reduction and relaxation techniques.
5. Develop situations in which the nursing assistant is close to crossing a professional boundary with a patient or family member. Have students work in pairs and role-play methods of handling the situation without a boundary violation.

Unit Review Answers

A. True/False

1. T	2. T	3. F	4. F	5. T
6. F	7. T	8. T	9. T	10. T
11. F	12. T	13. F	14. F	15. T
16. F	17. T	18. F	19. T	20. F
21. F	22. T	23. T	24. T	25. T

B. Matching

26. d	27. f	28. b	29. a
30. h	31. g	32. c	33. e

C. Multiple Choice

34. d	35. b	36. a	37. d	38. c
39. d	40. d	41. d	42. b	43. d
44. d	45. a	46. b		

D. Nursing Assistant Challenge

47. Eyes closed, throws water pitcher.
48. Yes—denial, displacement (throwing pitcher).
49. Be calm, caring, discuss appropriate approaches with nurse.
50. Screamed as walked in room. Picked up water pitcher and threw it.
51. Answer call light promptly, answer questions, explain procedures, do not avoid him.

UNIT 31 Caring for the Bariatric Patient

Instructor Objectives

When using this unit, you will be able to teach students to:
- Spell and define terms.
- Define overweight, obesity, and morbid obesity, and explain how these conditions differ from each other.
- Explain why weight affects life span (longevity) and health.
- Define comorbidities and explain how they affect a person's health.
- Briefly state how obesity affects the cardiovascular and respiratory systems.

- Explain how stereotyping and discrimination affect persons with obesity.
- List some team members and their responsibilities in the care of the bariatric patient.
- Explain why environmental modifications are needed for bariatric patient care.
- Describe observations to make and methods of meeting the bariatric patients' ADL needs.
- List precautions to take when moving and positioning bariatric patients.
- List at least five complications of immobility in bariatric patients.
- Describe nursing assistant responsibilities in the postoperative care of patients who have had bariatric surgery.

Suggested Activities

1. Review vocabulary terms.
2. Role-play various obese-patient situations in which the patient is struggling or unable to perform an activity, such as tying the shoes. Describe appropriate nursing assistant actions. Have students practice addressing these sensitive situations without offending or upsetting the patient.
3. Role-play or discuss a situation in which the patient is so obese that he or she cannot maintain personal cleanliness. (The patient cannot reach everywhere that needs washing because of size or because he or she lacks the range of motion and flexibility necessary.) The patient has been refusing personal care because of embarrassment, but now has developed an offensive odor.
4. Invite a nurse, social worker, or advocate who works with bariatric patients to speak with the class about the unique problems and needs of bariatric patients.
5. Obtain bariatric equipment and have students practice using it.
6. Tour the bariatric unit of the local hospital, if available. Create a list of questions for students to answer during the tour. Discuss the answers when you return to the classroom.

Unit Review Answers

A. True/False

1. F	2. T	3. F	4. F	5. T
6. F	7. T	8. F	9. F	10. F

B. Matching

11. e	12. i	13. f	14. j	15. a
16. h	17. c	18. b	19. g	20. d

C. Multiple Choice

21. c	22. b	23. b	24. a	25. a
26. d	27. c	28. d	29. b	30. c

D. Nursing Assistant Challenge

31. Check to see if a larger cuff is available. If not, consult the nurse.
32. Check to make sure the bladder size fits the patient's arm. Recheck it with another cuff. If the elevated reading persists, notify the nurse promptly.
33. Use a different cuff. If none is available, borrow one from another unit (return promptly when done), or follow protocol to obtain another cuff.

34. Notify the nurse. Wash the area with gentle soap, such as baby shampoo, and a gentle washcloth and towel. Gently pat dry. Follow the nurse's instructions. Use bath blankets or flannel to pad the skin.

35. Teach coughing and deep breathing, splinting the incision, and leg exercises. Inform her that you will be checking her vital signs frequently.

UNIT 32 Death and Dying

Instructor Objectives

When using this unit, you will be able to teach students to:
- Spell and define terms.
- Describe how different people handle the process of death and dying.
- Describe the nursing assistant's responsibilities for providing supportive care.
- Describe the spiritual preparations for death practiced by various religious denominations.
- Describe the hospice philosophy and method of care.
- List the signs of approaching death.
- Demonstrate the following procedure:
  #86—Giving postmortem care

Suggested Activities

1. Review vocabulary terms.
2. Invite clergy members from different religions to speak to the class.
3. Invite a hospice representative to speak to the class.
4. Encourage students to explore their personal feelings about dying.
5. Encourage students to discuss their experiences with the death of a loved one.

Unit Review Answers

A. True/False

1. F	2. F	3. T	4. F	5. T
6. T	7. T	8. T	9. F	10. T

B. Matching

11. c	12. e	13. f	14. b	15. a

C. Multiple Choice

16. c	17. b	18. c	19. d	20. b

D. Nursing Assistant Challenge

21. Yes.
22. Happy—comments "I'm glad I don't have cancer": denial. Refusal to follow staff suggestions, irritated, hostile: anger. If live to see granddaughter get married, will be hospital volunteer: bargaining.
23. Ask her to tell you about her granddaughter and the wedding plans.
24. Hospice will benefit her because she will be assured of supportive care, adequate pain relief, flexibility of routine, flexibility with visitors.
25. Do not touch the body 8 to 30 minutes after death, if possible. Do not wash the body unless death occurs on the Jewish sabbath. Remove water from room. Cover mirrors,

if family desires. Family member may wish to remain in room. Asking patient or family about their practices and beliefs is not offensive.

SECTION 10 OTHER HEALTH CARE SETTINGS
UNIT 33 Care of the Elderly and Chronically Ill

Instructor Objectives

When using this unit, you will be able to teach students to:
- Spell and define terms.
- List the federal requirements for nursing assistants working in long-term care facilities.
- Identify the expected changes of aging.
- Identify residents who are at risk of malnutrition and list measures to promote adequate food intake.
- Explain why elderly individuals are at risk of dehydration and list nursing assistant actions to prevent dehydration.
- List the actions a nursing assistant can take to prevent infections in the long-term care facility.
- Define delirium. List potential causes and signs and symptoms of delirium to report.
- Describe actions to use when working with residents who have dementia.
- Describe the management of wandering residents.

Suggested Activities

1. Review vocabulary terms.
2. Discuss the aging experience. Ask students to think of elderly people they know and discuss the differences between them.
3. Visit a long-term care facility, unless students are already having clinical practice in one.
4. Prepare the skills lab area with unacceptable conditions before students arrive. For example, place a bottle of chemicals on the table. Make the mock unit look untidy, with linen on the floor. Place a urinal on the overbed table, and food on the shelf with the bedpan in the bedside stand. Create as many realistic, unfavorable conditions as possible. Tell students the number of incorrect conditions. Have them tour the area, writing down as many problems as possible. Discuss the problems and identify them as a group, then relate the scenario to nursing assistant responsibilities within the job description and state regulations.

Unit Review Answers

A. True/False

1. T	2. T	3. F	4. T	5. F
6. T	7. F	8. F	9. F	10. T

B. Matching

11. c	12. d	13. b	14. a	15. e

C. Multiple Choice

16. b	17. b	18. b	19. b	20. d
21. b	22. a	23. c	24. a	25. c
26. d	27. a	28. b	29. c	30. a

D. Nursing Assistant Challenge

31. Skin is drier, less elastic, bruises easily, less oil secretion.
32. Pressure ulcers, skin tears.
33. Repositioning at least every 2 hours, make sure skin surfaces do not rub together, avoid pressure from any source, do range-of-motion exercises routinely, encourage adequate nutrition and fluid intake, keep dry, keep linens smooth, give lotion massages, protect arms and legs, check skin frequently for signs of redness, bruising.
34. Constipation.
35. Signs of infection, deterioration.

UNIT 34 The Organization of Home Care: Trends in Health Care

Instructor Objectives

When using this unit, you will be able to teach students to:
- Spell and define terms.
- Briefly describe the history of home care.
- Describe the benefits of working in home care.
- Identify members of the home health team.
- List guidelines for avoiding liability while working as a home health assistant.
- Describe the types of information a home health assistant must be able to document.
- Identify several time management techniques.
- List ways in which the home health assistant can work successfully with clients' families.

Suggested Activities

1. Review vocabulary terms.
2. Invite a nurse manager from a home health agency to speak with the class.

Unit Review Answers

A. True/False

1. F   2. T   3. F   4. F   5. T
6. T   7. F   8. T   9. T   10. F

B. Multiple Choice

11. a   12. c   13. a   14. b   15. b   16. b

C. Nursing Assistant Challenge

Home Care: Advantages: Caring for only one patient at a time, opportunity to know the patient and family, more flexibility in routine, may be less strenuous physically, probably will not have to work weekends or holidays.

Disadvantages: May need to drive several miles between patients, lack of camaraderie with other workers, may need to improvise due to lack of equipment that is normally available in a facility, may not have full-time work, will not have ready access to a supervisor.

Hospital: Advantages: May have more benefits, will have needed equipment and supplies readily available, will care for a variety of patients, enjoy relationships with other workers, ready access to supervisor.

Disadvantages: More patients to care for, may be more physically demanding, will be working weekends and holidays.

UNIT 35 The Nursing Assistant in Home Care

Instructor Objectives

When using this unit, you will be able to teach students to:
- Spell and define terms.
- Describe the characteristics that are especially important to the nursing assistant providing home care.
- List at least 10 methods of protecting your personal safety when working as a home care assistant in the community.
- Describe the duties of the nursing assistant who works in the home setting.
- Describe the duties of the homemaker assistant.
- Carry out home care activities needed to maintain a safe and clean environment.

Suggested Activities

1. Review vocabulary terms.
2. Invite a home health assistant to speak with the class.
3. Ask students to think about their own homes and to identify modifications or adaptations that would have to be made if a member of their family required home care.
4. Discuss how these modifications or adaptations can be made.

Unit Review Answers

A. True/False

1. T   2. F   3. T   4. F   5. F
6. T   7. F   8. F   9. T   10. T

B. Multiple Choice

11. a   12. b   13. a   14. b   15. a

C. Nursing Assistant Challenge

1. Do range-of-motion exercises before patient arises, to limber up. Assist patient to bathroom. Do oral care. Take vital signs.
2. Prepare breakfast and serve.
3. Prepare lunch and put in refrigerator while patient is eating breakfast.
4. Make bed and straighten bedroom while patient is eating. Allow patient to rest a few minutes after eating. During this time, clean up kitchen.
5. Do bath and personal care, dressing.
6. Let patient rest. While patient is resting, clean up bathroom. Do laundry if necessary.
7. Pick up prescriptions and return to patient. Finish laundry if necessary. Do documentation.

UNIT 36 Subacute Care

Instructor Objectives

When using this unit, you will be able to teach students to:
- Spell and define terms.
- Describe the purpose of subacute care.
- List the differences between acute care, subacute care, and long-term care.

- Describe the responsibilities of the nursing assistant when caring for patients receiving special treatments in subacute care.
- Demonstrate the following procedures:
  #87—Checking capillary refill.
  #88—Using a pulse oximeter.

Suggested Activities

1. Review vocabulary terms.
2. Collect as many pieces of equipment found in subacute care as possible: various IV equipment, feeding tubes, oximeter, etc. Explain the uses of the equipment.
3. Invite a nurse or nursing assistant from a subacute care unit to speak with the class.

Unit Review Answers

A. Multiple Choice

1. a	2. c	3. c	4. b	5. b
6. b	7. c	8. d	9. c	10. a
11. a	12. b	13. a	14. c	15. a
16. c	17. c	18. d	19. a	20. b
21. d	22. b	23. c	24. a	

B. Word Choice

25. transitional care	26. dialysis
27. pulse oximetry	28. piggyback
29. hyperalimentation	30. enteral
31. narcotic	32. transcutaneous electrical nerve stimulation (TENS)
33. multisensory stimulation	34. exacerbation
35. spasticity	36. Kelly
37. hypoxemia	38. continuous ambulatory peritoneal dialysis (CAPD)

C. Nursing Assistant Challenge

39. Depends on the types of patients cared for. Will need keen observation skills specific to problems of particular types of patients.
40. Will need new skills for operating equipment and doing different procedures. Will need to be knowledgeable about the reasons for the patient's admission (rehabilitation, orthopedics, cancer, etc.).
41. Staff development, reading, watching videos.

UNIT 37 Alternative, Complementary, and Integrative Approaches to Patient Care

Instructor Objectives

When using this unit, you will be able to teach students to:
- Spell and define terms.
- Define alternative medicine.
- Differentiate alternative practices from complementary and integrative practices.
- List five categories of alternative and complementary therapies.
- Define holistic care.
- List at least three ways in which the nursing assistant supports patients' spirituality.

Suggested Activities

1. Review vocabulary terms.
2. Ask a practitioner of various alternative and complementary therapies to speak with the class about the action, use, benefits, and precautions.
3. Have students each draw a slip of paper from an envelope listing alternative or complementary therapies studied in this unit or used in this area. Each student should prepare a five-minute presentation describing how the CAM practice is used, and nursing assistant responsibilities relating to it, to present at the next class session.
4. Discuss herbs, supplements, and other CAM therapies. Describe how they evolved from alternative into mainstream use.

Unit Review Answers

A. True/False

1. T	2. F	3. T	4. T
5. T	6. T	7. F	8. F
9. F	10. T	11. T	12. T

B. Matching

13. g	14. h	15. k	16. i
17. c	18. b	19. a	20. j
21. l	22. e	23. f	24. d

C. Multiple Choice

25. b	26. c	27. a	28. d	29. b

D. Nursing Assistant Challenge

30. Provide privacy and leave the room so as not to interrupt meditation and break her concentration.
31. Arrive in the room on time to assist the patient with meditation. Ask her what time she would like you to arrive, and be there at that time. Assist the patient into a comfortable position. Adjust the room temperature and lighting according to her wishes. Provide privacy, but make sure the call signal is within reach. When leaving the room, ask her what time she would like you to return.
32. Check the care plan or with the nurse. Ask the patient what she needs.
33. The meditation will help the patient relax and relieve stress. It may relieve pain. It is a personal experience for some people and may help the patient to get in touch with her inner self. Meditation may benefit the patient in personal growth and becoming more tolerant of others. It may help the patient channel awareness into a more positive direction.

SECTION 11 BODY SYSTEMS, COMMON DISORDERS, AND RELATED CARE PROCEDURES

UNIT 38 Integumentary System

Instructor Objectives

When using this unit, you will be able to teach students to:
- Spell and define terms.
- Review the location and function of the skin.

- Describe some common skin lesions.
- List three diagnostic tests associated with skin conditions.
- Describe nursing assistant actions relating to care of patients with specific skin conditions.
- Identify persons at risk for the formation of pressure ulcers.
- Describe measures to prevent pressure ulcers.
- Describe the stages of pressure ulcer formation and identify appropriate nursing assistant actions.
- List nursing assistant actions in caring for patients with burns.

Suggested Activities

1. Review the vocabulary terms.
2. Obtain and show an assortment of mechanical devices used to avoid pressure ulcer formation.
3. Obtain and show an assortment of different types of dressings used for pressure ulcers.

Unit Review Answers

A. True/False
1. T	2. T	3. T	4. F	5. T	6. F
7. F	8. T	9. T	10. T	11. F	12. F
13. F	14. F	15. T	16. T		

B. Matching
17. b	18. e	19. g	20. a	21. c
22. l	23. j	24. m	25. h	26. i

C. Multiple Choice
27. b	28. d	29. a	30. c	31. a
32. b	33. a	34. d	35. c	36. b

D. Completion
37. a. Observation and reporting, find out whether bathing and lotion are permitted.
    b. Wear gloves, do not remove crusts.
    c. Handle gently, avoid rubbing.
38. a. Scraping examination.
    b. Culture.
    c. Sensitivity testing.
39. a. Elderly.
    b. Obese.
    c. Immobile and/or with impaired circulation.
    d. Incontinent or frequent contact with other sources of moisture.
    e. Disoriented.
    f. Dehydrated.
40. a. Elbows.   b. Heels.   c. Shoulders.
    d. Sacrum.   e. Hips.
    Also ankles, ears, behind or beside the knee.
41. The patient needs extra protein for repair of body tissues.

E. Nursing Assistant Challenge
42. 15	43. 30	44. 2	45. twice

UNIT 39 Respiratory System

Instructor Objectives

When using this unit, you will be able to teach students to:
- Spell and define terms.
- Review the location and function of the respiratory organs.

- Describe some common diseases of the respiratory system.
- List five diagnostic tests used to identify respiratory conditions.
- Describe nursing assistant actions related to the care of patients with respiratory conditions.
- Identify patients who are at high risk of poor oxygenation.
- Describe the care of patients with a tracheostomy, laryngectomy, and chest tubes.
- List five safety measures for the use of oxygen therapy.
- Demonstrate the following procedures:
  #89—Collecting a sputum specimen

Suggested Activities

1. Review the vocabulary terms.
2. Demonstrate procedures and have students return demonstrations.
3. Invite a nurse to speak to the class about breathing techniques taught to patients with chronic obstructive pulmonary disease.
4. Invite a speaker from the American Cancer Society to discuss smoking and its relationship to lung diseases.
5. Use balloons to demonstrate an inability to expel air from the alveoli.
6. Have students breathe through a cocktail straw for a minute while holding their noses. This compares with the intake of a patient with COPD. Discuss their findings.

Unit Review Answers

A. True/False
1. T	2. F	3. T	4. F	5. T
6. T	7. T	8. T	9. F	10. F

B. Matching
11. c	12. a	13. d	14. f	15. b

C. Multiple Choice
16. a	17. c	18. d	19. b	20. b

D. Nursing Assistant Challenge
21. 2 L/min	22. is not	23. may not
24. 5 feet	25. weekly	

UNIT 40 Circulatory (Cardiovascular) System

Instructor Objectives

When using this unit, you will be able to teach students to:
- Spell and define terms.
- Review the location and functions of the organs of the circulatory system.
- Describe some common disorders of the circulatory system.
- Describe nursing assistant actions related to care of patients with disorders of the circulatory system.
- List five specific diagnostic tests for disorders of the circulatory system.

Suggested Activities

1. Review vocabulary terms.
2. Invite an EKG technician to demonstrate taking an EKG to students.

3. Invite a nurse to speak to the class about cardiac rehabilitation after a heart attack.

Unit Review Answers

A. True/False
1. F   2. T   3. T   4. F   5. T
6. F   7. T   8. T   9. F   10. T

B. Matching
11. e   12. c   13. f   14. a   15. h

C. Multiple Choice
16. a   17. a   18. b   19. c   20. c

D. Completion
21. a. Blood chemistry tests   b. EKG
c. Cardiac catheterization, angiogram   d. Ultrasound
e. CBC
22. a. Hypertension   b. Diabetes   c. Overweight
d. Heredity   e. Smoking   f. Stress
Also lack of exercise, high cholesterol, high-fat diet.

E. Nursing Assistant Challenge
23. high   24. temporary, brain   25. sodium
26. discouraged   27. stroke   28. exercise
29. blurred vision   30. hypertension

UNIT 41 Musculoskeletal System

Instructor Objectives

When using this unit, you will be able to teach students to:
- Spell and define terms.
- Describe the location and functions of the musculoskeletal system.
- Describe some common conditions of the musculoskeletal system.
- Describe nursing assistant actions related to the care of patients with conditions and diseases of the musculoskeletal system.
- List seven specific diagnostic tests for musculoskeletal conditions.
- Demonstrate the following procedures:
  #90—Procedure for continuous passive motion
  #91—Performing passive range-of-motion exercises

Suggested Activities

1. Review the vocabulary terms.
2. Demonstrate procedure 91, passive range-of-motion exercises, and have students return demonstrations.
3. Invite a physical therapist or occupational therapist to demonstrate other exercises to students, such as stretching and active range-of-motion exercises.
4. Ask a physical therapist to bring a lower extremity prosthesis to class and demonstrate its application.
5. Invite a prosthestist to class to discuss his or her work.
6. Arrange for students to observe in a physical therapy department such procedures as gait training for a new amputee or a patient with a new hip arthroplasty.

Unit Review Answers

A. True/False
1. F   2. T   3. T   4. F   5. T
6. F   7. T   8. T   9. T   10. F
11. T   12. F   13. F   14. F   15. T

B. Matching
16. f   17. d   18. b   19. g   20. a

C. Multiple Choice
21. c   22. a   23. c   24. a   25. c
26. b   27. d   28. c   29. a   30. d

D. Nursing Assistant Challenge
31. You need to know:
- How she is supposed to transfer out of bed.
- If she is able to ambulate, and if she does, can she bear full weight?
- Is she to use an assistive device when she is ambulating?
- Which positions should she avoid in bed and when completing the activities of daily living, such as adduction and internal and external rotation?

UNIT 42 Endocrine System

Instructor Objectives

When using this unit, you will be able to teach students to:
- Spell and define terms.
- Review the location and functions of the endocrine system.
- Review five specific diagnostic tests associated with conditions of the endocrine system.
- Describe some common diseases of the endocrine system.
- Recognize the signs and symptoms of hypoglycemia and hyperglycemia.
- Describe nursing assistant actions related to the care of patients with disorders of the endocrine system.
- Perform blood tests for glucose levels if facility policy permits.
- Perform the following procedure:
  #92—Obtaining a fingerstick blood sugar

Suggested Activities

1. Review vocabulary terms.
2. Invite a dietitian to speak to the class about diabetic diets.
3. Invite a registered nurse who does diabetic patient teaching to speak to the class about what these patients have to learn.
4. Demonstrate glucose testing and have students return the procedure.

Unit Review Answers

A. True/False
1. F   2. T   3. T   4. F   5. T
6. F   7. T   8. T   9. T   10. T

B. Matching
11. e   12. g   13. a   14. c   15. d
16. b   17. h   18. f   19. j   20. i

C. Multiple Choice

21. b   22. a   23. a   24. d   25. a

D. Nursing Assistant Challenge

26. Ms. Sakowski: polyuria, polydipsia, polyphagia, glycosuria
    Ms. Young: fatigue, skin infections, slow healing, itching, burning on urination, pain in fingers and toes, vision changes, obesity

27. Ms. Sakowski will receive insulin and will need to have frequent blood glucose monitoring—at least twice a day or more often. Ms. Young will control her diabetes with diet or will take hypoglycemic oral drugs. Ms. Sakowski will be more at risk for the complications of diabetes.

28. Both women should be able to live normal lives but will have to be cautious about diet, personal hygiene, and exercise. Ms. Sakowski may have concerns about pregnancy and should seek counseling before becoming pregnant.

29.

Hypoglycemia	Hyperglycemia
Rapid onset	Slower onset
Due to:	Due to:
• too much insulin	• not enough insulin
• too little food	• too much food
• too much exercise	• too little exercise
Shallow, rapid breathing	Deep breathing
Rapid, weak pulse	Full, bounding pulse
Hunger	Thirst
Pale, moist skin	Flushed, dry, hot skin
Low blood sugar	High blood sugar

UNIT 43 Nervous System

Instructor Objectives

When using this unit, you will be able to teach students to:

• Spell and define terms.
• State the location and functions of the organs of the nervous system.
• List five diagnostic tests used to determine conditions of the nervous system.
• Describe 15 common conditions of the nervous system.
• Describe nursing assistant actions related to the care of patients with conditions of the nervous system.
• Explain the proper care, handling, and insertion of an artificial eye.
• Explain the proper care, handling, and insertion of a hearing aid.
• Demonstrate the following procedures:
  #93—Caring for the eye socket and artificial eye.
  #94—Warm or cool eye compresses

Suggested Activities

1. Review vocabulary terms.
2. Invite a person with one of the neurological diseases to speak to students about the way the disease affects his or her lifestyle.

3. Invite an audiologist to speak to students about how hearing tests are conducted, how hearing aids are prescribed, and how hearing aids should be handled.
4. Demonstrate all procedures and have students return demonstrations.

Unit Review Answers

A. True/False

1. F   2. F   3. T   4. T   5. T
6. T   7. T   8. F   9. T

B. Multiple Choice

10. a   11. c   12. c   13. d   14. b
15. b   16. c   17. a   18. a   19. a
20. c   21. b   22. c   23. d   24. c
25. a   26. b   27. b   28. c   29. a
30. d   31. b

C. Matching

32. c   33. f   34. a   35. b
36. d   37. h   38. g

D. Nursing Assistant Challenge

39. Left side.
40. The entire right side of his body is paralyzed.
41. He will have difficulty either understanding language or expressing language or both. He may become very frustrated in his attempts to communicate verbally.
42. He is at risk for contractures, pressure ulcers, pneumonia, and blood clots. Preventive measures include appropriate positioning in bed and chair, range-of-motion exercises, keeping him dry, and encouraging fluid and appropriate food intake. Transfer and ambulate the patient if ordered. If splints and orthoses are ordered, apply them correctly.
43. Mr. Johnson may be disoriented as to time, place, and/or person. He may be unable to complete a task because he lacks the ability to concentrate and to pay attention.

Unit 44 Gastrointestinal System

Instructor Objectives

When using this unit, you will be able to teach students to:

• Spell and define terms.
• Review the location and functions of the organs of the gastrointestinal system.
• List specific diagnostic tests associated with disorders of the gastrointestinal system.
• Describe some common disorders of the gastrointestinal system.
• Describe nursing assistant actions related to the care of patients with disorders of the gastrointestinal system.
• Identify different types of enemas and state their purposes.
• Demonstrate the following procedures:
  #95—Collecting a stool specimen
  #96—Giving a soap-solution enema
  #97—Giving a commercially prepared enema
  #98—Inserting a rectal suppository

Suggested Activities

1. Review vocabulary terms.
2. Give students time to handle and inspect the equipment used in the procedures.
3. Obtain different types of nasogastric tubes and gastrostomy tubes for display.
4. Demonstrate all procedures in the text and have students return demonstrations.

Unit Review Answers

A. True/False
1. F   2. T   3. T   4. T   5. T
6. T   7. T   8. F   9. F

B. Matching
10. b   11. g   12. f   13. a   14. c

C. Multiple Choice
15. b   16. c   17. c   18. c   19. b

D. Completion
20. oil retention   21. cleanse the lower bowel of feces

E. Nursing Assistant Challenge
22. Hydrochloric acid.   23. No.   24. Cleansing enema.
25. Swallow.   26. Yes.

UNIT 45 Urinary System

Instructor Objectives

When using this unit, you will be able to teach students to:
- Spell and define terms.
- Review the location and function of the urinary system.
- List five diagnostic tests associated with conditions of the urinary system.
- Describe some common diseases of the urinary system.
- Describe nursing assistant actions related to the care of patients with urinary system diseases and conditions.
- Demonstrate the following procedures:
  #99—Collecting a routine urine specimen
  #100—Collecting a clean-catch urine specimen
  #101—Collecting a 24-hour urine specimen
  #102—Routine drainage check
  #103—Giving indwelling catheter care
  #104—Emptying a urinary drainage unit
  #105—Disconnecting the catheter
  #106—Applying a condom for urinary drainage
  #107—Connecting a catheter to a leg bag
  #108—Emptying a leg bag

Suggested Activities

1. Review vocabulary terms.
2. Gather and display all equipment identified in this unit.
3. Tour a hemodialysis unit, if possible, or invite a nurse from the unit to speak with students.
4. Inflate the balloon of an indwelling catheter so the students can envision the internal fixation of the catheter.
5. Demonstrate and have students return demonstrations of all procedures in the text.

Unit Review Answers

A. True/False
1. F   2. T   3. T   4. T   5. F
6. T   7. T   8. F   9. T   10. T

B. Matching
11. f   12. d   13. a   14. c   15. b

C. Multiple Choice
16. c   17. b   18. a   19. c   20. b

D. Completion
21. Wipe the ends of the catheter and the drainage tube with antiseptic and reconnect. Report to nurse. Change the bed if it is wet.
22. • Signs of irritation or urinary discomfort
    • Tubing secure
    • Catheter is intact and drainage tube is intact and not too coiled
    • Catheter strap is in place
    • Drainage bag is below level of bladder but not touching floor
    • Amount, color, and character of urine

E. Nursing Assistant Challenge
23. yes   24. rolling it down toward the base   25. leave

UNIT 46 Reproductive System

Instructor Objectives

When using this unit, you will be able to teach students to:
- Spell and define terms.
- Review the location and functions of the organs of the male and female reproductive systems.
- Describe some common disorders and conditions of the male reproductive system.
- Describe some common disorders and conditions of the female reproductive system.
- List six diagnostic tests associated with conditions of the male and female reproductive systems.
- Describe nursing assistant actions related to the care of patients with conditions and diseases of the reproductive system.
- State the nursing precautions required for patients who have sexually transmitted diseases.
- Demonstrate the following procedure:
  #109—Giving a nonsterile vaginal douche

Suggested Activities

1. Review vocabulary terms.
2. Obtain the model examination breast from the American Cancer Society so female students can practice breast examination.
3. Demonstrate and have students return demonstrations for vaginal douche.
4. Invite a nurse from a public health clinic to speak to students about sexually transmitted diseases.

Unit Review Answers

A. True/False
1. T   2. T   3. F   4. T   5. T
6. F   7. T   8. T   9. F

B. Matching
10. e   11. f   12. a   13. b   14. d

C. Multiple Choice
15. c   16. c   17. b   18. c

D. Completion
19. standard precautions   20. every year   21. monthly

E. Nursing Assistant Challenge
22. Excessive vaginal bleeding during her period and difficult, painful periods.
23. No.
24. Low back pain.
25. Vagina, incision.
26. Slowing of blood supply to pelvis may result in clot formation.

SECTION 12 EXPANDED ROLE OF THE NURSING ASSISTANT
UNIT 47 Caring for the Patient with Cancer

Instructor Objectives

When using this unit, you will be able to teach students to:
- Spell and define terms.
- List methods of reducing the risk of cancer.
- Explain the importance of good nutrition in cancer prevention and treatment.
- List seven signs and symptoms of cancer.
- Describe three types of cancer treatment.
- Describe nursing assistant responsibilities when caring for patients with cancer.

Suggested Activities

1. Review vocabulary terms.
2. Write modifiable risk factors for cancer on individual pieces of paper. Have each student draw a paper and prepare a five-minute report to the class on the risk factor and preventive health care.
3. Ask a dietitian to speak to the class about reducing cancer risk through dietary intervention. Ask the dietitian to address ways of maintaining good nutrition in patients who are receiving cancer treatment.
4. Ask a nurse or hospice worker to speak to the class about cancer treatment and palliative care.
5. Cover an area of the wall with flip-chart paper. At the end of the unit, ask students to write comments in each of the following categories: a) How I feel about cancer; b) Best idea I got from this material; c) One way I will use this information right away. Discuss each comment with the group.

Unit Review Answers

A. True/False
1. F   2. T   3. F   4. T   5. T

B. Matching
6. b   7. d   8. a   9. e   10. c

C. Multiple Choice
11. d   12. c   13. c   14. b   15. a
16. c   17. b   18. a   19. d   20. c

D. Nursing Assistant Challenge
21. He is upset about his condition and may be in pain or feeling ill because of the treatment.
22. No.
23. Inform the nurse.
24. Report the behavior exactly. "The patient refused to speak when I took his vital signs. When I served his tray, he pushed it onto the floor and said he was not hungry. He told me to get out of the room and to leave him alone."
25. No. The patient still needs care. Consult the nurse and follow his or her instructions.

UNIT 48 Rehabilitation and Restorative Services

Instructor Objectives

When using this unit, you will be able to teach students to:
- Spell and define terms.
- Compare and contrast rehabilitation and restorative care.
- Identify five members of the interdisciplinary team.
- Describe the role of the nursing assistant in rehabilitation and restorative care.
- Describe the principles of rehabilitation.
- List the elements of successful rehabilitation/restorative care.
- List six complications resulting from inactivity.
- Identify four perceptual deficits.
- Describe four approaches used for restorative programs.
- List the guidelines for implementing restorative programs.

Suggested Activities

1. Visit the rehabilitation department of a long-term care facility.
2. Have students role-play with simulated disabilities. Write several different disabilities on slips of paper and have each student draw one. Examples: right hemiplegia, left hemiplegia, paraplegia, quadriplegia, vision and/or hearing impairment, arthritis, etc. Obtain needed equipment such as wheelchairs, crutches, canes, walkers. Give students a list of tasks to complete while disabled: getting a drink of water, going to the restroom, using a pay phone, getting in and out of a car, etc.

Unit Review Answers

A. True/False
1. F   2. T   3. T   4. F   5. F

B. Multiple Choice
6. a   7. c   8. d   9. a
10. b   11. c   12. c

C. Completion
13. rehabilitation   14. mobility skills
15. activities of daily living   16. disability
17. handicap   18. geriatric
19. physiatrist   20. contracture

21. Atrophy
23. embolus
25. verbal cues

22. disuse osteoporosis
24. self-care deficit

D. Nursing Assistant Challenge

26. Patients who have had orthopedic surgery, injuries, or stroke and who need to relearn certain tasks.
27. Hemiplegia, quadriplegia, paraplegia, head injuries.
28. Diseases, injuries, vision impairment, emotional illness.
29. Decreased strength, lack of endurance, limited range of motion, depression, disorientation, perceptual deficits.
30. Rehabilitation is more aggressive and intense.
31. Know what the patient's self-care deficits are and what caused them; know what the goals and approaches are and follow the approaches exactly as written; use assistive or adaptive devices correctly.

UNIT 49 Obstetrical Patients and Neonates

Instructor Objectives

When using this unit, you will be able to teach students to:
- Spell and define terms.
- Assist in prenatal care of the normal pregnant woman.
- List reportable observations of patients in the prenatal period.
- Define *doula* and identify the role and responsibilities of the doula as a member of the childbirth team.
- Assist in care of the normal postpartum patient.
- Properly change a perineal pad.
- Recognize reportable observations of patients in the postpartum period.
- Recognize reportable signs and symptoms of urine retention in the postpartum patient.
- Assist in care of the normal newborn.
- Demonstrate three methods of safely holding a baby.
- List measures to prevent inadvertent switching, misidentification, and abduction of infants.
- Assist in carrying out the discharge procedures for mother and infant.
- Demonstrate the following procedures:
  #110—Changing a diaper
  #111—Bathing an infant

Suggested Activities

1. Invite a mother and small baby to class and demonstrate bathing, diapering, and feeding.
2. Invite a nurse from a clinic to discuss prenatal care.

Unit Review Answers

A. True/False

1. T	2. T	3. T	4. F	5. F
6. T	7. T	8. T	9. F	10. T
11. T	12. T			

B. Matching

13. f	14. h	15. e	16. b	17. a

C. Nursing Assistant Challenge

18. Mother will report: absence of menstrual period, nausea and vomiting, swelling and tenderness of breasts, frequent urination, constipation.
19. Scales, equipment for vital signs, urine specimen cup.
20. Weight gain, abdominal enlargement, stretch marks on abdominal skin, breast enlargement; mother may report feeling quickening.
21. Edema of ankles, varicose veins; mother may report backaches, indigestion, insomnia, shortness of breath, and feeling painless uterine contractions.
22. Weight, vital signs, urine specimen, examination by nurse practitioner.
23. Persistent headache, elevated blood pressure, vaginal bleeding, complaints of dizziness, swelling of hands and feet.

UNIT 50 Pediatric Patients

Instructor Objectives

When using this unit, you will be able to teach students to:
- Spell and define terms.
- Describe how to foster growth and development of hospitalized pediatric patients.
- Describe how to maintain a safe environment for the pediatric patient.
- Discuss the problem of childhood obesity and identify special problems and complications that occur as a result of this condition.
- Discuss the role of parents and siblings of the hospitalized pediatric patient.
- Demonstrate the following procedures:
  #112—Admitting a pediatric patient
  #113—Weighing the pediatric patient
  #114—Changing crib linens
  #115—Changing crib linens (infant in crib)
  #116—Measuring temperature
  #117—Determining heart rate (pulse)
  #118—Counting respiratory rate
  #119—Measuring blood pressure
  #120—Bottle-feeding an infant
  #121—Burping an infant
  #122—Collecting a urine specimen from an infant

Suggested Activities

1. Review vocabulary terms.
2. Demonstrate and have students return demonstrations for all procedures in the text.

Unit Review Answers

A. True/False

1. T	2. T	3. T	4. F	5. F
6. F	7. T	8. F	9. F	10. T
11. T	12. F	13. T	14. F	15. F
16. T	17. T	18. F	19. F	20. T
21. F	22. T	23. F	24. T	25. T

B. Matching

26. f   27. d   28. g   29. b

30. c   31. e   32. a

C. Nursing Assistant Challenge

33. electronic, rectal

34. electronic, rectal

35. electronic, axillary (or oral if policies permit and child can follow instructions)

36. electronic, axillary

37. electronic, oral

38. electronic, oral

UNIT 51 Special Advanced Procedures

Instructor Objectives

When using this unit, you will be able to teach students to:
- Spell and define terms.
- State the reasons for removing an indwelling catheter as soon as possible.
- List the guidelines for caring for an ostomy.
- List at least six procedures in which sterile technique is used.
- State nursing assistant responsibilities for the care of patients with advanced airways.
- Demonstrate the following procedures:
  #123—Testing for occult blood using Hemoccult and developer
  #124—Collecting a urine specimen through a drainage port
  #125—Removing an indwelling catheter
  #126—Giving routine stoma care (colostomy)
  #127—Routine care of an ileostomy (with patient in bed)
  #128—Setting up a sterile field using a sterile drape
  #129—Adding an item to a sterile field
  #130—Adding liquids to a sterile field
  #131—Applying and removing sterile gloves
  #132—Using transfer forceps

Suggested Activities

1. Review vocabulary terms.
2. Discuss the opportunities for and the restrictions on nursing assistants performing advanced procedures.
3. Demonstrate the procedures in the text and have students return demonstrations.

Unit Review Answers

A. True/False

1. F	2. F	3. T	4. F	5. T
6. T	7. F	8. T	9. T	10. F
11. F	12. T	13. T	14. F	15. F
16. T	17. F	18. T		

B. Matching

19. c	20. e	21. b	22. a	23. d

C. Multiple Choice

24. b	25. b	26. c	27. c	28. b
29. d	30. d	31. b	32. b	33. a
34. c	35. c	36. b	37. a	38. d
39. c	40. d			

D. Nursing Assistant Challenge

41. Yes.

42. Toilet tissue, then soap and water.

43. Too much lotion will interfere with the seal of the ostomy bag.

44. With a belt.

45. Leakage, odor, irritation of skin.

SECTION 13 RESPONSE TO BASIC EMERGENCIES

UNIT 52 Response to Basic Emergencies

Instructor Objectives

When using this unit, you will be able to teach students to:
- Spell and define terms.
- Recognize emergency situations that require urgent care.
- Evaluate situations and determine the sequence of appropriate actions to be taken.
- List and describe the 11 standardized types of codes.
- Describe how to maintain the patient's airway and breathing during respiratory failure and respiratory arrest.
- Recognize the need for CPR.
- List the benefits of early defibrillation.
- Identify the signs, symptoms, and treatment of common emergency situations such as cardiac arrest, choking, bleeding, shock, fainting, heart attack, brain attack (stroke), seizure, vomiting and aspiration, thermal injuries, poisoning, and known or suspected head injury.
- Demonstrate the following procedures:
  #133—Head-tilt, chin-lift maneuver
  #134—Jaw-thrust maneuver
  #135—Mask-to-mouth ventilation
  #136—Positioning the patient in the recovery position
  #137—Heimlich maneuver—abdominal thrusts
  #138—Assisting the adult who has an obstructed airway and becomes unconscious
  #139—Obstructed airway: infant
  #140—Child with foreign body airway obstruction

Suggested Activities

1. Review vocabulary terms.
2. Demonstrate and have students return demonstrations for all the procedures in the text.

Unit Review Answers

A. True/False

1. F	2. T	3. F	4. T	5. T
6. F	7. T	8. T	9. F	10. F

B. Matching

11. c	12. f	13. d	14. h	15. b

C. Multiple Choice

16. d	17. c	18. c	19. b	20. c
21. d	22. c	23. b	24. a	25. a
26. b	27. a	28. a	29. a	30. a
31. b	32. d	33. b	34. a	

D. Nursing Assistant Challenge

36. a. Check everyone for consciousness and injuries.

b. Remain with the passenger in the car that ran the stop sign. Hold the head so the person does not aspirate vomitus. Check bleeding, apply clean cloth, apply pressure if bleeding is heavy.

SECTION 14 MOVING FORWARD
UNIT 53 Employment Opportunities and Career Growth

Instructor Objectives

When using this unit, you will be able to teach students to:

- Spell and define terms.
- List nine objectives to be met in obtaining and maintaining employment.
- Follow a process for self-appraisal.
- Name sources of employment for nursing assistants.
- Prepare a résumé and a letter of resignation.
- List the steps for a successful interview.
- List the requirements that must be met when accepting employment.
- List steps for continuing development in your career.

Suggested Activities

1. Conduct mock interviews in class. Have students critique one another.
2. Have students complete application-for-employment forms. Provide suggestions for improvement, if necessary.
3. Ask students to bring in the want ads from newspapers and discuss and compare the ads.
4. Have each student write out a résumé and a resignation. Provide suggestions for improvement, if necessary.
5. Have each student complete a self-appraisal as suggested in the text.
6. Discuss opportunities for career development.
7. Invite a director of nursing to speak with the class about interviewing techniques.

Unit Review Answers

A. True/False

1. F	2. F	3. F	4. T	5. T
6. T	7. F	8. T	9. T	10. T

B. Multiple Choice

11. b	12. d	13. a	14. d	15. a

C. Nursing Assistant Challenge

16. Social security number; date of birth, address, and phone number; addresses and phone numbers of references; dates, names, and addresses of past employers and name of supervisor; dates, names, and addresses of educational institutions attended.
17. Social security card, driver's license, pen.
18. Clean and well-groomed, simple clothing in good repair, very little jewelry.
19. Ask the interviewer what the starting salary is. Ask if there are benefits.

Section 1
SELF-EVALUATION

A. Multiple Choice. Choose the phrase that best completes each of the following sentences by circling the proper letter.

1. Functions of a health care facility include
   a. immunizing the community to prevent disease.
   b. analyzing water to ensure that it is safe to drink.
   c. providing radio and television to relieve boredom.
   d. providing services for the ill and injured.

2. Health care has changed because
   a. fewer people are requiring health care.
   b. there are many more ethics questions.
   c. the government now pays for all health care.
   d. many patients require technology that is not available.

3. Your daily assignment is usually given to you by the
   a. assistant.
   b. director of nursing.
   c. team leader or charge nurse.
   d. physician.

4. The Patients' Bill of Rights includes the right to know that
   a. orders will be acknowledged.
   b. privacy will be preserved.
   c. you may withhold health information.
   d. the bill must be paid on time.

5. Which of the following is *not* a part of your job?
   a. Starting IVs
   b. Collecting specimens
   c. Assisting patients to ambulate
   d. Giving enemas

6. Personal information about patients
   a. may be discussed during coffee break.
   b. must never be discussed outside the hospital.
   c. may be discussed with other patients.
   d. may be used for your personal advantage.

7. When a patient offers you a tip for your services, you should
   a. refuse in a firm, courteous manner.
   b. accept the tip and share it with the other team members.
   c. refuse and act shocked that the offer was ever made.
   d. accept and then return the tip to a member of the patient's family.

8. A case of negligence would arise if a patient
   a. who has bathroom privileges falls when the nursing assistant is out of the room.
   b. falls because water on the floor was not wiped up.
   c. develops an infection because the nursing assistant performed a procedure that had not been taught.
   d. develops an important symptom that he does not report to the nursing team.

9. A case of negligence would arise if a patient were injured because you
   a. followed the care plan and left the side rails down at night.
   b. carried out a special procedure in which you had not been instructed.
   c. wiped up some water on the floor.
   d. reported a defective electrical wire.

10. When caring for a patient whose religious beliefs differ from your own, you are obliged to
    a. help the patient understand your faith.
    b. show the patient how wrong her faith is.
    c. respect his religious beliefs.
    d. arrange to have your clergyperson make a visit.

11. Important characteristics for the nursing assistant include
    a. knowing all there is to know.
    b. good grooming and interest in others.
    c. having a cell phone and pager.
    d. having experience in all areas of the hospital.

12. Part of good grooming includes
    a. cleaning shoes every week.
    b. keeping fingernails long and polished.
    c. taking a bath or shower daily.
    d. wearing expensive jewelry.

13. Lines of authority are important. Your immediate line of authority is
    a. another nursing assistant.
    b. a staff LVN/LPN or registered nurse.
    c. the administrator.
    d. the physician.

14. You protect the patient's privacy by
    a. exposing the patient.
    b. listening to personal telephone calls.
    c. always staying when visitors are present.
    d. knocking before entering a patient's room.

15. You learn something personal about a patient from her chart. You should
    a. keep quiet about the information.
    b. share it with other patients.
    c. share it with coworkers during coffee break.
    d. let the patient know what you have learned.

16. You observe a coworker stealing supplies and fail to report it. You are guilty of
    a. malpractice.   b. aiding and abetting.
    c. negligence.   d. loyalty.

17. A patient tells you he is worried about being able to pay his bill. You should
    a. talk to his wife about the problem.
    b. call the physician.
    c. share the information with a coworker.
    d. report to your team leader/supervisor.

18. When the patient's clergyperson comes for a visit, you should
    a. move other patients out of the room.
    b. ask the patient's visitor to remain.
    c. draw the curtains for privacy.
    d. stay with the patient.

19. Nursing assistant responsibilities include
    a. giving injections and oral medications.
    b. making observations and reporting them.
    c. simple treatments and dressing changes.
    d. taking physician orders for assigned patients.

20. The service that you give to a patient is determined by the patient's
    a. need.   b. race.   c. desire.   d. ability to pay.

B. **Matching.** Match Column I with Column II.

Column I

21. _____ medical department
22. _____ surgical department
23. _____ pediatric department
24. _____ obstetrical unit
25. _____ emergency department

Column II

a. cares for pregnant women and newborns
b. cares for children
c. cares for trauma victims
d. cares for patients with medical conditions
e. cares for patients with surgical conditions

C. **True/False.** Mark the following true or false by circling T or F.

26. T F Patients have the right to considerate and respectful care.
27. T F Patients must participate in any treatment their physician feels is necessary.
28. T F It is all right to discuss patients' treatment in front of their family members.
29. T F Patients have the right to refuse to participate in research programs that might help them.
30. T F Information about patients' bills is not discussed with patients because it is sent to the insurance company.
31. T F Skilled care facilities provide care for critically ill persons.
32. T F Patient-focused care means that each person is considered a unique individual with different needs.

33. T F Informed consent means that the consumer gives permission for care or procedures after full disclosure and explanation of the treatment or procedure.
34. T F The rights of health care consumers are important only to patients in hospitals.
35. T F The outcome of patient care is the total responsibility of the physician and the nurses.

D. **Completion**

36. List five actions you can take to ensure that your practice remains within legal guidelines.

    _____
    _____
    _____
    _____
    _____

Section 2
SELF-EVALUATION

A. **Definitions.** Define the following words.

1. cell _____
2. organ _____
3. system _____
4. neoplasm _____
5. etiology _____

B. **Matching.** Match Column I with Column II.

Column I

6. _____ above
7. _____ back
8. _____ structure
9. _____ divides the body into right and left sides
10. _____ away from the midline
11. _____ front
12. _____ divides the body into upper and lower parts
13. _____ divides the body into back and front

Column II

a. midline   b. transverse   c. frontal   d. posterior
e. anterior   f. inferior   g. superior   h. anatomy
i. physiology j. lateral   k. medial   l. dorsal

C. **Multiple Choice.** Choose the phrase that best completes each of the following sentences by circling the proper letter.

14. The tissue that carries messages is called
    a. epithelial. b. connective. c. muscular. d. nervous.
15. The tissue that protects, secretes, and absorbs is called
    a. epithelial. b. connective. c. muscular. d. nervous.
16. Included in the gastrointestinal system is/are
    a. kidneys. b. ovaries. c. stomach. d. adrenals.
17. Included in the respiratory system is/are
    a. lungs.   b. stomach. c. ovaries. d. liver.
18. Included in the urinary system is/are
    a. gallbladder. b. kidneys. c. spinal cord. d. uterus.
19. Included in the nervous system is/are
    a. oil glands. b. larynx. c. joints. d. brain.

20. The small intestine is found in the
    a. abdominal cavity.   b. pelvic cavity.
    c. spinal cavity.   d. thoracic cavity.

D. Matching. Match Column I with Column II.

Column I

21. _____ an inadequate blood flow to an area
22. _____ an abnormal condition that is present at birth
23. _____ a condition that progresses rapidly and lasts a relatively short period
24. _____ a condition that persists over a long time
25. _____ a condition made more serious by another already existing condition

Column II

a. chronic   b. acute   c. complication
d. congenital   e. ischemia

E. Completion. Complete the following statements correctly.

26. Ultrasound is frequently performed on the uterus to give information about _____.
27. When a patient undergoes MRI, he will experience _____.
28. The examiner directly observes the _____ by using a proctoscope.
29. During a barium swallow, the patient swallows a barium solution while _____ are being taken.
30. Besides providing emotional support for patients during diagnostic procedures, the nursing assistant should:

F. Word Choice. Select the correct spelling by circling the word.

31. vane vein vien vene
32. lateral leteral laterale laterel
33. neoplasm nioplasm neoplasme neoplasem
34. carsinoma carcinoma karsinoma karcinoma
35. troma trauma tromma traumer
36. protosols protachols protocols protokols

G. Definitions. For each term in Section F, write a definition.

37. _____
38. _____
39. _____
40. _____
41. _____
42. _____

H. Matching. Match each abbreviation with its meaning.

43. _____ GI   a. transient ischemic attack
44. _____ CVA   b. low back pain
45. _____ FX   c. aneurysm
46. _____ TIA   d. cerebral vascular accident
47. _____ LBP   e. gastrointestinal
                      f. temporary incomplete attachment
                      g. fracture

I. Word Choice. Select the best answer to complete each statement.

48. The brain is found in the _____ cavity.
    (spinal) (cranial)

49. The heart is found in the _____ cavity.
    (abdominal) (thoracic)
50. The stomach is found in the _____ cavity.
    (abdominal) (pelvic)
51. The liver is found in the _____ cavity.
    (peritoneal) (thoracic)
52. The lungs are found in the _____ cavity.
    (spinal) (thoracic)

J. Brief Answers

The patient suffers from meningitis. Answer the following questions.

53. What are the meninges?
54. Where are they located?
55. What do they cover?
56. What does the suffix "itis" mean?
57. What does meningitis mean?

Section 3
SELF-EVALUATION

A. Matching. Match the observations in Column I with the systems in Column II. (Each may be used more than once.)

Column I

1. _____ orientation to time and place
2. _____ shortness of breath
3. _____ frequent urination
4. _____ diarrhea
5. _____ scars
6. _____ dryness
7. _____ cough
8. _____ increased pulse rate
9. _____ inability to see
10. _____ ability to move

Column II

a. circulatory   b. musculoskeletal   c. urinary
d. nervous   e. respiratory   f. digestive
g. integumentary

B. Multiple Choice. Choose the phrase that best completes each of the following sentences by circling the proper letter.

11. One example of nonverbal communication is
    a. spoken words.   b. pictures.
    c. written words.   d. body language.
12. A key to successful relationships is to remember
    a. all patients react to stress in the same way.
    b. words alone communicate feelings and thoughts.
    c. people always say exactly what they mean.
    d. each person is unique.
13. The spiritual needs of people
    a. are lessened when they are sick.
    b. may be disregarded because physical needs come first.
    c. are usually greater when they are sick.
    d. do not change when they are sick.

14. If a patient expresses a desire for a visit from the clergy, you should
    a. call your rabbi.
    b. let the nurse know.
    c. tell the patient he is going to get better and does not really need a clergyperson.
    d. call the clergy.
15. An objective observation is
    a. what you think or feel.
    b. something the patient tells you.
    c. factual or measurable.
    d. identified by the physician.
16. Breathing needs can be aided by
    a. positioning the patient properly.
    b. keeping the patient flat.
    c. withholding oxygen.
    d. making the patient ambulate more.
17. Your patient is having trouble sleeping. You may help by
    a. giving medication for pain.
    b. allowing the patient to talk with you.
    c. disconnecting the IV.
    d. giving the patient a full meal.
18. Patients consider their problems
    a. less important than your own concerns.
    b. equally important to the problems of roommates.
    c. most important.
    d. less important than the concerns of other staff members.
19. The organizational chart is
    a. a procedure manual.
    b. a guide for communication among staff members.
    c. used for making patient care assignments.
    d. used to ensure patients' rights.
20. The purpose of staff development is to
    a. inform the staff of new developments in health care.
    b. provide patient education.
    c. provide staff with recreational benefits.
    d. develop unit schedules and assignments.
21. The patient's care plan provides information for
    a. nursing procedures.
    b. employee benefits.
    c. emergency procedures.
    d. nursing assistant assignments.
22. The patient's medical record is
    a. used only by the physician.
    b. used by all health care workers.
    c. destroyed when the patient is discharged.
    d. a record of the nursing assistant's competencies.
23. Assessment requires the
    a. collection of data.
    b. identification of solutions to patient problems.
    c. the formulation of goals.
    d. a list of nursing diagnoses.
24. The purpose of the nursing process is to
    a. make a medical diagnosis.
    b. make assignments.
    c. achieve patient-focused care.
    d. cure illness.

25. Classifying individuals according to shared physical characteristics such as skin color, hair, and facial features is classifying by
    a. class.   b. culture.   c. religion.   d. race.
26. Spirituality is
    a. a sense of connection with the world and a higher power.
    b. a belief in God or a power greater than oneself.
    c. passed on in families and largely based on ethnicity and race.
    d. rituals and traditions practiced by persons of some cultures.
27. The way a particular group views the world and passes traditions from one generation to the next is
    a. personal space. b. culture. c. ethnicity. d. ritualism.

C. Matching. Identify the age group with its characteristic by matching Column I and Column II. (Each may be used more than once.)

Column I

28. _____ gradual loss of vitality and stamina
29. _____ rapid growth and system stabilization
30. _____ careers and families established
31. _____ associated with final career advancement
32. _____ desire for independence and security; a turbulent period
33. _____ period of beginning physical sexual changes
34. _____ become aware of right and wrong

Column II

a. infancy   b. toddler   c. preschool
d. school age   e. preadolescent   f. adolescent
g. adulthood   h. middle age   i. later maturity
j. old age

D. Short Answer

35. List three ways the nursing assistant can support the nurse for each of the steps of the nursing process.

Step of Nursing Process	Nursing Assistant Action
Assessment	a. _____ b. _____ c. _____
Planning	a. _____ b. _____ c. _____
Implementation	a. _____ b. _____ c. _____
Evaluation	a. _____ b. _____ c. _____

E. True/False. Mark the following true or false by circling T or F.

36. T F   Intimacy is a feeling of closeness experienced with another human being.
37. T F   All intimate relationships are sexual in nature.

38. T F Touching another person is a form of expressing intimacy.
39. T F Skin contact is an important way of receiving and giving pleasure and satisfaction.
40. T F Human intimate sexual expression may take many forms.
41. T F Masturbation is self-stimulation for sexual pleasure and must not be permitted.
42. T F The homosexual is sexually attracted to members of the opposite sex.
43. T F Sexual preference is a personal matter and may or may not conform to the personal preference of the nursing assistant.
44. T F Intimate relationships include an element of commitment between two persons.
45. T F Standing too close to someone can be interpreted as invading personal space.
46. T F Flow sheets are special record forms that are used when patients are progressing well and only a few notations are needed.
47. T F Printed nursing care protocols need to be individualized for each patient.
48. T F All documentation is done exactly the same in every facility.
49. T F Spiritual beliefs are often a strong guide to patient reactions and behaviors.
50. T F Documentation must conform to the policy for each facility.
51. T F Only authorized persons may read patient records.
52. T F Questions about patients may be discussed with visitors.
53. T F It is permissible to try to convince a patient that your personal beliefs are correct.
54. T F Culture has no real influence over a patient's responses to illness and treatment.
55. T F Cultural mores influence the way people interact.
56. T F Standards are established by a group based on their values and beliefs.
57. T F Direct eye contact with another person is always appropriate.
58. T F If the patient says, "I have a headache," this is an example of an objective observation.
59. T F Nursing assistants are not responsible for the development or implementation of the care plan.
60. T F The patient's medical record is considered a legal document.

Section 4
SELF-EVALUATION

A. **Definitions.** Define the following words:

1. protozoa _____
2. bacteria _____
3. contamination _____
4. fomite _____
5. vectors _____

B. **Matching.** Match Column I with Column II.

Column I

6. _____ disease-causing organisms
7. _____ arranged in pairs
8. _____ arranged in chains
9. _____ hard-to-destroy forms of microbes
10. _____ poisons
11. _____ grow on living organisms
12. _____ arranged in clusters

Column II

a. staphylococcus   b. pathogens   c. toxins
d. drug-resistant   e. streptococcus   f. diplococcus
g. parasites   h. carrier

C. **Multiple Choice.** Choose the phrase that best completes each of the following sentences by circling the proper letter.

13. Using proper handwashing technique, you should
    a. rinse with fingertips pointed up.
    b. use very hot water.
    c. not include the fingernails at this time.
    d. turn faucets off with a paper towel.
14. If the seal on a commercially prepared sterile package of gauze is broken, you will
    a. consider the package contaminated.
    b. use it anyway if the contents look clean.
    c. know that the condition of the seal is not important.
    d. know that the seal has to be broken before use anyway.
15. When a patient is in isolation,
    a. equipment can be moved in and out without special precautions.
    b. frequently used equipment remains in the patient unit.
    c. one person can move equipment safely in and out of the unit.
    d. contaminated equipment is labeled "clean."
16. Standard precautions are infection control actions used for
    a. patients with certain skin conditions only.
    b. only patients with diarrhea caused by spores.
    c. all patients receiving care regardless as diagnosis.
    d. only patients with upper respiratory infections.
17. When isolation technique is being used, a sign will be placed on the door which might read
    a. stop and report to nurse.   b. keep clear.
    c. universal precautions.   d. barrier-free gone.

D. **Completion.** Complete the following statements correctly.

18. One very important way to control the spread of bacteria is by proper _____.
19. The special way of caring for patients with easily transferable diseases is called _____.
20. The portal of entry for salmonellosis is the _____ tract.
21. Gonorrhea is primarily transmitted by way of the _____ tract.
22. Droplet transmission is _____ from coughing, sneezing, or talking.

23. Contact transmission is through _____ contact by a person with the source of pathogens.
24. Airborne transmission occurs when small _____ remain suspended in the air and move with air currents.
25. Some organisms may be transmitted in _____ than one way.

E. Short Answer. Provide short answers to the following questions.

26. Write five procedures included in standard precautions.
    a. _____
    b. _____
    c. _____
    d. _____
    e. _____
27. List the three developmental stages of an infectious organism in a host.
    a. _____
    b. _____
    c. _____
28. List four risk factors that make a person more susceptible to infection.
    a. _____
    b. _____
    c. _____
    d. _____
29. List two other factors that play a role in the progression of infectious disease.
    a. _____
    b. _____
30. List four natural protective body defenses.
    a. _____
    b. _____
    c. _____
    d. _____
31. Name four types of PPE.
    a. _____
    b. _____
    c. _____
    d. _____

F. True/False. Mark the following true or false by circling T or F.

32. T F Carriers cannot transmit infectious disease.
33. T F The normal flora are different in different parts of the body.
34. T F Toxins produced by microbes have little effect on the body.
35. T F An elevated body temperature is believed to increase the body's ability to fight infection.
36. T F Phagocytes help destroy infectious organisms.
37. T F Cohorting is practiced when patients with different infections share a single room.
38. T F You should wear gloves if you have a cut or rash on your hand.
39. T F Used sharps may be disposed of by wrapping them in paper towels and placing in a wastepaper basket.

40. T F All laboratory specimens should be considered potentially infectious.
41. T F Eating is prohibited in work areas where there may be exposure to infectious materials.
42. T F Infection with *Escherichia coli* 0157:H7 can be transmitted in undercooked ground beef.
43. T F *Escherichia coli* 0157:H7 infection may cause renal failure.
44. T F *Clostridium difficile* is a friendly bacterium that resides in the colon.
45. T F *Clostridium difficile* may be picked up on the hands on environmental surfaces, such as faucets, doorknobs, and bed rails.
46. T F Pseudomembranous colitis is a disease that is spread through the air and causes severe dehydration.
47. T F Hantavirus is spread by rodents and transmitted by direct contact.
48. T F The use of biological agents, such as pathogenic organisms or agricultural pests, for terrorist purposes is called chemical warfare.
49. T F The nursing assistant should avoid touching environmental surfaces with used gloves.
50. T F Handwashing is not necessary after patient care if gloves were worn during the contact.
51. T F Position the clean linen cart and soiled linen hamper next to each other in the hallway so they are conveniently located.
52. T F Waterless hand cleaner may be used in place of handwashing unless hands are visibly soiled.
53. T F Waterless hand cleaners are not as effective as using soap and water.
54. T F People who have not had chickenpox should not enter the room of a patient in isolation for shingles.
55. T F The object of infection control is to disrupt the chain of infection.
56. T F *Listeriosis* is caused by inhaling *Listeria monocytogenes* bacteria.
57. T F *Acinetobacter baumannii* was eradicated during the Vietnam War.
58. T F *Aspergillosis* is a fungal infection that affects patients with weak immune systems.
59. T F Infection with *Streptococcus B* is the most common cause of necrotizing fasciitis.
60. T F An abscess is a collection of pus in the tissue, usually in a confined space.
61. T F Spores are microscopic reproductive bodies that cannot live long once separated from the human host.
62. T F SARS is a highly contagious respiratory illness caused by a coronavirus.
63. T F SARS can be picked up on environmental surfaces on the hands and introduced into the host's body.
64. T F Nits are yellow-white in color and easily removed.
65. T F Scabies is highly contagious and is spread by direct and indirect contact.
66. T F Bedbugs are imaginary pests in children's stories.
67. T F Bedbugs must have a blood meal each day to survive.

68. T F The scabies rash does not go away immediately after treatment.
69. T F Head lice hop or fly from person to person.

Section 5
SELF-EVALUATION

A. Multiple Choice. Choose the phrase that best completes each of the following sentences by circling the proper letter.

1. Concurrent cleaning refers to
   a. daily dusting and mopping.
   b. annual redecorating of patient rooms.
   c. cleaning that is done when the patient is discharged.
   d. the sterilization of supplies and equipment.
2. Ergonomics refers to
   a. immunizations given to prevent disease.
   b. the rights of patients in the hospital.
   c. adapting the job to the worker.
   d. the use of standard precautions.
3. Material Safety Data Sheets (MSDS) are required to include information that
   a. describes where to store the chemical in the facility.
   b. explains whether you need PPE when using the product.
   c. instructs the user on how to dilute the chemical.
   d. describes how to repackage the chemical into a smaller container.
4. An example of correct body mechanics is to
   a. hold the load away from your body.
   b. keep your knees locked when lifting.
   c. use the muscles of your legs when lifting.
   d. keep your feet close together when lifting.
5. OSHA is a federal agency that is concerned with the
   a. rights of patients in hospitals.
   b. safety of patients in hospitals.
   c. ethics of health care workers.
   d. safety of employees.
6. Environmental safety is the responsibility of
   a. the maintenance department.
   b. all employees.
   c. the housekeeping department.
   d. the administrator.
7. Alternatives to the use of restraints include
   a. chairs with locking trays across the lap.
   b. belts and straps.
   c. exercise and activities.
   d. tucking the blanket in tightly.
8. Body alignment is maintained by
   a. using physical restraints.
   b. administering chemical restraints.
   c. moving, turning, and positioning patients.
   d. positioning the legs and arms.
9. When transferring patients, you should
   a. have the patient place his hands on your shoulders during the transfer.
   b. place your hands under the patient's shoulders while lifting.
   c. place the bed in high position.
   d. use a transfer belt unless it is contraindicated.
10. A person's gait is not affected by
    a. wearing a prosthesis.   b. a neuromuscular disability.
    c. orthopedic surgery.   d. the doctor's orders.
11. A cane is an example of
    a. an assistive device.   b. an orthosis.
    c. a prosthesis.   d. a supportive device.
12. Which instructions are correct for a patient who has had surgery on the right hip and is using a three-point gait and walker?
    a. Move walker, then right leg, then left leg
    b. Move right leg, then walker, then left leg
    c. Move walker and right leg together, then left leg
    d. Move walker and left leg together and then right leg

B. Short Answer. Indicate what each of the letters means in the following acronyms.

13. R _____
    A _____
    C _____
    E _____
14. P _____
    A _____
    S _____
    S _____

C. True/False. Mark the following true or false by circling T or F.

15. T F An incident is any unexpected situation that disrupts normal unit operations.
16. T F Ergonomics is important only when lifting heavy loads.
17. T F Chemical restraints are appropriate when a patient frequently calls out.
18. T F Side rails may be considered a restraint.
19. T F Restraints should be released every 8 hours.
20. T F Aspiration means the accidental entry of food into the trachea.
21. T F Physical restraints are an example of a supportive device.
22. T F An underhand grasp should be used when using a transfer belt.
23. T F You should always transfer the patient toward her or his weakest side.
24. T F There should always be two people working together when a mechanical lift is being used.
25. T F Mechanical lifts are frequently used for persons with no weight-bearing ability.

D. Matching. Choose the correct word from the list in a–j to match the terms in questions 26–35.

26. _____ contracture
27. _____ Fowler's position
28. _____ lateral position
29. _____ orthopneic position
30. _____ orthosis
31. _____ pressure ulcer

32. _____ prone
33. _____ spasticity
34. _____ supine
35. _____ trochanter roll
a. prevents external rotation of the hip
b. positioned on the abdomen
c. a device used to hold an extremity in position
d. involuntary muscle contractions
e. positioned on the side
f. positioned on the back
g. positioned with backrest elevated
h. position used for patients who have difficulty breathing
i. caused by unrelieved pressure on bony prominence
j. stiffness and shortening of the muscles around a joint

Section 6
SELF-EVALUATION

A. Multiple Choice. Choose the phrase that best completes each of the following sentences by circling the proper letter.

1. To read a glass thermometer properly, you should
   a. hold it straight up and down.   b. hold it by the bulb.
   c. hold it at eye level.   d. turn it rapidly.
2. When a patient has just finished a cool drink, it is best to
   a. wait 15 minutes to take her temperature.
   b. take the temperature right away.
   c. omit the temperature until next time.
   d. take the temperature by the axillary method.
3. To take the patient's pulse accurately, you will need
   a. pencil and pad.   b. a watch with a second hand.
   c. oral thermometer.   d. lubricant.
4. When you take a rectal temperature, remember to
   a. hold the thermometer in place.
   b. insert the thermometer 3 inches into the rectum.
   c. use a thermometer with a blue tip.
   d. wait 5 minutes if the patient has had a drink.
5. When taking a tympanic temperature in an adult,
   a. insert the probe cover into the ear as far as it will comfortably go.
   b. pull the earlobe down and forward before inserting the thermometer.
   c. leave the thermometer in place for at least 3 minutes.
   d. rotate the handle of the thermometer to align it with the jaw.
6. To take an axillary temperature accurately, the thermometer must be in place
   a. 2 minutes.   b. 20 minutes.
   c. 3 minutes.   d. 10 minutes.
7. Respirations are best counted
   a. without letting the patient know.
   b. while the patient is eating.
   c. while the patient is talking.
   d. after telling the patient what you plan to do.
8. The most common place to take the pulse is at the
   a. temple.   b. bend in the elbow.
   c. wrist.   d. knee.

9. The pulse of an adult male patient is 72 beats per minute. You know that this rate is
   a. too fast and must be reported.
   b. about average for an adult.
   c. too slow and must be reported.
   d. about average for a young child.
10. One function of respiration is
    a. to circulate blood.
    b. to transmit nerve impulses.
    c. to rid the body of carbon dioxide.
    d. take in carbon monoxide.
11. When taking blood pressure, it is important that the
    a. gauge be at eye level.
    b. armband be smooth and loose.
    c. stethoscope be placed over the radial artery.
    d. gauge be tilted.

B. Short Answer. Read the temperature on each thermometer in the accompanying figure and record the value on the proper line.

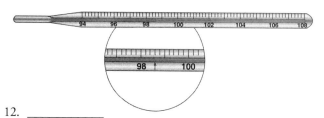

12. _____

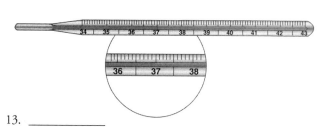

13. _____

C. Short Answer. Complete the following statements.

14. To indicate on a graphic chart that the temperature has been taken other than orally, you should

_____.
_____.

15. The following equipment is needed to determine vital signs:

_____.
_____.

16. Four sites, other than the wrist, where the pulse may be taken are

_____.
_____.
_____.
_____.

17. Three types of clinical thermometers in general use are

_____.
_____.
_____.

18. Height may be recorded in feet and inches or

_____.

19. Weight may be recorded in pounds or

_____.

D. Matching. Choose the correct term from Column II to match the phrases in Column I.

Column I

20. _____ moist, bubbling respirations
21. _____ abnormally slow pulse rate
22. _____ highest blood pressure reading
23. _____ difficult respirations

Column II

a. bradycardia   b. systolic   c. diastolic
d. tachycardia   e. dyspnea   f. apnea
g. gurgles

E. Short Answer. Identify four times when the nursing assistant should report a blood pressure reading:

24. _____
25. _____
26. _____
27. _____

Section 7
SELF-EVALUATION

A. Multiple Choice. Choose the phrase that best completes each of the following sentences by circling the proper letter.

1. When making an occupied bed, remember
   a. that the unit must be screened.
   b. that the side rails should both be up, to prevent falls.
   c. one side of the bottom is made at a time.
   d. to alternate from one side to the other.
2. During the patient's bed bath,
   a. the patient is completely uncovered.
   b. the water is changed to maintain warmth.
   c. the unit is not screened.
   d. the top linen remains in place.
3. Oral hygiene should be performed
   a. three times each day.   b. only in the morning.
   c. only in the afternoon.   d. before dinner.
4. When admitting a patient, remember to
   a. allow the patient to keep large amounts of money at the bedside.
   b. tell the family to leave because you have work to do.
   c. be courteous and helpful to both the patient and family.
   d. ask the nurse what to do.
5. During the admission procedure, you will
   a. take at least three sets of vital signs.
   b. list the patient's medications.
   c. put the patient to bed with side rails up.
   d. observe the patient carefully.
6. When a patient wears dentures, you are responsible for
   a. storing the dentures in the closet.
   b. storing the dentures in mouthwash.
   c. using great care when handling dentures.
   d. brushing the dentures without removing from the mouth.

7. An open bed is made by
   a. fanfolding the top bedclothes to the foot of the bed.
   b. adding an extra pillow.
   c. leaving the top bedding off.
   d. padding the bottom linen.
8. When gathering linen to make a bed,
   a. put the spread on the top of the pile.
   b. include a bath blanket.
   c. include a draw sheet.
   d. stack linen in order of use.
9. When making an unoccupied bed,
   a. make the entire bottom of the bed first.
   b. change the pillowcase first.
   c. make one entire side first.
   d. place the bottom sheet even with the head of the mattress.
10. The whirlpool bath is beneficial for patients because the temperature can be regulated at an optimum temperature of
    a. 95°F.   b. 97°F.   c. 105°F.   d. 110°F.
11. Before leaving the patient after making an occupied bed, be sure that
    a. the bed is in the lowest horizontal position.
    b. the top linen is tucked in tightly on both sides of the bed.
    c. the bed is in the highest horizontal position with both side rails up.
    d. the head of the bed is elevated at least 45°.
12. When bathing a patient, you may
    a. lower an IV bag below the level of the infusion site.
    b. gently stress tubing as long as it does not become disconnected.
    c. raise drainage tubing above the drainage site.
    d. never put stress on the tubing.
13. When using the waterless bathing system,
    a. add liquid soap to the package.
    b. heat the package in the microwave for at least 5 minutes.
    c. save as many washcloths as possible.
    d. date the package when opening and discard unused cloths after 72 hours.
14. The temperature of the bath water should be about
    a. 97°F.   b. 100°F.   c. 105°F.   d. 110°F.
15. When transferring a patient to another unit in the hospital, the nursing assistant should
    a. take the patient to the new room, then quickly return to the assigned unit.
    b. leave the chart and medications on the original unit for the nurse to transfer.
    c. introduce the patient to the staff and make sure she has the call signal before leaving the room.
    d. ask the patient to pack her belongings and carry them to the new unit.
16. When asking visitors to leave,
    a. tell them abruptly that they cannot stay.
    b. let them know how long you will be.
    c. there is no need to tell them about a refreshment area or lounge.
    d. ask them to return the next day.

17. When discharging a patient,
    a. allow the patient to walk from the unit to the outside.
    b. throw all disposables away.
    c. call the doctor to check the patient's order.
    d. gather the patient's belongings and assist with packing.
18. Your best action when a patient feels weak in a shower is
    a. turn the shower to cold water to stimulate the patient.
    b. use the call bell to get assistance.
    c. help the patient immediately out of the shower.
    d. get help by leaving the patient.
19. A good backrub should take about
    a. 1 minute.   b. 3 to 5 minutes.
    c. 10 minutes.   d. 20 minutes.
20. When not in the patient's mouth, dentures should be
    a. left on the bed.
    b. placed on the bedside table.
    c. placed in a marked container.
    d. left on the bathroom shelf.
21. When giving a bedpan or urinal, always
    a. pad the receptacle.   b. provide privacy.
    c. allow visitors to remain.   d. disconnect the call bell.
22. To wake a patient,
    a. rap loudly on the door.
    b. call the patient's name loudly.
    c. gently place your hand on the patient's arm.
    d. shake the patient vigorously.
23. When shampooing a patient in the shower, you should
    a. use a large amount of shampoo.
    b. cover the patient's eyes when rinsing.
    c. massage the scalp vigorously.
    d. let the hair air-dry.
24. When giving the patient a backrub, the nursing assistant should
    a. squeeze the lotion onto the back from the bottle.
    b. warm the lotion before applying it to the patient's skin.
    c. use alcohol to stimulate the circulation.
    d. massage red and open areas well to prevent further breakdown.
25. Identify the patient by asking her name and
    a. checking her chart.
    b. asking a visitor.
    c. asking the nurse.
    d. checking the identification bracelet.
26. Valuables brought with the patient to the hospital should be listed and left
    a. in the patient's locker.   b. at the bedside.
    c. in the hospital safe.   d. on the patient.
27. The proper temperature of bath water is
    a. 90°F.   b. 105°F.   c. 115°F.   d. 120°F.
28. Nursing assistants are responsible for completing the patient's bathing if
    a. they feel like it.
    b. the supervisor tells them.
    c. the patient cannot.
    d. the patient is tired.
29. When giving a bed bath, expose
    a. the entire body at one time.
    b. the part to be washed.
    c. both legs at one time.
    d. one whole side of the body.
30. You are assigned to give Mr. Lee a partial bath. You know this means to wash the
    a. face, abdomen, legs, underarms, and feet.
    b. face, hands, underarms, back, and perineum.
    c. face, arms, hands, perineum, and legs.
    d. face, underarms, perineum, and feet.
31. If the patient is receiving an IV and his gown must be changed, the assistant will
    a. discontinue the IV.
    b. call the team leader to disconnect the IV.
    c. remove the gown using the proper technique.
    d. not change the gown.
32. Patients should be encouraged to help as much as possible during morning care because
    a. the work will be done faster.
    b. it stimulates the patient's general outlook.
    c. you do not want the patient to get too tired.
    d. maintaining independence is good for self-esteem.
33. Before the bath procedure,
    a. tighten the bottom bedding.
    b. loosen the top bedding.
    c. place two pillows under the patient's head.
    d. remove the laundry hamper from the room.
34. When preparing to give a bed bath, include in your supplies
    a. bed linen and gown.   b. sphygmomanometer.
    c. emesis basin.   d. socks and underwear.
35. Which of the following is *not* true about wearing gloves during the bathroom procedure?
    a. Gloves are worn for the entire procedure.
    b. Gloves are changed immediately before contact with nonintact skin.
    c. Gloves are changed immediately before performing perineal care.
    d. Gloves should be changed if they become heavily soiled.
36. When assisting the female resident with perineal care, wash
    a. from back to front.   b. in a back-and-forth motion.
    c. in a circular motion.   d. from front to back.
37. You are assigned to bathe Mrs. Lloyd. You notice that her toenails are long and dirty. You should
    a. clean and cut the nails.
    b. clean the nails and consult the nurse.
    c. do nothing about it, as you are not allowed to care for nails.
    d. clean the nails and file them with an emery board.

B. Matching. Choose the correct item from Column II to match the words in Column I.

Column I

38. _____caries   39. _____halitosis
40. _____dentures   41. _____foot drop
42. _____early (AM) care

Column II

a. artificial teeth   b. toes involuntarily point down
c. dental cavities   d. care given before breakfast
e. care given before bedtime f. unpleasant breath

C. True/False. Mark the following true or false by circling
T or F.

43. T F Nail care is not part of the routine morning care.
44. T F If a patient feels faint while taking a shower, stay
         and signal for help.
45. T F The bathtub need only be rinsed between patients.
46. T F Bed shampoos may be given without a physician's
         order.
47. T F A patient going to surgery at 8 AM should be wakened
         for breakfast.
48. T F Adjust the bed to comfortable working height
         before starting an in-bed procedure.
49. T F Daily shaving of the face is a routine for most male
         patients.
50. T F Handwashing need only be performed after
         completing a patient care procedure.
51. T F A used bedpan need not be covered when carrying
         it to the patient's bathroom.
52. T F When a bedpan is properly placed under a patient, the
         buttocks should rest on the rounded shelf of the pan.
53. T F The only purpose of bed cradles is to keep the
         weight of the bedding off the patient's feet.
54. T F Gloves should be worn when shaving a patient.
55. T F A trochanter roll should extend from above the
         shoulders to below the waist of the patient.
56. T F Unconscious patients do not require oral care.
57. T F If a person is dehydrated, oral care is especially
         important.
58. T F Gloves should be worn when giving male or female
         perineal care.
59. T F Perineal care should be performed each time a
         patient is incontinent.
60. T F It is important to provide privacy during perineal care.
61. T F The washcloth should be rinsed after each side of
         the labia has been washed.

D. Short Answer. Write short answers to the following.

62. How might a female patient who cannot separate her legs
    sufficiently for perineal care be positioned?

    _____

    _____

63. When a male patient has not been circumcised, what
    special precaution must you take with respect to the
    foreskin during perineal care?

    _____

    _____

Section 8
SELF-EVALUATION

A. Matching. Choose the correct phrase from Column II to
match each item in Column I.

Column I

1. _____ gastrostomy tube   2. _____ carbohydrates
3. _____ proteins   4. _____ roughage
5. _____ f.f.   6. _____ gavage
7. _____ feces   8. _____ fats

Column II

a. tube feeding
b. important nutrient for body building and repair
c. stored form of energy
d. solid body wastes
e. feeding tube inserted surgically through the abdominal wall
   into the stomach
f. encourage fluid intake
g. called "energy" foods
h. cellulose

B. Multiple Choice. Choose the phrase that best
completes each of the following sentences by circling
the proper letter.

9. Foods that contain the greatest amount of carbohydrates
   come from
   a. eggs.   b. milk.   c. fruits.   d. nuts.
10. Your patient has an order for a regular diet. This means
    a. more calories than usual must be supplied.
    b. only liquids may be consumed.
    c. a basic normal diet will be provided.
    d. salt must be omitted.
11. Your patient has been nauseated and has been placed on a
    clear liquid diet. You would
    a. offer coffee with cream and sugar.
    b. offer 7-Up or ginger ale.
    c. offer tomato juice.
    d. offer vegetable soup.
12. Your patient has dentures that fit poorly. His nutritional
    needs would best be met with a
    a. regular diet.   b. full liquid diet.
    c. salt-free diet.   d. mechanically altered diet.
13. Your patient is on a full liquid diet. When the tray arrives
    and you check it, you discover one of the following that
    does not belong:
    a. soup (strained).   b. sherbet.
    c. eggnog.   d. crackers.
14. You are assigned to pass nourishments. One patient's
    name has a "withhold." You will
    a. offer only solids.
    b. remember to measure intake.
    c. offer an extra portion of juice.
    d. not offer that patient nourishments.
15. Your patient is blind but able to feed himself. You will
    a. feed him; it's faster.
    b. explain the tray compared with the face of a clock.
    c. place all food in a straight line across the overbed
       table.
    d. explain the tray arrangement by putting all hot
       foods toward the tray top and cold toward the tray
       bottom.

16. You filled Mrs. Tsai's water pitcher at 8:00 AM. The pitcher contained 1,000 mL of water and ice. At 2:30 PM, when you collect the intake and output, there is 335 mL remaining in the pitcher. You will record Mrs. Tsai's water intake for your shift as
    a. 856 mL   b. 665 mL   c. 765 mL   d. 586 mL

17. A diabetic diet would *not* include
    a. bread and butter.   b. baked chicken.
    c. vegetable soup.   d. jam or jelly.

18. Your patient took in 240 mL of juice and 180 mL of sherbet. The total intake would be
    a. 8 ounces.   b. 320 mL.   c. 10 ounces.   d. 420 mL.

19. Your patient put out 16 ounces of urine. You will record this as
    a. 460 mL.   b. 480 mL.   c. 500 mL.   d. 520 mL.

20. Nutritional supplements
    a. are ordered by the physician.
    b. are served with meals.
    c. must be high in protein.
    d. are given only to diabetics.

21. A low-sodium diet means the diet is low in
    a. salt.   b. cholesterol.   c. sugar.   d. potassium.

22. Mr. Palu-ay is on a clear liquid diet. For lunch, he drank 4 ounces of cranberry juice. He ate 100% of a 4-ounce bowl of gelatin. He drank a 6-ounce cup of tea. You will record his oral intake as
    a. 420 mL.   b. 446 mL.   c. 680 mL.   d. 820 mL.

C. Matching. The daily servings from each of the food groups should include:

Group
23. _____ fruits   24. _____ vegetables
25. _____ grains   26. _____ fats, oils, sweets

Servings
a. sparingly   b. 2 cups   c. 2–5 cups   d. 1-2
e. 6 ounces

D. Short Answer. Write short answers to the following.

27. Name five foods permitted on a low-fat/low-cholesterol diet.
    a. _____
    b. _____
    c. _____
    d. _____
    e. _____

28. Explain the term *fluid balance.*
    _____

29. Explain how a patient may assist in accounting for fluid intake.
    _____

30. List five patients who might require more careful monitoring of their intake and output.
    a. _____
    b. _____

c. _____
d. _____
e. _____

Section 9
SELF-EVALUATION

A. Multiple Choice. Choose the phrase that best completes each of the following sentences by circling the proper letter.

1. The nurse instructs you to prepare a patient so she can apply the aquathermia blanket. You will
   a. remove all the patient's clothing and cover him with a bath blanket.
   b. assist the patient to change to a hospital gown and make sure no snaps or other metal contact the skin.
   c. take the patient's temperature every 5 minutes for 30 minutes.
   d. apply a thin coat of water-soluble lubricant to the patient's arms and legs to protect the skin.

2. The disposable cold pack
   a. provides continuous cold for 3 hours.
   b. is activated by striking or squeezing.
   c. does not need to be covered.
   d. should be checked every 30 minutes once it is in place.

3. If you are assigned to surgically prep the patient,
   a. always use a safety razor.
   b. shave hair opposite to the direction of growth.
   c. do not use soap, because a dry shave is best.
   d. do not wash the shave area.

4. When a patient is allowed to dangle or ambulate for the first time,
   a. help the patient sit up rapidly.
   b. watch closely for signs of vertigo or fatigue.
   c. stay with the patient, walking a long way.
   d. take his temperature before assisting the patient up.

5. When a patient returns from surgery, you should check
   a. range of motion.   b. vital signs.
   c. lung sounds.   d. ability to move.

6. After which type of anesthesia is a patient most apt to be nauseated?
   a. Local   b. Spinal   c. Intravenous   d. Inhalation

7. Description of postoperative shock includes
   a. elevated blood pressure.   b. weak, rapid pulse.
   c. bounding pulse.   d. flushed face.

8. Patients are often required to lie flat following spinal anesthesia in order to reduce the chance of
   a. nausea.   b. headache.
   c. blood clots.   d. abdominal pain.

9. Refusing to acknowledge unacceptable thoughts and feelings is called
   a. suppression.   b. repression.   c. denial.   d. fantasy.

10. When working with demanding patients, it is best to
    a. explain to the patient that you can't be everywhere at once.
    b. ask the supervisor if the patient can be moved to another unit.

c. maintain open communications.

d. ignore the signal light if the patient keeps calling.

11. Effects of alcohol on the body include

    a. impaired mental judgment.   b. hallucinations.

    c. delirium.   d. tremors.

12. Signs and symptoms of depression include

    a. disorientation.   b. increased physical activity.

    c. elevated temperature.   d. fatigue.

13. When learning of a terminal diagnosis, the first response of the patient usually is

    a. anger.   b. denial.   c. depression.   d. acceptance.

14. Signs that death is approaching include

    a. increase of general muscle tone.

    b. pupils constrict.

    c. extremities cool as circulation slows down.

    d. pulse becomes rapid and bounding.

15. When a patient is in the final stages of life,

    a. leave the patient alone.

    b. you do not have to be careful of what you say.

    c. check on the patient frequently.

    d. mouth care is no longer needed.

16. When giving postmortem care,

    a. remove dentures.

    b. leave equipment in the room.

    c. bathe as necessary.

    d. place the body in a natural sitting position.

B. Short Answer. Name the piece of equipment pictured in the accompanying figure.

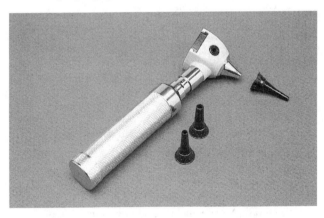

17. _____

C. Short Answer. Name the following examination positions.

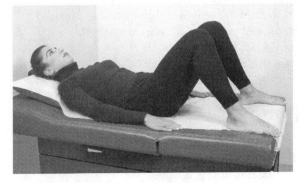

18. _____

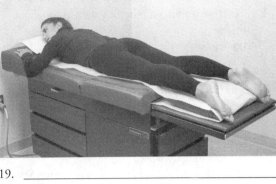

19. _____

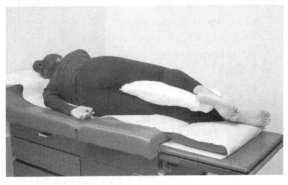

20. _____

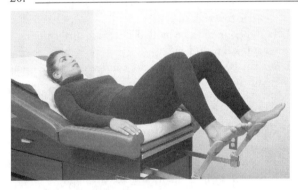

21. _____

D. True/False. Mark the following true or false by circling T or F.

22. T   F   An anxiety disorder is not a recognized mental illnesses.

23. T   F   People with panic disorder may be so fearful that they are unable to function.

24. T   F   OCD is an anxiety disorder.

25. T   F   An example of compulsive behavior is washing hands many times each day.

26. T   F   PTSD is always a response to a recent event.

27. T   F   A phobia is an unfounded, recurring thought that may or may not cause fear.

28. T   F   Affective disorders may also be called mood disorders.

29. T   F   People with schizoaffective disorder maintain contact with reality and do not hallucinate.

30. T   F   Symptoms of SAD usually begin in spring or early summer.

31. T F Patients with BPD can be very manipulative to family, friends, and health care workers.
32. T F People with anorexia purge regularly throughout the day.
33. T F Anorexia and bulimia occur only in females.
34. T F A patient with bulimia may appear skeletal, but view his or her body as fat.
35. T F DTs are part of alcohol withdrawal syndrome.
36. T F DTs usually begin 48 to 96 hours after taking the last drink.
37. T F Suicide precautions are needed only if a patient attempts to harm herself.
38. T F Approximately 67% of adults in the United States are overweight.
39. T F Obesity is well understood.
40. T F Environment does not affect obesity.
41. T F A fat baby is a healthy baby.
42. T F Bariatrics is a field of medicine that focuses on the study of obesity, including its causes, prevention, and treatment, as well as medical conditions and diseases associated with obesity.
43. T F Patients weighing more than 350 pounds should not use a wall-mounted toilet.
44. T F To obtain an accurate weight, transport the bariatric patient to the laundry, loading dock, or maintenance department, and use a freight scale to weigh them.
45. T F A person must be morbidly obese to qualify for surgical treatment.
46. T F The BMI is only one factor considered in diagnosing obesity.
47. T F Comorbidities are diseases and medical conditions that are caused by or contribute to morbid obesity.
48. T F Persons with obesity have about the same risk of cancer as persons of normal weight.
49. T F Overweight people often feel deep emotional pain caused by insensitivity and stereotyping.
50. T F Overweight people usually lack self-discipline, overeat, and are unclean.
51. T F Patients do not choose to be overweight.
52. T F Bariatric patients often sweat profusely, and often feel as if they are chronically short of breath.
53. T F A thigh blood pressure cuff will fit most bariatric patients.
54. T F Some bariatric patients cannot maintain their own personal hygiene because they cannot reach all areas of the body.
55. T F The bariatric patient is usually an expert in knowing what works with his or her own care.
56. T F Obese people cannot develop malnutrition.
57. T F Excessive moisture from perspiration in skin folds creates a risk for yeast infection.
58. T F One staff person should never lift or move more than 35 pounds of body weight without extra help or a mechanical device.
59. T F Using the Trendelenburg position for a brief time makes it easier to move the patient up in bed.

60. T F There is no need to support the obese patient's arms and legs, because of their size.

Section 10
SELF-EVALUATION

A. Multiple Choice. Choose the phrase that best completes each of the following sentences by circling the proper letter.

1. Long-term care may be needed by
   a. a 23-year-old male who had an appendectomy.
   b. a 55-year-old female who had a myocardial infarction and is critically ill.
   c. a 35-year-old male who has had multiple sclerosis for 10 years and requires maximum assistance.
   d. a 72-year-old female who is a newly diagnosed noninsulin-dependent diabetic.
2. Assisted living is appropriate for persons who
   a. require monitoring and may need help with medications.
   b. need extensive rehabilitation.
   c. require specialized nursing care.
   d. have an acute health problem.
3. Subacute care is appropriate for the person who
   a. is elderly, can ambulate, and can do activities of daily living independently.
   b. has a stable health problem but needs assistance with activities of daily living.
   c. requires critical care.
   d. has an unstable health problem.
4. The Omnibus Budget Reconciliation Act (OBRA) of 1987 is federal legislation called the
   a. Self-Determination Act.
   b. Standard Precautions Act.
   c. Nursing Home Reform Act.
   d. Patients' Bill of Rights.
5. Elderly persons may have decreased appetites due to
   a. increased acid production.
   b. decreased smell and taste.
   c. decreased peristalsis.
   d. heartburn and indigestion.
6. Persons with Alzheimer's disease who wander should be
   a. placed in physical restraints.
   b. given chemical restraints.
   c. instructed to remain in their rooms.
   d. allowed to wander in a safe environment.
7. The skilled nursing care facility
   a. provides care for premature babies.
   b. provides acute care.
   c. cares for persons with long-term needs.
   d. provides only custodial care.
8. Elderly persons are characterized by
   a. graying of the hair.
   b. confusion and disorientation.
   c. lack of interest in activities.
   d. incontinence.

9. Foot care for the elderly should include
   a. daily washing and inspection.
   b. heavy use of powder to keep the skin dry.
   c. applications of alcohol.
   d. clipping nails and trimming calluses.
10. Measures to control pain include
   a. increased fluid intake.
   b. vigorous activity.
   c. electrical current stimulation.
   d. immobility and isolation.
11. Homemaker duties usually include
   a. washing windows.   b. shampooing carpets.
   c. mowing the lawn.   d. preparing meals.
12. The nursing assistant working on a subacute care unit
   a. may care for patients receiving complicated treatments.
   b. will administer medications.
   c. may take physician orders for patients.
   d. will learn to change complex wound dressings.
13. A catheter inserted into a vein near the patient's collar bone is called a
   a. piggyback.
   b. peripheral intravenous central catheter.
   c. central venous catheter.
   d. enteral feeding.
14. Continuous medication infusion into the epidural space is commonly done
   a. to relieve pain.
   b. for cancer treatment.
   c. to lower blood pressure.
   d. for hydration management.
15. The client you are caring for at home is unable to report your conduct. Therefore, it is all right to
   a. talk to friends on the phone.
   b. stop for frequent coffee breaks.
   c. watch your favorite television programs.
   d. carry out your work efficiently.
16. Which of the following would *not* be a part of your responsibilities when caring for a client at home as a home care nursing assistant?
   a. Settling family disputes
   b. Assisting with activities of daily living
   c. Carrying out range-of-motion exercises
   d. Shopping for meals
17. When working in home health care, your personal safety is
   a. not a concern if you work for an agency.
   b. always a concern to which you should be alert.
   c. your client's responsibility.
   d. not an issue unless you are in a bad neighborhood.
18. When caring for the client's kitchen,
   a. clean up once a day so dishes can be washed all at once.
   b. rearrange the cupboards to make it easier to make meals.
   c. take any leftover food home with you so it does not go to waste.
   d. wash soiled dishes and put them away promptly.

B. True/False. Mark the following true or false by circling T or F.
19. T F Most expenses for long-term care are paid for by Medicare.
20. T F According to the OBRA legislation, nursing assistants are required to participate in 24 hours of in-service education annually.
21. T F The joints of elderly people become less flexible.
22. T F The diet of an elderly person should include increased amounts of sugar, salt, and fat.
23. T F Side rails are a frequent cause of falls in the elderly.
24. T F Elderly people are at risk for developing infections.
25. T F The elderly should be discouraged from exercising.
26. T F Mental deterioration is an expected change of aging.
27. T F The nursing assistant working in home care is responsible for doing the client assessment.
28. T F A physical therapist may be a member of the home care team.
29. T F The nursing assistant in home care must be a self-starter.
30. T F Incontinence is a normal part of aging.
31. T F Epidural catheters are used for dialysis.
32. T F Patients with tracheostomies should be observed for changes in respiratory rate, depth, and quality.

C. Matching. Choose the correct item from Column II to match each question in Column I.

Column I
33. _____ alopecia
34. _____ anorexia
35. _____ chemotherapy
36. _____ dialysis
37. _____ epidural catheter
38. _____ narcotic
39. _____ oncology
40. _____ patient-controlled analgesia
41. _____ pulse oximetry
42. _____ radiation
43. _____ TENS
44. _____ tracheostomy
45. _____ PICC

Column II
a. the study of cancer
b. cancer treatment using medication
c. cancer treatment using X-rays
d. use of electricity for pain management
e. loss of scalp hair
f. treatment to cleanse blood of liquid wastes
g. drug used for pain relief
h. surgical opening in windpipe
i. loss of appetite
j. catheter inserted near spinal cord
k. measurement of arterial oxygen
l. pain management under control of the patient
m. peripherally inserted central catheter

Section 11
SELF-EVALUATION

A. Matching. Choose the correct term from Column II to match each phrase in Column I.

Column I

1. _____ break in a bone
2. _____ ovaries and testes
3. _____ simple sugar
4. _____ bringing the arm toward the midline
5. _____ chemical messengers
6. _____ scabs
7. _____ color less than normal
8. _____ cerebrovascular accident
9. _____ carry blood toward the heart

Column II

a. flexion	b. abduction	c. pallor
d. adduction	e. crusts	f. fracture
g. hormones	h. stroke (brain attack)	i. gonads
j. veins	k. glucose	l. cyanosis

B. Multiple Choice. Choose the phrase that best completes each of the following sentences by circling the proper letter.

10. Patients in traction require special care. Remember to
    a. allow weights to rest on the floor.
    b. allow the patient's feet to rest on the foot of the bed.
    c. adjust the belt and straps smoothly and snugly.
    d. remove the weight when repositioning the patient.

11. The best position for the patient with respiratory problems is
    a. lithotomy.   b. high Fowler's.   c. prone.   d. Sims'.

12. You may be asked to weigh the cardiac patient daily because
    a. decreased appetite may cause weight loss.
    b. increased appetite may cause weight gain.
    c. fluid tends to collect in the tissues, increasing weight.
    d. urine output is increased, causing weight loss.

13. Remember in caring for patients with arteriosclerosis that
    a. hot water bottles may cause serious burns.
    b. injuries heal well.
    c. circulation is very adequate.
    d. a cool room is most comfortable.

14. The patient who has suffered a CVA usually
    a. is paralyzed.
    b. speaks clearly.
    c. is able to assist in his own care.
    d. has a short convalescence.

15. Fractures of children's bones are frequently incomplete. These fractures are called
    a. compound.   b. simple.
    c. comminuted.   d. greenstick.

16. A patient with skin lesions must
    a. be washed off with soap and water.
    b. have crusts removed daily.
    c. have frequent backrubs with alcohol.
    d. be handled gently.

17. A bed patient may develop pressure ulcers if
    a. her position is not changed at least every 2 hours.
    b. the bed is kept dry and clean.
    c. the patient is bathed frequently.
    d. pressure areas are not frequently massaged.

18. The patient with emphysema has respiratory problems because
    a. he cannot inhale completely.
    b. he cannot exhale completely.
    c. he inhales more deeply than usual.
    d. he exhales more deeply than usual.

19. In caring for patients receiving oxygen, remember
    a. no smoking is permitted in the area.
    b. electric call bells may be used.
    c. woolen blankets are used for warmth.
    d. electrical equipment may be used without discontinuing the oxygen.

20. Following a thyroidectomy, check your patient carefully for
    a. signs of dehydration.   b. inability to speak.
    c. nausea.   d. fatigue.

21. All males should perform testicular self-examination
    a. yearly.   b. before showering.
    c. with soapy fingers.   d. using the palms of the hands.

22. Your patient has anemia. You should carry out which of the following nursing procedures?
    a. Oxygen by cannula   b. Special mouth care
    c. Vital signs   d. Urine measurement

23. You are assigned to care for a convalescing patient who has suffered a stroke. You will pay particular attention to
    a. skin care.   b. exercise and activity.
    c. ambulation.   d. need to void.

24. When a patient is aphasic, you can communicate with her best if you
    a. raise your voice.
    b. leave the patient alone much of the time.
    c. ask lengthy questions.
    d. speak in short, concise sentences.

25. Patients at risk for pressure ulcers are those who are
    a. well nourished.   b. young.
    c. incontinent.   d. up and about.

26. The nursing assistant helping to care for the burn patient should
    a. give medication for pain.
    b. restrict fluids.
    c. assist in preventing infection.
    d. keep the door to the room closed.

27. The nursing assistant caring for the diabetic patient
    a. may give nourishments freely.
    b. knows the signs of diabetic coma and insulin shock.
    c. cuts the patient's toenails.
    d. need not monitor how much food is eaten.

28. When the patient has an arterial-venous shunt for renal dialysis,
    a. use the arm with the shunt to measure an accurate blood pressure.
    b. do not use the shunted arm to determine pulse rate.

c. do not use the shunted arm to measure blood pressure.

d. it is not necessary to measure ordered intake and output.

29. During which of the following procedures should the nursing assistant wear disposable gloves?
    a. Complete bed bath
    b. Giving perineal care
    c. Measuring intake
    d. Repositioning patients

30. Food is absorbed through the walls of the
    a. pancreas.
    b. stomach.
    c. large intestine.
    d. small intestine.

31. When caring for a patient with a spinal cord injury, the nursing assistant should
    a. recognize that pain and pressure will be felt more acutely.
    b. realize that the patient requires extra care to prevent contractures.
    c. know the patient will not need skin care because voluntary movement will not be impaired.
    d. use a hurried approach to care to stimulate the patient into action.

32. The nursing assistant preparing a patient for an 8:00 AM gastrointestinal series might expect to find as part of the instructions
    a. a high-calorie breakfast.
    b. enemas until clear in the morning of test.
    c. surgical prep of abdomen.
    d. no visitors the night before the test.

33. To make insertion of a rectal tube easier, the nursing assistant might suggest that the patient
    a. take a breath and bear down.
    b. exhale as the tube is inserted.
    c. lie with legs extended.
    d. cross the legs.

34. When preparing to give a prepackaged chemical enema, the nursing assistant knows
    a. water must be added.
    b. approximately 500 mL of solution will be used.
    c. to handle the fluid-filled glass container carefully.
    d. the tip of the container is prelubricated.

35. The eye and ear are part of which system?
    a. Endocrine
    b. Cardiovascular
    c. Nervous
    d. Digestive

36. The female nursing assistant who is 52 years old should have a mammogram
    a. yearly.
    b. every other year.
    c. every three years.
    d. every five years.

37. Frequent herpes simplex II outbreaks
    a. put females at less risk of cancer of the cervix.
    b. put females at greater risk of miscarriage.
    c. make vaginal delivery the preferred route.
    d. cannot affect a newborn in any way.

38. Membranes that line body cavities that open to the outside are called
    a. mucous membranes.
    b. mucus membranes.
    c. serifs membranes.
    d. filirous membranes.

39. Syphilis and gonorrhea are diseases that are commonly sexually transmitted. Other sexually transmitted diseases include
    a. MRSA.
    b. VRE.
    c. HIV.
    d. Hantavirus.

Section 12
SELF-EVALUATION

A. Multiple Choice. Choose the phrase that best completes each of the following sentences by circling the proper letter.

1. Your patient has just delivered a baby. She is pale, complains of being cold, and begins to shiver. You suspect that she is
    a. excited about having the baby.
    b. tired.
    c. in danger of shock.
    d. hungry.

2. When removing and replacing a perineal pad,
    a. both sides may be handled.
    b. draw it forward before lifting.
    c. gloves need not be used.
    d. lift from the body from front to back.

3. When assisting the nursing mother,
    a. recommend a tight brassiere.
    b. breast pads are not necessary.
    c. assist with handwashing before feeding the baby.
    d. give the mother milk suppression medication.

4. When giving routine ileostomy care, you should
    a. not wear gloves.
    b. use sterile technique.
    c. use alcohol to clean the stoma.
    d. observe the drainage.

5. Diarrhea is
    a. multiple loose, watery stools.
    b. similar to fecal impaction.
    c. a stool with abnormal color.
    d. a single loose, watery stool.

6. Which of the following are nursing assistant responsibilities when caring for an infant?
    a. Maintaining a safe environment
    b. Caring for the circumcision
    c. Caring for the umbilical cord
    d. Applying silver nitrate to the eyes

7. When collecting a urine specimen from a patient with a urinary catheter,
    a. withdraw the urine from the sampling port using a syringe.
    b. empty the urine from the spout in the drainage bag.
    c. clamp the catheter, then collect urine from the drainage tubing.
    d. insert a needle into the side of the catheter and withdraw with a syringe.

8. Keys to successful restorative nursing care are
    a. turning the patient every 2 to 3 hours.
    b. ambulating the patient with a gait belt.
    c. consistency and continuity of care.
    d. providing emotional support to the family.

9. A disability exists when a person has
    a. any chronic illness.
    b. an inability to perform a normal activity for a person of that age.
    c. a health problem requiring daily medication.
    d. any mental or emotional problem.

10. A handicap exists when a person
    a. cannot fulfill a role that is normal for that person.
    b. has a prosthesis.
    c. is hearing impaired.
    d. cannot walk.
11. A disability may result from
    a. acute infection.   b. multiple sclerosis.
    c. dehydration.   d. delirium.
12. A physician who specializes in rehabilitation is called a
    a. psychiatrist.   b. dermatologist.
    c. neurosurgeon.   d. physiatrist.
13. Nursing assistants who work in rehabilitation may be responsible for
    a. teaching the patient gait training for mobility.
    b. assessing patients in bowel and bladder training.
    c. doing passive range-of-motion exercises.
    d. discharge planning.
14. Inactivity may result in
    a. sore throat.   b. osteoporosis.
    c. headache.   d. aphasia.
15. The activities of daily living include
    a. driving a car.
    b. managing personal finances.
    c. using the telephone.
    d. personal hygiene and grooming.
16. An example of a self-care deficit is
    a. disease.   b. trauma.
    c. emotional illness.   d. inability to dress.

B. Matching. Choose the correct term from Column II to match each phrase in Column I.

Column I

17. _____ occult
18. _____ ostomy
19. _____ episiotomy
20. _____ lochia
21. _____ colostrum
22. _____ postpartum
23. _____ excessive blood loss
24. _____ thrombus
25. _____ embolus
26. _____ verbal cue
27. _____ atrophy
28. _____ adaptive device
29. _____ tetraplegia

Column II

a. hemorrhage
b. incision in perineum
c. first breast milk
d. vaginal discharge
e. hidden
f. after birth
g. artificial opening
h. inability to complete an ADL
i. orally prompting the patient to complete an ADL
j. blood clot
k. paralysis of arms and legs
l. blood clot that moves throughout circulatory system
m. item used for helping patients complete ADLs
n. muscle deterioration

C. True/False. Mark the following true or false by circling T or F.

30. T F   A colostomy is a surgical opening in the stomach.
31. T F   Contamination must be prevented when collecting a urine specimen through a drainage port.
32. T F   The Hemoccult test is used to determine the presence of blood in the stool.
33. T F   The toddler stage includes children from 3 to 6 years of age.
34. T F   Children in the toddler stage should be able to read.
35. T F   The normal heart rate for a preschooler is 80 to 110 beats per minute.
36. T F   The Apgar score is an evaluation of the mother after childbirth.
37. T F   Massaging the uterus after childbirth stimulates uterine muscles to contract.
38. T F   Disabilities are always permanent.
39. T F   Disabled people cannot contribute to society.
40. T F   A speech therapist may evaluate patients for swallowing ability.
41. T F   The physical therapist teaches patients gait training.
42. T F   The patient's inability to organize a task such as dressing is called a perceptual deficit.
43. T F   Hand-over-hand is a technique used in restorative care.
44. T F   Rehabilitation is generally a waste of time for elderly patients.

Section 13
SELF-EVALUATION

A. Multiple Choice. Choose the phrase that best completes each of the following sentences by circling the proper letter.

1. You observe someone having a seizure. You should
   a. restrain her movements.
   b. force something between her teeth to prevent her from biting her tongue.
   c. move articles away that the patient might strike.
   d. encourage the patient to walk around as soon as the seizure is over.
2. The Heimlich maneuver is used for persons who are
   a. having cardiac arrest.   b. choking.
   c. having a seizure.   d. having an insulin reaction.
3. The *B* in the ABCs of emergencies stands for
   a. breathing. b. bleeding. c. burns. d. breakdown.
4. When an emergency occurs, the first thing you should check is the patient's
   a. degree of consciousness.   b. airway/breathing ability.
   c. heart rate.   d. blood pressure.
5. Risk factors for heart attack include
   a. being underweight.   b. exercising frequently.
   c. smoking.   d. eating a low-fat diet.

B. True/False. Mark the following true or false by circling T or F.

6. T F   CPR is not used for people over 60 years of age.
7. T F   Adults should be hit firmly between the shoulder blades if they are choking.
8. T F   The patient loses consciousness during a grand mal seizure.
9. T F   A strain is an injury to a ligament.
10. T F   Emergency treatment for burns includes putting petroleum jelly on the burned area.
11. T F   Reinsert the oral airway promptly if a patient pulls it out.
12. T F   The most common cause of airway obstruction is spasm of the vocal cords.
13. T F   Apply the principles of standard precautions when caring for patients who use oral and nasal airways.
14. T F   A nasal airway must never be used in a conscious patient.
15. T F   A nasal airway will be in place if the patient has a nasal deformity.
16. T F   Endotracheal intubation provides complete control over the airway.
17. T F   Patients who are intubated often require restraints to prevent them from removing the tube.
18. T F   You may turn the ventilator alarm off when working at the bedside.
19. T F   When monitoring the vital signs of patients using mechanical ventilation, count only the ventilator-delivered breaths.
20. T F   Empty condensation in the ventilation tubing backward into the humidifier.
21. T F   The bag-valve-mask should always be visible and available in the ventilator patient's room.
22. T F   The Yankauer catheter is used only for oral suctioning.
23. T F   Suctioning is not a routine nursing assistant responsibility.
24. T F   Suctioning should be done at fixed intervals, such as every hour.
25. T F   Patients who are mechanically ventilated are usually totally dependent on staff to meet their needs.

Section 14
SELF-EVALUATION

A. Multiple Choice. Choose the phrase that best completes each of the following sentences by circling the proper letter.

1. Nursing assistants may find employment in
    a. hospitals.   b. convenience stores.
    c. day care centers.   d. social service agencies.
2. A résumé should include your
    a. age.   b. religion.
    c. marital status.   d. educational history.
3. You would list as a reference, on a job application, your
    a. mother.   b. best friend.   c. instructor.   d. sister.

4. During the interview, it is appropriate to
    a. eat a snack if you did not have time for lunch.
    b. chew gum to relieve your nervousness.
    c. refer to a list of questions you want to ask.
    d. discuss personal problems.
5. Orientation to a new job is
    a. only for experienced nursing assistants.
    b. only for nursing assistants working day shift.
    c. done to ensure safe performance of your duties.
    d. generally, a waste of time.
6. As a new employee, you will be expected to
    a. get an X-ray.
    b. receive a two-step Mantoux test.
    c. refuse immunization for hepatitis B.
    d. work every weekend.
7. Some employers may require
    a. you to have a phone or pager.
    b. drug testing.
    c. you to attend orientation on your own time.
    d. a one-year contract.
8. If you are told during the interview that you will have to work every other weekend, and you do not wish to do this, you should
    a. call in sick when it is your weekend to work.
    b. tell the interviewer you expect to work Monday through Friday.
    c. not accept the position, if offered.
    d. tell the interviewer you must attend church on the weekends.
9. When you decide to leave a position, you should
    a. not come to work any more.
    b. give two weeks notice.
    c. give a two-day notice.
    d. leave in the middle of the shift.
10. To maintain employment, you will need to
    a. work whenever you want.
    b. attend nursing classes.
    c. maintain an excellent attendance record.
    d. finish your assignment quickly.

ANSWER KEYS FOR SECTION SELF-EVALUATIONS
Section 1
SELF-EVALUATION

A. Multiple Choice

1. d	2. b	3. c	4. b	5. a
6. b	7. a	8. b	9. a	10. c
11. b	12. c	13. b	14. d	15. a
16. b	17. d	18. c	19. b	20. a

B. Matching

21. d	22. e	23. b	24. a	25. c

C. True/False

26. T	27. F	28. F	29. T	30. F
31. F	32. T	33. T	34. F	35. F

D. Completion

36. Stay within the scope of practice.
- Do only what you have been taught to do.
- Carry out procedures as taught and according to facility policy.
- Request guidance from the proper person before taking action in questionable situations.
- Keep safety and well-being of patients foremost in mind—act accordingly.
- Understand directions for care.
- Perform according to facility policy.
- Stay within OBRA guidelines.
- Maintain in-services required by OBRA.
- Do no harm to the patient.
- Respect patients and their belongings.

Section 2
SELF-EVALUATION

A. Definitions
1. Basic unit of body.
2. Different tissues.
3. Organs working together.
4. Tumor, new growth.
5. Cause of illness or abnormality.

B. Matching
6. g   7. d   8. h   9. a   10. j
11. e   12. b   13. a

C. Multiple Choice
14. d   15. a   16. c   17. a   18. b
19. d   20. a

D. Matching
21. e   22. d   23. b   24. a   25. c

E. Completion
26. the fetus   27. no sensations
28. rectum   29. X-rays.
30. assist with the correct preparation of patients

F. Word Choice
31. vein   32. lateral   33. neoplasm
34. carcinoma   35. trauma   36. protocols

G. Definitions
37. Blood vessel that takes blood back to the heart.
38. Farther away from the midline.
39. Tumor.   40. Malignant tumor.
41. Injury.   42. Standards of procedures and care.

H. Matching
43. e   44. d   45. g   46. a   47. b

I. Word Choice
48. cranial   49. thoracic   50. abdominal
51. peritoneal   52. thoracic

J. Brief Answers
53. Covering of brain and spinal cord.
54. In the cranial and spinal cavities.
55. Brain and spinal cord.

56. Inflammation of.
57. Inflammation of meninges.

Section 3
SELF-EVALUATION

A. Matching
1. d   2. e   3. c   4. f   5. g
6. g   7. e   8. a   9. d   10. b

B. Multiple Choice
11. d   12. d   13. c   14. b   15. c
16. a   17. b   18. c   19. b   20. a
21. d   22. b   23. a   24. c   25. d
26. a   27. b

C. Matching
28. j   29. a   30. g   31. h   32. f
33. e   34. b

D. Short Answer
35.
Assessment
   a. collect observations
   b. report observations
   c. document observations
Planning
   a. collect, report, document observations
   b. inform nurse of any problems noted with care plan
   c. participate in planning care if possible
Implementation
   a. carry out care plan and assignment as instructed
   b. inform nurse of any problems noted with approaches
   c. continue to make and report observations
Evaluation
   a. report to nurse if approaches are not working
   b. determine whether approaches are helping patient to reach goals
   c. report to nurse if you note reasons why patient may not be reaching goals

E. True/False
36. T   37. F   38. T   39. T   40. T
41. F   42. F   43. T   44. T   45. T
46. F   47. T   48. F   49. T   50. T
51. T   52. F   53. F   54. F   55. T
56. T   57. F   58. F   59. F   60. T

Section 4
SELF-EVALUATION

A. Definitions
1. One-celled organisms that cause diseases such as malaria.
2. One-celled organisms that are classified according to shape and arrangement.
3. The process of an object coming into contact with infectious material.
4. An object that comes into contact with excretions or secretions of an infected person.
5. Insects or animals that carry pathogens that can be transmitted to humans.

B. Matching

6. b   7. f   8. e   9. d   10. c
11. g   12. a

C. Multiple Choice

13. d   14. a   15. b   16. c   17. a

D. Completion

18. handwashing   19. transmission-based precautions
20. digestive   21. reproductive
22. spread or transmission   23. direct or indirect
24. pathogens   25. more

E. Short Answer

26. a. Handwashing.
    b. Use of gloves.
    c. Use of other personal protective equipment.
    d. Proper disposal of sharps.
    e. Proper handling of waste and soiled linen.
27. a. Organism enters body.
    b. Organism grows and multiplies in body.
    c. Symptoms are noted.
28. a. Number and strength of infectious organism.
    b. General health of individual.
    c. Age, sex, heredity of individual.
    d. Condition of person's immune system.
29. a. Emotional stress.
    b. Fatigue.
30. a. Mucous membranes.
    b. Cilia.
    c. Coughing and sneezing.
    d. Hydrochloric acid in stomach.
    e. Tears.
31. a. Gloves.   b. Gowns.   c. Masks.   d. Goggles.

F. True/False

32. F   33. T   34. F   35. T   36. T
37. F   38. T   39. F   40. T   41. T
42. T   43. T   44. F   45. T   46. F
47. F   48. F   49. T   50. F   51. F
52. T   53. F   54. T   55. T   56. F
57. F   58. T   59. F   60. T   61. F
62. T   63. T   64. F   65. T   66. F
67. F   68. T   69. F

Section 5
SELF-EVALUATION

A. Multiple Choice

1. a   2. c   3. b   4. c   5. d
6. b   7. c   8. c   9. d   10. d
11. a   12. a

B. Short Answer

13. Remove patient.   Activate alarm.
    Contain fire.   Extinguish fire.
14. Pull the pin.
    Aim the nozzle at the base of the fire.
    Squeeze the handle.
    Sweep back and forth along base of fire.

C. True/False

15. T   16. F   17. F   18. T   19. F
20. T   21. F   22. T   23. F   24. T
25. T

D. Matching

26. j   27. g   28. e   29. h   30. c
31. i   32. b   33. d   34. f   35. a

Section 6
SELF-EVALUATION

A. Multiple Choice

1. c   2. a   3. b   4. a   5. d   6. d
7. a   8. c   9. b   10. c   11. a

B. Short Answer

12. 98.6°F   13. 37°C

C. Short Answer

14. indicate the method in parentheses, for example, (ax)
15. thermometer, watch with second hand,
    sphygmomanometer, stethoscope
16. brachial, carotid, femoral, popliteal
17. glass, electronic, tympanic, plastic, digital
18. centimeters
19. kilograms

D. Matching

20. g   21. a   22. b   23. e

E. Short Answer

24. B/P is higher than previous reading.
25. B/P is lower than previous reading.
26. Site of reading is other than brachial artery.
27. Cannot hear it.

Section 7
SELF-EVALUATION

A. Multiple Choice

1. a   2. b   3. a   4. c   5. d
6. c   7. a   8. d   9. c   10. b
11. a   12. d   13. d   14. c   15. c
16. b   17. d   18. b   19. b   20. c
21. b   22. c   23. b   24. b   25. d
26. c   27. b   28. c   29. b   30. b
31. c   32. d   33. b   34. a   35. a
36. d   37. b

B. Matching

38. c   39. f   40. a   41. b   42. d

C. True/False

43. F   44. T   45. F   46. F   47. F
48. T   49. T   50. F   51. F   52. T
53. F   54. T   55. F   56. F   57. T
58. T   59. T   60. T   61. T

D. Short Answer

62. Place patient on her side with legs flexed.
63. Foreskin must be moved up to clean the penis and must
    be gently moved back down into position after cleaning.

Section 8
SELF-EVALUATION

A. Matching
1. e   2. g   3. b   4. h   5. f
6. a   7. d   8. c

B. Multiple Choice
9. c   10. c   11. b   12. d   13. d
14. d   15. b   16. b   17. d   18. d
19. b   20. a   21. a   22. a

C. Matching
23. b   24. c   25. e   26. a

D. Short Answer
27. a. fruits
    b. vegetables
    c. pasta
    d. lean baked or broiled meat, especially poultry or fish
    e. whole-grain breads and cereals
28. Fluid balance is the ratio of fluid intake to fluid output.
29. Alert patients may write down the amount each time they drink.
30. a. dehydrated   b. vomiting
    c. with IVs running   d. with Foley catheter
    e. with fluid retention problems or on diuretics

Section 9
SELF-EVALUATION

A. Multiple Choice
1. b   2. b   3. a   4. b   5. b   6. d
7. b   8. b   9. a   10. c   11. a   12. d
13. b   14. c   15. c   16. c

B. Short Answer
17. otoscope

C. Short Answer
18. dorsal recumbent position
19. prone position
20. Sim's position
21. dorsal lithotomy position
22. F   23. T   24. T   25. T   26. F
27. F   28. T   29. F   30. F   31. T
32. F   33. F   34. T   35. T   36. T
37. F   38. T   39. F   40. F   41. F
42. T   43. T   44. F   45. F   46. T
47. T   48. F   49. T   50. F   51. T
52. T   53. F   54. T   55. T   56. F
57. T   58. T   59. T   60. F

Section 10
SELF-EVALUATION

A. Multiple Choice
1. c   2. a   3. d   4. c   5. b
6. d   7. c   8. a   9. a   10. c
11. d   12. a   13. c   14. a   15. d
16. a   17. b   18. d

B. True/False
19. F   20. F   21. T   22. F   23. T
24. T   25. F   26. F   27. F   28. T
29. T   30. F   31. F   32. T

C. Matching
33. e   34. i   35. b   36. f   37. j
38. g   39. a   40. l   41. k   42. c
43. d   44. h   45. m

Section 11
SELF-EVALUATION

A. Matching
1. f   2. i   3. k   4. d   5. g
6. e   7. c   8. h   9. j

B. Multiple Choice
10. c   11. b   12. c   13. a   14. a
15. d   16. d   17. a   18. b   19. a
20. b   21. c   22. b   23. a   24. d
25. c   26. c   27. b   28. c   29. b
30. d   31. b   32. b   33. a   34. d
35. c   36. a   37. b   38. a   39. c

Section 12
SELF-EVALUATION

A. Multiple Choice
1. c   2. d   3. c   4. d   5. a   6. a
7. a   8. c   9. b   10. a   11. b   12. d
13. c   14. b   15. d   16. d

B. Matching
17. e   18. g   19. b   20. d   21. c
22. f   23. a   24. j   25. l   26. i
27. n   28. m   29. k

C. True/False
30. F   31. T   32. T   33. F   34. F
35. T   36. F   37. T   38. F   39. F
40. T   41. T   42. F   43. T   44. F

Section 13
SELF-EVALUATION

A. Multiple Choice
1. c   2. b   3. a   4. b   5. c

B. True/False
6. F   7. F   8. T   9. F   10. F
11. F   12. F   13. T   14. F   15. F
16. T   17. T   18. F   19. F   20. F
21. T   22. T   23. T   24. F   25. T

Section 14
SELF-EVALUATION

A. Multiple Choice
1. a   2. d   3. c   4. c   5. c
6. b   7. b   8. c   9. b   10. c

COMPREHENSIVE FINAL EVALUATION

A. Multiple Choice. Choose the phrase that best completes each of the following sentences by circling the proper letter.

1. Special health services offered in the community include
   a. health insurance.
   b. activities of daily living.
   c. immunization procedures.
   d. critical care.

2. All of these health care facilities provide short-term care *except*
   a. hospitals.
   b. outpatient clinics.
   c. skilled care facilities.
   d. subacute care units.

3. Nursing assistants are most often employed by
   a. long-term care facilities.
   b. local health departments.
   c. the World Health Organization.
   d. state sanitation departments.

4. The immediate supervisor of the nursing assistant is
   a. another nursing assistant.
   b. a licensed nurse.
   c. the director of nursing.
   d. an MD.

5. A nursing assistant failed to check the temperature of an enema solution and the patient was burned. This is a case of
   a. malpractice.
   b. abuse.
   c. neglect.
   d. aiding and abetting.

6. The nursing assistant fails to raise a side rail and the patient falls out of bed and breaks a hip. This is a case of
   a. neglect.
   b. aiding and abetting.
   c. libel.
   d. negligence.

7. Responsibilities of the nursing assistant include
   a. starting intravenous feeding.
   b. giving personal care to patients.
   c. administering medications.
   d. completing physical assessments.

8. The patient offers the nursing assistant a little extra money for the care received. The nursing assistant should
   a. accept and say nothing.
   b. accept and share with other team members.
   c. refuse courteously.
   d. pretend not to hear the offer.

9. The nursing assistant learns that the patient has several bank accounts. The assistant should
   a. inform the charge nurse.
   b. tell the family this information.
   c. inform the patient's physician.
   d. keep this information confidential.

10. The nursing assistant learns that the patient is concerned about the cost of hospitalization. The assistant should
    a. inform the nurse.
    b. tell the family this information.
    c. keep this information confidential.
    d. inform the patient's physician.

11. The patient is terminal and begs the nursing assistant to "pull the plug." The assistant should
    a. do as asked so the patient will not suffer any longer.
    b. explain that God makes those decisions and tell the patient to pray.
    c. report the incident to the nurse.
    d. tell the family.

12. Patients are responsible for
    a. keeping health information confidential.
    b. providing information to the physician and other caregivers.
    c. trusting the doctor to manage their health.
    d. designating a nurse on the unit to have power of attorney.

13. Another nursing assistant asks you to help move a patient up in bed. You should
    a. agree to help but be annoyed.
    b. say you are doing more than your share already.
    c. agree only if the other assistant will help with your assignment.
    d. agree in a courteous manner.

14. Your team leader needs a specimen taken to the laboratory "stat" and asks you do to so.
    a. You ask another nursing assistant to take the specimen.
    b. You follow directions but give a patient status report to your team leader before leaving.
    c. You take the specimen and deliver it upon completion of your assignment.
    d. You take the specimen and leave the floor immediately without reporting.

15. Your patient is very irritable this morning and complains about how slow you are. You know that
    a. people sometimes direct their frustrations about their illness toward other people.
    b. you had better rush the care.
    c. you had better get help to finish the care.
    d. the patient is being unfair and you tell him so.

16. Which of the following could act as a fomite?
    a. A patient sneezing   b. A mouse
    c. A roach   d. Soiled linen
17. In carrying out the handwashing procedure,
    a. it is all right to remove suds with a paper towel.
    b. rinse hands with fingertips down.
    c. rinse hands with fingertips straight up.
    d. use very hot water.
18. The best temperature for the patient's room is about
    a. 60°F.   b. 48°F.   c. 72°F.   d. 88°F.
19. A patient is being visited by her clergy. You should provide privacy by
    a. drawing the privacy curtain.
    b. asking the other patients to leave.
    c. asking the other patients not to listen.
    d. telling the cleric to speak softly.
20. Your attitude is reflected in your
    a. speed.   b. technical ability.
    c. documentation.   d. tact.
21. Nursing assistants communicate their feelings by
    a. body language.   b. reporting.
    c. documentation.   d. adherence to procedures.
22. Your patient has difficulty sleeping. You should consider
    a. asking the nurse to give a sleeping pill.
    b. pain the patient may be having.
    c. turning off the hallway light.
    d. telling the roommate not to make noise.
23. The nursing assistant can increase the patient's sense of security by
    a. hanging his clothes in the closet.
    b. providing opportunities for the patient to talk.
    c. taking every remark by the patient personally.
    d. doing every aspect of care that the patient could do.
24. The nursing assistant demonstrates proper body mechanics by
    a. using the right muscles to do the job.
    b. using the back muscles to lift heavy objects.
    c. bending from the waist when picking up objects.
    d. keeping feet close together when picking up an object.
25. The nursing assistant will turn patients frequently when they are unable to change their own position
    a. to prevent complaints.
    b. to improve behavior.
    c. to prevent pressure ulcers.
    d. only if ordered by the doctor.
26. The safest way to transfer a heavy patient who is dependent and unable to bear weight is to
    a. use a mechanical lift.
    b. use a two-person transfer and gait belt.
    c. leave the patient in bed to avoid staff injuries.
    d. cradle-lift the patient out of bed.
27. People of different cultures often differ in their
    a. basic needs.   b. need for personal space.
    c. feelings.   d. emotions.
28. The proper temperature for bath water is
    a. 85°F.   b. 95°F.   c. 105°F.   d. 115°F.

29. During the bath procedure, other care is given, which includes
    a. dressing.   b. ambulation.   c. transfer.   d. shaving.
30. Your patient will be most likely to require special mouth care if
    a. he is unconscious.   b. he drinks lots of fluids.
    c. he is receiving an IV.   d. he cannot get out of bed.
31. To protect the patient's dentures,
    a. leave them uncovered in the bedside table.
    b. use hot water to clean the dentures.
    c. use a heavy stream of water and toothpaste.
    d. store them in a labeled denture cup.
32. A patient on a diabetic diet would not be given
    a. bread and butter.   b. broiled chicken.
    c. toast with strawberry jam.   d. dill pickles.
33. The patient orders read "NPO after 4 PM." This means that the nursing assistant will
    a. withhold all food and fluids after 4:00 PM.
    b. force fluids after 4:00 PM.
    c. encourage the patient to ambulate.
    d. do range-of-motion exercises.
34. The patient has an order for a clear liquid diet. Which of the following would you omit from the tray?
    a. Coffee with cream   b. Ginger ale
    c. Gelatin   d. Tea with sugar
35. The patient on a low-sodium diet would not be given
    a. mashed potatoes.   b. fresh peaches.
    c. dill pickles.   d. green beans.
36. You are assigned to give postmortem care. You assemble equipment to
    a. assist with elimination.   b. give afternoon (PM) care.
    c. determine vital signs.   d. care for the body after death.
37. Which is the most accurate temperature reading?
    a. Oral   b. Vaginal   c. Axillary   d. Tympanic
38. A temperature of 98.6°F is equal to
    a. 32°C.   b. 35°C.   c. 37°C.   d. 39°C.
39. An oral thermometer should be left in place before reading for
    a. 1 minute.   b. 2 minutes.   c. 3 minutes.   d. 4 minutes.
40. When measuring a blood pressure,
    a. apply the cuff 4 inches above the elbow.
    b. first determine the palpated systolic pressure.
    c. pump the gauge up quickly to 180 mm Hg and then release.
    d. place the stethoscope bell over the radial artery.
41. A blood pressure of 80/30 should be reported because the patient is probably suffering from
    a. bradycardia.   b. tachycardia.
    c. hypertension.   d. hypotension.
42. The nursing assistant would record vital signs on the
    a. physician's progress report.   b. graphic chart.
    c. physical and history.   d. laboratory report.
43. Your patient is to be transferred to ICU. You would assist in transporting her to the
    a. isolation care unit.   b. intermediate care unit.
    c. intensive care unit.   d. isotope unit.

44. Your patient is to have f.f. and receive solids ad. lib. You will
    a. encourage the patient to eat but withhold liquids.
    b. place an NPO sign on the bed.
    c. caution the patient to limit his drinking to 2 glasses of water every 8 hours.
    d. encourage fluids and let the patient eat what he wishes.
45. When giving an oral report, include the patient's
    a. name, age, weight.
    b. name, marital status, diagnosis.
    c. name, location, vital signs.
    d. location, diagnosis, age.
46. Charting is important because the patient's medical record
    a. is a communication tool.
    b. is read only by nurses.
    c. is destroyed upon discharge.
    d. shows that you completed your assignment.
47. Important rules to remember about charting include
    a. erasures are permitted.   b. each entry must be signed.
    c. spaces may be left safely.   d. errors must be obliterated.
48. The time 1:00 PM is expressed in international time as
    a. 0100.   b. 0101.   c. 1000.   d. 1300.
49. The most effective way to communicate with hearing-impaired patients is to
    a. speak as loudly as you can.
    b. face the patient.
    c. avoid speaking if at all possible.
    d. teach them how to lip-read.
50. Which of the following represents normal body defenses?
    a. Unbroken skin   b. Urine
    c. Fecal matter   d. Red blood cells
51. The patient is on her abdomen with arms flexed and hands under her face, which is turned to one side. This position is
    a. semi-Fowler's.   b. Sims'.   c. prone.   d. supine.
52. The patient is going to surgery. Which of the following would you check?
    a. The laboratory records
    b. Wearing glasses and socks
    c. Bed rails in low position
    d. Patient wearing an ID band
53. Elastic stockings are used postoperatively to
    a. support the operative area.
    b. support the leg veins.
    c. reduce the flow of blood to the legs.
    d. reduce the risk of infection.
54. The physical examination helps the physician
    a. determine the need for nursing care.
    b. get to know the family better.
    c. evaluate the patient's current status.
    d. write the advance directive.
55. The patient with emphysema is receiving oxygen by nasal cannula. Which of the following precautions should be followed?
    a. No smoking allowed
    b. Use only woolen blankets

c. Turn O₂ off for meals and baths.
    d. Limit fluid intake
56. The patient is recovering from an attack of congestive heart failure. Which of the following applies?
    a. Weigh the patient three times a day.
    b. Carefully monitor I&O.
    c. Give a mechanical soft diet.
    d. Assist the patient to ambulate every hour.
57. Your patient has a fractured femur and is currently in traction. Which of the following applies?
    a. Check for areas of pressure or irritation
    b. Allow feet to press gently against end of bed
    c. Keep weights balanced on the floor
    d. Periodically remove traction to relieve pressure
58. Your patient has diabetes mellitus. Which of the following nursing care will you give?
    a. Strain all urine
    b. Restrict fluids
    c. Serve a high-carbohydrate diet
    d. Check the FSBS as ordered.
59. According to Maslow's hierarchy of needs,
    a. all physical needs have priority over other types of needs.
    b. elderly people have fewer needs than young people.
    c. self-esteem needs are not important when a person is ill.
    d. safety needs can always be met by raising side rails.
60. The stoma of a colostomy may be in the
    a. pancreas.   b. transverse colon.
    c. distal ileum.   d. stomach.
61. Your patient has a douche ordered. You know that
    a. the temperature of the solution is 85°F.
    b. the procedure is simple and will not require draping.
    c. the perineum should be cleansed.
    d. the patient should assume the prone position.
62. To be successfully employed, you should
    a. only be late for work occasionally.
    b. perform your work as you were taught.
    c. remember that you have learned all you will ever have to know.
    d. set your own rules of ethical conduct.
63. When resigning from employment, you should
    a. stop going to work; there is no need to notify anyone.
    b. call and tell the nurse you will not be returning.
    c. write a letter of resignation and give notice.
    d. ask a coworker to tell them you will not be back.
64. Which of the following is *not* a stereotype of the patient in a long-term care facility? They
    a. are not competent to make decisions.
    b. have no interest in sex.
    c. are all old.
    d. have health needs requiring assistance.
65. You can give your best care to a long-term care patient by recognizing that
    a. admission is permanent.
    b. a reversion to childlike behavior is to be expected.
    c. the patient needs to be permitted to make choices.
    d. the patient must not participate in his own care.

66. When providing care for older persons, you should remember that they may
    a. sleep less at night but need naps during the day.
    b. have a more rapid sensory response to stimuli.
    c. have more acute hearing as they age.
    d. experience a gradually increasing appetite.

67. Which of the following is *not* a psychological need?
    a. Need to be loved
    b. Need to eliminate regularly
    c. Need to be recognized as worthy
    d. Need to be physically and financially secure

68. The elderly patient who is at greatest risk of malnutrition and weight loss is
    a. Mr. Martinez, who eats 90% of each meal.
    b. Miss Kosmacek, who is confused, weak, and needs prompting and assistance at mealtime.
    c. Dr. Shams, who is bedfast but may be up in a chair three times a day for meals.
    d. Mrs. Ling, a 47-year-old patient who feeds herself with her left hand.

69. You may receive a home care assignment
    a. from a private agency that employs you.
    b. because the hospital sends you to a patient's house.
    c. because the doctor refers patients to you.
    d. because you work in assisted living.

70. Which characteristics will be most helpful when working in a private home? Being
    a. a self-starter.
    b. one who needs constant supervision.
    c. rigid in your approach to how things should be done.
    d. critical.

71. Which duties would be part of your responsibilities as a nursing assistant?
    a. Washing windows
    b. Waxing floors
    c. Preparing meals for the client
    d. Moving heavy furniture

72. Which duties would *not* be part of your functions as a nursing assistant?
    a. Making financial decisions for a client
    b. Light housekeeping
    c. Assisting the client in carrying out ADLs
    d. Maintaining a safe environment

73. Sources of danger in the home to be avoided include
    a. allowing clutter to develop.
    b. washing dishes and air-drying them.
    c. using a three-prong plug.
    d. refrigerating leftovers.

74. To help a conscious adult person with an obstructed airway, you should
    a. give the person a drink of water.
    b. begin CPR immediately.
    c. hit the person on the back.
    d. do abdominal thrusts.

75. If you come upon an accident, remember to
    a. speak quickly and excitedly.
    b. allow onlookers to form a protective circle.
    c. keep calm.
    d. take care of the person closest to you first.

76. The national emergency number to call is
    a. 911.   b. 468.   c. 555.   d. 742.

77. The most common cause of airway obstruction is
    a. eating too fast.
    b. ill-fitting dentures.
    c. the tongue falling into the throat.
    d. respiratory arrest.

78. Nursing assistant duties when caring for a pregnant woman in the first trimester would include
    a. checking the level of the fundus.
    b. weighing the patient.
    c. advising the patient about proper diet.
    d. listening for fetal heart sounds.

79. Signs and symptoms in a pregnant woman that must be reported include
    a. blood pressure of 124/68.
    b. vaginal bleeding.
    c. fetal movement.
    d. 3-pound weight gain in 4 weeks.

80. A patient who has received medication to relieve the discomfort of labor and delivery by epidural route will, when returned to the postpartum floor,
    a. be able to move her legs.
    b. not be able to void.
    c. not be able to feel her legs.
    d. not be able to move her toes.

81. The pregnant woman may undergo a cesarean section if the
    a. mother is overdue.
    b. parents want to select the birth date.
    c. membranes are intact.
    d. fetus is in distress.

82. Patients on a subacute care unit may include
    a. patients who require rehabilitation.
    b. women who have just given birth.
    c. patients recovering from the anesthesia of surgery.
    d. patients requiring intensive care.

83. Which of the following represents a major stress factor?
    a. A visit from a grandchild   b. Loss of a spouse
    c. Getting a new job   d. Getting a promotion

84. The person who involuntarily excludes a painful experience from memory is using the defense mechanism of
    a. denial. b. suppression. c. projection. d. repression.

85. A nursing assistant is reprimanded for displaying an uncaring attitude and explains to his coworkers that it is really the patient's fault for being so grouchy. He is using the defense mechanism of
    a. projection.   b. reaction formation.
    c. denial.   d. repression.

86. You best relate to a demanding patient by
    a. telling her she will get care when it is her turn.
    b. trying to establish a personal rapport with her.
    c. ignoring her because all patients get that way sometimes.
    d. being just as demanding as she is.

87. Your patient is constantly by the sink washing his hands. You know he has been found guilty of child abuse. You might think he is using the defense mechanism of
   a. conversion.   b. rationalization.
   c. compensation.   d. undoing.

88. Pathogenic microbes can enter the body through
   a. the hair.   b. unbroken skin.
   c. breaks in the skin. d. broken fingernails.

89. Perineal care means to wash
   a. under the arms.   b. from shoulder to waist.
   c. the genitals and anus.   d. under the breasts.

90. When giving male perineal care,
   a. gloves are not needed.
   b. reposition the foreskin after cleansing the uncircumcised penis.
   c. do not wash the scrotum.
   d. use a large amount of liquid soap.

91. When giving female perineal care, the nursing assistant should
   a. use gloves.
   b. use heavy soap application.
   c. cleanse the vulva from anus toward urethra.
   d. scrub back and forth.

92. A trochanter roll helps prevent
   a. internal hip rotation.   b. foot contractures.
   c. pressure ulcers.   d. lateral hip rotation.

93. After the amputation of an extremity, it is common for the patient to
   a. have hallucinations.   b. be comatose.
   c. experience phantom pain. d. develop pneumonia.

94. When inserting a lubricating suppository, the patient should be
   a. sitting upright.   b. positioned in Sims' position.
   c. sitting on the toilet. d. in the prone position.

95. When using a gait belt, the nursing assistant should
   a. be sure the belt is very tight.
   b. adjust the belt just under the axilla.
   c. be able to slip two fingers between patient and belt.
   d. hold the belt with an overhand grasp.

96. The tympanic thermometer measures temperature of the
   a. ear.   b. oral cavity.   c. rectal cavity.   d. axilla.

97. To help prevent falls in a long-term care facility,
   a. increase noise and activity.
   b. help residents to get up quickly.
   c. encourage residents to use wheelchairs.
   d. use tub or shower chairs.

98. To prevent thermal injuries,
   a. follow procedures accurately.
   b. allow food to get cold before feeding.
   c. post oxygen signs at the nurses' station.
   d. use microwave ovens to heat food.

99. When handling soiled linen in an isolation unit, the nursing assistant should
   a. shake the linen.
   b. put soiled linen on the floor.
   c. fold the dirtiest side outward.
   d. fold the dirtiest side inward.

100. Isolation cover gowns should be
   a. made of moisture-resistant material.
   b. used in airborne precautions.
   c. used routinely in droplet precautions.
   d. used routinely if a patient is coughing.

101. In which situation should the nursing assistant use gloves?
   a. Serving food
   b. Giving an enema
   c. Giving a routine backrub
   d. Carrying out range-of-motion exercises

102. Which of the following applies to immunization?
   a. Vaccines exist for all infectious diseases.
   b. Vaccine is available for hepatitis B.
   c. Vaccine is unavailable for rubella.
   d. Vaccines make people more susceptible to an infection.

103. Which of the following are at greatest risk for infections?
   a. Middle-aged adults
   b. Patients with fractures
   c. Patients with migraine headaches
   d. Those infected with HIV

104. An important way to protect yourself from pathogens is to
   a. keep active and get little sleep.
   b. stay on a calorie-limited diet.
   c. manage stress.
   d. limit fluids to 1,000 mL daily.

105. The patient reports feeling anxious, is dyspneic, cyanotic, and has a feeling of heaviness in his chest. The nursing assistant should
   a. let the patient get up to ambulate.
   b. report immediately to the nurse.
   c. lower the head of the bed.
   d. encourage the patient to take deep breaths.

106. The symptoms of an insulin reaction include
   a. vomiting.   b. dry, flushed skin.
   c. pale, perspiring skin. d. drowsiness.

107. Tuberculosis is often seen today among those who are
   a. janitorial workers.   b. debilitated.
   c. middle-aged.   d. diabetic.

108. When delivering oxygen by nasal cannula, the nursing assistant should
   a. be sure straps are very tight.
   b. check for signs of irritation where prongs touch patient.
   c. clean the cannula every 2 hours.
   d. fill the humidifier every 2 hours.

109. The odometer of the nursing assistant's car read 45061 when leaving one client's home and 45068 on arrival at the second client's home. The total mileage traveled should be recorded as
   a. 3 miles.   b. 5 miles.   c. 6 miles.   d. 7 miles.

110. The basic guidelines for reality orientation include
   a. speaking clearly and directly.
   b. calling patients by pet names.
   c. eliminating clocks and calendars.
   d. speaking loudly so patients will better understand.

111. Validation therapy is a technique that
    a. helps disoriented people feel good about themselves.
    b. denies feelings and memories.
    c. denies people based in reality.
    d. reminds the patient of time and season.
112. When caring for the patient with dementia, the nursing assistant should
    a. use logic to reason with the patient.
    b. keep the environment stimulating.
    c. provide a structured but flexible routine.
    d. avoid eye contact with the patient.
113. A catastrophic reaction may be signaled by
    a. decreased physical activity.
    b. increased talking or mumbling.
    c. excessive thirst.
    d. incontinence.
114. To help decrease "sundowning," the nursing assistant might
    a. feed the evening meal 2 to 3 hours before bedtime.
    b. increase activity before bedtime.
    c. increase the level of caffeine in the diet.
    d. watch a stimulating TV program.
115. When caring for the disoriented patient, the nursing assistant should
    a. speak slowly and clearly.
    b. give two instructions at the same time.
    c. use negative comments to change behavior.
    d. frequently change the routine so it will not be boring.
116. Patients have the right to
    a. play the radio loudly at night.
    b. choose their caregivers.
    c. full information about health care planning.
    d. withhold health information.
117. The validation therapy process is utilized with
    a. psychotic patients.
    b. elderly, disoriented patients.
    c. pediatric patients recovering from surgery.
    d. new mothers.
118. Under OBRA regulations, nursing assistants must
    a. pass a competency test within 4 attempts.
    b. complete a 10-hour course.
    c. complete a 50-hour course.
    d. complete a written and skill test.
119. The Omnibus Budget Reconciliation Act of 1987 is federal legislation which is also called the
    a. Hemodialysis Safety Act.
    b. Nursing Home Reform Act.
    c. Acute Care Facility Act.
    d. Nursing Assistant Registration Act.
120. One way to keep track of wandering residents is to
    a. use a restraint jacket.
    b. apply a sensor around the patient's wrist.
    c. keep the patient in bed.
    d. paint the exit doors bright red.
121. Immobility can cause
    a. pressure ulcers.   b. hunger.
    c. thirst.   d. increased sensory awareness.
122. When restraints *must* be used,
    a. check patients at least every 2 hours.
    b. release the restraints every 4 hours.
    c. keep the patient in a sitting position.
    d. apply restraints according to manufacturer's directions.
123. The nursing assistant can be an effective member of the interdisciplinary team by
    a. socializing with coworkers.
    b. making and reporting observations.
    c. making decisions for patients.
    d. getting to know the doctor.
124. It is important to follow techniques that prevent infection transmission in a long-term care facility, because the elderly
    a. are more susceptible to infection.
    b. have bladders that empty more efficiently.
    c. have a stronger cough reflex.
    d. pay close attention to their diets.
125. The nursing assistant can help prevent infections by helping patients
    a. limit fluid intake.
    b. maintain proper nutrition.
    c. exercise monthly.
    d. dress and undress independently.
126. The risk of a patient falling is increased when
    a. the patient wears glasses.
    b. the environment is well lit.
    c. the patient is disoriented.
    d. the patient is ambulatory.
127. People with Alzheimer's disease may live
    a. only briefly.   b. only one year.
    c. up to 2 years.   d. up to 20 years.
128. Alzheimer's disease is
    a. the least common form of dementia.
    b. a condition that only affects people aged 25 to 35 years.
    c. progressive and cannot be cured.
    d. known to be caused by a virus.
129. Which of the following is sexually transmitted?
    a. Chlamydia   b. Hantavirus
    c. Tuberculosis   d. MRSA
130. When the patient is receiving a tube feeding, the nursing assistant should keep the
    a. head of the bed elevated during the feeding.
    b. patient flat during the feeding.
    c. tubing open between feedings.
    d. feeding flowing readily by using force.
131. The nursing assistant should take which action if the patient is receiving fluids through an infusion pump and the alarm sounds?
    a. Notify the nurse
    b. Call the doctor
    c. Do nothing; the alarms often go off
    d. Stop the infusion
132. The daily calcium requirement for postmenopausal women is
    a. 1,000 mg.   b. 1,200 mg.
    c. 1,500 mg.   d. 2,500 mg.

133. When feeding a patient who has had a stroke,
     a. give no liquids.
     b. direct food toward the unaffected side.
     c. give only thick liquids.
     d. direct food to the affected side.
134. Which of the following foods would be limited in a low-fat diet?
     a. Vegetables and fruits   b. Jam, jellies
     c. Cereal, pasta   d. Butter and margarine

B. True/False. Mark the following true or false by circling T or F.

You have been assigned to a patient who is terminally ill. Questions 135 to 139 apply to this assignment.

135. T F When in the denial stage of grieving, the patient accepts that her death is inevitable.
136. T F The patient who says "You are not really trying to help me" is probably in the stage of anger.
137. T F The patient who is writing her will may have reached the stage of bargaining.
138. T F Patients with a terminal diagnosis move through the process of grieving in an orderly manner, one step at a time.
139. T F The family and staff also move through the same stages of grieving as the patient, but not necessarily at the same rate.

The nurse has asked you to set up sterile supplies and assist with a sterile dressing change of a large wound. Questions 140 to 142 apply to this assignment.

140. T F It is permissible to reach over a sterile field when adding sterile sponges.
141. T F If a sterile towel placed on an unsterile surface becomes wet, it is considered contaminated and must be replaced.
142. T F Always check to see that the color-coded autoclave tape has changed color before considering a package sterile.

You have been asked to prepare an isolation unit. Questions 143 to 146 apply to this assignment.

143. T F Place the proper sign on the door.
144. T F Stock a table or cart just outside the anteroom with isolation gowns.
145. T F Line the wastepaper basket inside the room with a plastic bag.
146. T F Prepare a soiled linen hamper and leave it in the room.
147. T F The infant is able to smile, laugh aloud, and show pleasure at familiar objects by the age of 4 months.
148. T F The 10-month-old infant can usually walk without help.
149. T F Sterile technique is not needed when collecting a sample of urine from a urinary drainage system that has a port.
150. T F The patient with a colostomy may experience problems of leakage, odor control, and irritation around the stoma.

151. T F Hospitalization is particularly traumatic for a child.
152. T F A toddler is safest in a crib with sides and top.
153. T F The teenager is most often hospitalized for accidents, such as sports injuries.
154. T F The disoriented person has impaired judgment, memory, and orientation.
155. T F Disposable gloves should be worn when handling wet, soiled linen.
156. T F All patients are shaved prior to surgery.
157. T F A urinary drainage tube should be coiled on the bed with a straight drop to the drainage bag.
158. T F The patient should be checked every 30 minutes after a lubricating suppository has been inserted.
159. T F An arm with an atrial-venous shunt for dialysis may be used to measure blood pressure.
160. T F Always use a gait belt if a patient has problems with balance, coordination, or strength.
161. T F Spasticity is common in paralyzed limbs.
162. T F All patients should be encouraged to let the nursing assistant complete most of the activities of daily living.
163. T F People who are obese always lack self-control.
164. T F When ambulating a patient, always stand on the patient's strongest side.
165. T F Medications sometimes act as chemical restraints.
166. T F Protection of the disoriented person is the nursing assistant's primary responsibility.
167. T F Sexuality is a characteristic that defines the maleness or femaleness of each person.
168. T F People over 65 have no interest in sexual activity.
169. T F A special sensor may be attached to the leg or wrist to keep track of a wandering patient.
170. T F Reminiscing is a waste of time.
171. T F Medicare is a government program that partially pays for health care for persons over the age of 65 and for those who are permanently disabled.
172. T F Passive range-of-motion exercises are usually carried out by the physical therapist or the registered nurse.
173. T F Obesity negatively affects every body system, increasing the risk for many serious medical conditions.
174. T F Persons with obesity experience discrimination and prejudice in social and employment situations.
175. T F Approximately 1 in 10 American adults is obese.
176. T F Patients who are morbidly obese have a BMI of 29 or higher and are 50 pounds or more over their ideal body weight.
177. T F Many obese patients hyperventilate because of the weight of the chest and the inability of the diaphragm to descend during inhalation.
178. T F The regular hydraulic mechanical lift on your unit can safely move a patient who weighs 678 pounds.
179. T F Bariatric patients require about 1,000 mL to 1,500 mL of oral fluid daily.
180. T F Bedfast bariatric patients need not be turned every 2 hours if a special low air loss bed is used.

C. Matching. I. Choose the correct phrase from Column II to match the words in Column I.

Column I

181. _____ bisexuality   182. _____ homosexuality
183. _____ fomite   184. _____ ombudsman
185. _____ DRG   186. _____ advance directive
187. _____ tympanic   188. _____ DNR
189. _____ care plan   190. _____ power of attorney

Column II

a. diagnosis related group
b. patient advocate
c. sexual attraction to members of both sexes
d. provides direction for giving care and resolving patient problems
e. relates to the eardrum
f. sexual attraction between members of the same sex
g. a contaminated item that can spread infection
h. a document giving one person the legal right to make decisions for another
i. a document signed before diagnosis of a terminal illness permitting a physician to respect a person's wishes regarding dying care
j. means no extraordinary measures should be used to resuscitate a person to prevent death

II.   Match the following phrases and terms.

191. _____ atelectasis   192. _____ rales
193. _____ dyspnea   194. _____ prosthesis
195. _____ hypochondriasis 196. _____ dementia
197. _____ receptive aphasia 198. _____ gait belt
199. _____ Hemovac drain 200. _____ expressive aphasia

a. difficult breathing
b. an artificial body part
c. transfer belt
d. inability to understand communication
e. closed drainage system
f. magnification of physical ailments
g. collapsed lung tissue
h. gurgles heard in the chest
i. set of symptoms affecting thinking, judgment, memory, and ability to reason
j. inability to properly form thoughts or express them coherently

III. Match the following phrases and terms.

201. _____ solid wastes
202. _____ abnormal shortening of muscle fibers
203. _____ intravenous infusions
204. _____ armpit area
205. _____ external reproductive organs
206. _____ intake and output
207. _____ area around nail beds
208. _____ an item that can be thrown away
209. _____ artificial teeth
210. _____ nutrient that provides energy

a. disposable   b. genitalia   c. carbohydrate   d. contracture
e. dentures   f. minerals   g. feces   h. I/O
i. IV   j. axilla   k. cuticle

IV. Match the following phrases and terms.

211. _____ poisons produced by microbes
212. _____ bacteria that grow in clusters
213. _____ procedures used to prevent germs from spreading
214. _____ one-celled microbes that cause malaria and diarrhea
215. _____ disease-producing microbes
216. _____ machine used to sterilize equipment
217. _____ organism that grows best in the absence of oxygen
218. _____ rod-shaped microbes
219. _____ damage-resistant forms of bacteria

a. anaerobe   b. spores   c. autoclave
d. aerobes   e. staphylococci f. medical asepsis
g. pathogens   h. bacteria   i. toxins
j. protozoa   k. bacilli

V. Match the following terms and definitions.

220. _____ language impairment
221. _____ used to listen to body sounds
222. _____ used to provide continuous, constant temperature
223. _____ cancer of the blood
224. _____ used to determine blood pressure

a. aphasia   b. sphygmomanometer
c. leukemia   d. stethoscope
e. Aquamatic K-Pad

D. Completion.

225. Complete the chart by listing observations related to each system:

System	Significant observations
a. Integumentary	_____
b. Musculoskeletal	_____
c. Circulatory	_____
d. Respiratory	_____
e. Nervous	_____
f. Urinary	_____
g. Digestive	_____

226. List 10 negative effects of immobility.

a. _____
b. _____
c. _____
d. _____
e. _____
f. _____
g. _____
h. _____
i. _____
j. _____

227. List four ways the nursing assistant can help relieve patient frustration.

a. _____

b. _____

c. _____

d. _____

228. List three basic steps to learning.

a. _____

b. _____

c. _____

229. List the steps in the nursing process and explain two actions a nursing assistant does to support the process.

Steps	Nursing assistant actions
a. _____	_____
	_____
b. _____	_____
	_____
c. _____	_____
	_____
d. _____	_____
	_____

230. Describe the attitude a nursing assistant should display.

_____

_____

_____

_____

231. List three articles usually carried in a home health assistant's kit.

a. _____

b. _____

c. _____

232. List three characteristics of each stage of Alzheimer's disease.

Stage	Characteristics
I	a. _____
	b. _____
	c. _____
II	d. _____
	e. _____
	f. _____
III	g. _____
	h. _____
	i. _____

233. Explain the relationship of the acronym RACE and fire control by indicating what each letter represents.

a. R _____

b. A _____

c. C _____

d. E _____

E. Yes/No. In each of the following situations, indicate if you believe the action taken by the nursing assistant was proper by circling a for Yes or b for No.

234. a b Because she felt tired in the morning, the nursing assistant did not take time to remove the bright red nail polish she had worn to a party last night before reporting to duty.

235. a b A nursing assistant overheard the social worker talking about a patient's dwindling financial reserves. He shared this information with coworkers at coffee break.

236. a b The patient being cared for is very irritable with the nursing assistant. The nursing assistant's response is, "We've all got problems."

237. a b The patient is receiving an intravenous feeding and the needle site looks red and swollen. The nursing assistant reports this fact immediately to the nurse.

238. a b The postsurgical patient's blood pressure has dropped from 118/80 to 98/50. The nursing assistant believes that this is all right because the patient is just back from surgery. The information is recorded but not reported.

239. a b The nursing assistant notices that a postural support seems too tight on a patient who is not part of her assignment. She feels that because this is someone else's patient, she can safely ignore the situation.

240. a b A nursing assistant makes it a routine part of the care he gives to offer water each time he contacts a patient, unless otherwise prohibited by the patient's condition or orders.

241. a b The nursing assistant observes another nursing assistant handling a patient in a rough manner. Because the other nursing assistant is her friend, she says nothing.

242. a b The nursing assistant learns that her patient had an abortion two years ago. Because the nursing assistant strongly disapproves of abortion, she visits this patient less often than her other patients.

243. a b The nursing assistant notices that a wheel on a patient's walker is loose but, because this is not his patient, does not report the observation to the nurse.

244. a b The patient is 12 years old and small in stature. The nursing assistant measures the patient's blood pressure with an adult blood pressure cuff.

245. a b The nursing assistant knows that her patient has tested positive for HIV but has not told his wife. Although the assistant sees the patient's wife daily, she makes no mention of this information to the wife.

246. a b The patient complains about a "heaviness" in her chest, but the nursing assistant overheard someone say that this patient is a hypochondriac, so she does not feel it is necessary to report the complaint to the nurse.

247. a b The disoriented patient believes that she is in school and that the nurse is her teacher. The patient becomes very agitated when the nursing assistant, trying to orient her to reality, argues with her.

ANSWER KEY FOR COMPREHENSIVE FINAL EVALUATION

A. Multiple Choice

1. c	2. c	3. a	4. b	5. a
6. d	7. b	8. c	9. d	10. a
11. c	12. b	13. d	14. b	15. a
16. d	17. b	18. c	19. a	20. d
21. a	22. b	23. b	24. a	25. c
26. a	27. b	28. c	29. d	30. a
31. d	32. c	33. a	34. a	35. c
36. d	37. d	38. c	39. c	40. b
41. d	42. b	43. c	44. d	45. c
46. a	47. b	48. d	49. b	50. a
51. c	52. d	53. b	54. c	55. a
56. b	57. a	58. d	59. a	60. b
61. c	62. b	63. c	64. d	65. c
66. a	67. b	68. b	69. a	70. a
71. c	72. a	73. a	74. d	75. c
76. a	77. c	78. b	79. b	80. a
81. d	82. a	83. b	84. d	85. a
86. b	87. c	88. c	89. c	90. b
91. a	92. d	93. c	94. b	95. c
96. a	97. d	98. a	99. d	100. a
101. b	102. b	103. d	104. c	105. b
106. c	107. b	108. b	109. d	110. a
111. a	112. c	113. b	114. a	115. a
116. c	117. b	118. d	119. b	120. b
121. a	122. d	123. b	124. a	125. b
126. c	127. d	128. c	129. a	130. a
131. a	132. c	133. b	134. d	

B. True/False

135. F	136. T	137. F	138. F	139. T
140. F	141. T	142. T	143. T	144. F
145. T	146. T	147. T	148. F	149. F
150. T	151. T	152. T	153. T	154. T
155. T	156. F	157. T	158. F	159. F
160. T	161. T	162. F	163. F	164. F
165. T	166. T	167. T	168. F	169. T
170. F	171. T	172. F	173. T	174. T
175. F	176. F	177. T	178. F	179. F
180. F				

C. Matching

I.

181. c	182. f	183. g	184. b	185. a
186. i	187. e	188. j	189. d	190. h

II.

191. g	192. h	193. a	194. b	195. f
196. i	197. d	198. c	199. e	200. j

III.

201. g	202. d	203. i	204. j	205. b
206. h	207. k	208. a	209. e	210. c

IV.

211. i	212. e	213. f	214. j	215. g
216. c	217. a	218. k	219. b	

V.

220. a	221. d	222. e	223. c	224. b

D. Completion

225. a. color, temperature, flexibility, dryness, clarity, moisture, areas of redness, scars, rashes, other abnormalities
  b. deformities; ability to walk, move, and sit; posture; twitching
  c. skin color, heart rate, character of pulse, blood pressure, color of nails and lower extremities, chest pain
  d. difficulty breathing, cyanosis, shortness of breath, noisy respirations, cough, nature and quantity of mucus
  e. orientation to time, place, and person; response to questions; condition of eyes and ears; level of consciousness; convulsions; dizziness; irritability
  f. frequency, amount, and character of urine; hematuria; dysuria; nocturia; distention
  g. appetite, tolerance to food, elimination problems, difficulty chewing or swallowing, nausea, vomiting, bleeding, pain

226. a. respiratory problems   b. contractures
  c. atrophy   d. congestion
  e. pressure ulcers   f. slow healing
  g. infection   h. loss of movement
  i. pneumonia   j. sensory deprivation

227. a. provide opportunities for patients to make choices
  b. provide patients with communication aids
  c. allow patient ample time to express himself or herself
  d. learn and appreciate underlying factors causing patient reactions

228. a. active listening   b. effective studying
  c. careful practicing

229. a. Assessment:
  • observe carefully
  • measure vital signs accurately
  • report findings to nurse
  • document if permitted
  b. Planning:
  • be informed of and follow plan
  • participate in planning conference
  • clarify the assignment
  c. Implementation:
  • carry out assignments correctly
  • be willing to cooperate and help other team members

d. Evaluation:
- report observations
- participate in team conferences
- review new care plans

230. courtesy, tact, cooperation, emotional control, sympathy, empathy, competence, positive, friendliness, honesty, integrity

231. a. plastic apron
b. disposable gloves
c. observational equipment, such as thermometer, stethoscope, and so forth

232. I. anxiety, depression, agitation, disorientation, poor judgment, poor concentration, delusions of persecution

II. short-term memory loss, more severe, perseveration phenomena, complete disorientation, poor sensory perception

III. totally dependent, may have seizures, verbally unresponsive

233. a. R = remove patient
b. A = activate alarm
c. C = contain fire
d. E = extinguish fire

E. Proper Actions

234. b 235. b 236. b 237. a 238. b
239. b 240. a 241. b 242. b 243. b
244. b 245. a 246. b 247. b

PART 4   Answers to Student Workbook Activities

Study Skills

Vocabulary Exercise
1. listening with personal involvement
2. questions and learning activities
3. making sense of what is being heard
4. stated expected outcomes
5. listing of words and their meanings

Completion
1. learning
2. listening, studying, practicing
3. interfere
4. effectively
5. glossary
6. Follow the maze.

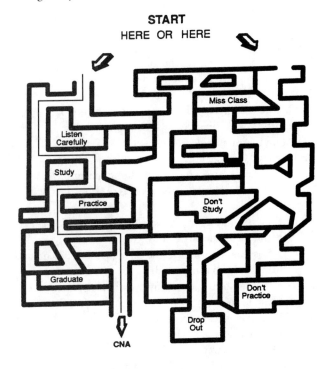

7. a. schematic lines   b. using numbers and letters
8. a.
I. Case History
   a. 8½ months pregnant   b. 3 young children
   c. Prenatal care clinic patient
II. Problems
   a. Fatigue   b. Pain   c. Abnormal clinical readings
   1. elevated BP 140/100
   2. elevated temperature 103°F
   3. swollen fingers and hands

III. Resolution
   a. Examination and evaluation
      1. nursing assistant
      2. registered nurse
      3. physician
   b. Admission to hospital
      1. treatment with antibiotics
      2. delivery of baby
      3. arrange child care
   b.

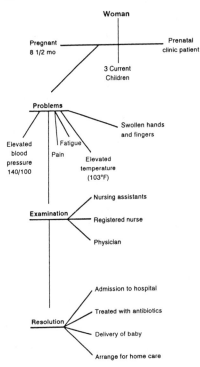

SECTION 1 INTRODUCTION TO NURSING ASSISTING
UNIT 1 Community Health Care

Vocabulary Exercise
1. A place in which health care is given.
2. Care provided to people who are dying.
3. Person receiving health care in a hospital.
4. Relating to children; health care of children.
5. People who live in a common area and share common health needs.

63

Completion

1. a. Provide services for the ill and injured.
    b. Prevention of disease.
    c. Promote individual and community health.
    d. Education of health care workers.
    e. Promote research in medicine and nursing.
2. Each patient is a unique individual and has different needs. Attention must be given to the physical, mental, and emotional needs of the patient.
3. people living longer and more advanced technology.
4. patient.
5. hospitals, long-term care facilities, hospices, urgent care facilities, surgicenters, outpatient clinics, psychiatric hospitals, physician offices, long-term acute care hospitals, subacute care facilities, transitional care facilities.
6. a. patient   b. resident   c. client
7. a. Prepare and dispense medications
    b. Care for patients with medical conditions such as diabetes or heart disease
    c. Diagnose and treat disease with X-rays and other imaging techniques
    d. Care of children
    e. Assist patients to regain mobility skills
8. a. Preparation of food and nutritional education for patients
    b. Cleanliness of facility
    c. Environmental concerns: plumbing, heating, electricity, repairs
    d. Patient billing, employee payroll, all financial concerns
9. a. Deliver mail and flowers   b. Run the gift shop
    c. Direct visitors   d. Raise funds for the facility
10. insurance, Medicare, Medicaid
11. establish the Medicare payment rate
12. review and evaluate the facility to ensure that acceptable standards of practice are maintained
13. protects the health and safety of employees

Word Search

1. a. Care of dying patients
    b. Period after childbirth
    c. Period in pregnancy from conception to labor
    d. Study of disease

e. A place where health care is given
f. A review and evaluation to ensure that facilities are maintaining acceptable standards of practice
g. Assisting an ill or injured person to attain his or her optimal level of function
h. A written notice that informs the facility of violations found by the survey agency
i. Long-term, unlikely to go away
j. The person who receives care in the hospital

UNIT 2 Role of the Nursing Assistant

Vocabulary Exercise

1. Behavior that reflects our experiences and feelings
2. Total mental, emotional, and sometimes physical exhaustion
3. Consisting of RNs, LPNs, LVNs, and nursing assistants, provides nursing care
4. Skills the nursing assistant is legally permitted to perform by state regulation
5. Assists with the care of patients under the direction and supervision of an LPN or RN
6. A method of providing care that involves pairing a registered nurse or primary nurse with a nursing assistant or other team member

Completion

1. a. honest   b. dependable
    c. accurate   d. respects coworkers
2. a. LPN, LVN   b. RN   c. Nursing assistant
3. Defines who gives assignments, who each employee reports to, who supervises which workers. It is a communication tool.
4. Discuss it with the nurse.
5. a. One nurse cares for a patient during the hospital stay—that nurse does assessments, plans the care, does patient teaching.
    b. Each person on team is assigned a specific task, such as baths, medications, or treatments.
    c. RN is team leader, plans the care, gives assignments and instructions to team members.
6. a. Limit number of people involved in the patient's care.
    b. Contain costs.
    c. Meet the patient's needs efficiently.
7. a. Dependable.   b. Honest.   c. Caring.
8. a. Daily bath/shower.
    b. Use deodorant; mouth care; hair care.
    c. Wear clean clothes daily.
9. Jewelry is unsafe because it carries microorganisms; it may get caught on equipment; a confused patient may grab the jewelry, causing injury.
10. A name pin and watch are considered part of the uniform. Other permissible jewelry items are a wedding ring and small, non-dangling earrings.
11. safety of patients
12. a. Fear of diagnosis, disfigurement, disability, death
    b. Pain
    c. Unrealistic perceptions of activities

d. Uncertainty about future, worries about family, loss of social support systems, dependence on others, financial concerns.

13. Mental, emotional, physical, social, spiritual

14. a. Remember each person has a specific role to fulfill and a job to do.
   b. Do not overstep authority or criticize others.
   c. Listen and understand instructions.
   d. Remember the tone of your voice and body language.
   e. Carry out orders promptly, report tasks that cannot be completed, help others, accept help when needed, be cheerful, have positive attitude, extend dignity and courtesy to all, keep the common goal in mind.

15. a. negative   b. positive   c. negative
   d. negative   e. negative   f. negative
   g. positive   h. negative   i. positive

16. The work is physically and emotionally demanding. To reduce stress, get adequate rest and nutrition, take time out—sit with feet up, take deep breaths, take warm baths, listen to music, exercise, drink a cup of tea, have a hobby, join a stress reduction program.

17. a. Multiskilled worker—health care provider who is trained to perform specific procedures from several different disciplines, such as health care assisting, phlebotomy, ECG, and respiratory care.
   b. Cross-training—the training required to enable the multiskilled worker to perform procedures from several different health care disciplines.

18. Refer to text Figure 2-4.

Matching

1. i   2. h   3. j   4. b   5. a
6. c   7. f   8. e   9. d   10. g

UNIT 3 Consumer Rights and Responsibilities in Health Care

Vocabulary Exercise

1. Patients' Bill of Rights   2. Clients' Rights
3. Residents' Rights   4. advance directives

Completion

1. federal   2. Patients' Bill of Rights
3. Clients' Rights   4. responsibility
5. honestly   6. past, medications
7. will not   8. accept
9. clarification   10. financial

True/False

1. T   2. F   3. F   4. F   5. T
6. T   7. F   8. T   9. T   10. F
11. T   12. T   13. F   14. T   15. T
16. F   17. F   18. T

Identification

1. I   2. I   3. C   4. I   5. I
6. I   7. C   8. C   9. I   10. C
11. C   12. C   13. I   14. C   15. I
16. C   17. C   18. I

UNIT 4 Ethical and Legal Issues Affecting the Nursing Assistant

Vocabulary Exercises

1. Keeping patient information private
2. Intentionally touching another person or threatening to do so
3. Carelessness
4. Making abusive threats or statements, calling names, using inappropriate language
5. Making a false, verbal statement
6. Failure to exercise the degree of care considered reasonable under the circumstances, resulting in an unintended injury to a patient
7. Failure to give care that is expected or required

Completion

1. moral
2. a. When is life gone for the patient on life support?
   b. How much should be done to extend the life of a patient who is terminally ill?
   c. When does human life begin?
   d. Questions regarding abortion, euthanasia, animals in research, organ transplants, use of marijuana for medical purposes
3. Stay within the scope of practice, do procedures in the manner you were taught and are qualified to do, avoid shortcuts, keep skills current, make sure you understand directions and request guidance if necessary, keep patient safety in mind, adhere to facility policies, stay within OBRA guidelines, attend in-services, protect patients from harm, respect patients' belongings; avoid negligence, theft, defamation, false imprisonment, assault and battery, abuse, and invasion of privacy
4. Tactfully refuse and kindly tell the patient that patients are not expected to tip.
5. Aiding and abetting
6. Refer her to the nurse.
7. cannot be removed by the patient, restricts movement, and does not allow the patient access to his or her own body.
8. nonaccidental
9. involuntary seclusion
10. Do unto others as you would have them do unto you.
11. Treat others the way they want to be treated.

True/False

1. F   2. T   3. T   4. T   5. T
6. T   7. T   8. F   9. T

Complete the Chart

1. sexual abuse   2. verbal abuse
3. verbal abuse   4. verbal abuse
5. physical abuse   6. psychological abuse
7. psychological abuse   8. psychological abuse
9. sexual abuse   10. physical abuse
11. psychological abuse   12. physical abuse
13. psychological abuse   14. sexual abuse
15. physical abuse   16. psychological abuse
17. psychological abuse   18. sexual abuse

SECTION 2 SCIENTIFIC PRINCIPLES
UNIT 5 Medical Terminology and Body Organization

Vocabulary Exercise
1. Word part added to the beginning of a word to change or add to its meaning
2. Word part added to the end of a word to change or add to its meaning
3. Shortened form of a word
4. Vowel added to end of word root
5. Foundation of a medical word

Completion
1. Medical dictionary
2. a. adenoma   tumor of gland
   b. colectomy   surgical removal of colon
   c. craniotomy   surgical opening of skull
   d. dentist   person licensed to practice dentistry
   e. hysterectomy   surgical removal of uterus
   f. myalgia   muscle pain
   g. nephrolithiasis   kidney stone (renal calculus)
   h. pneumonectomy   surgical removal of lung
   i. thoracotomy   surgical opening of chest
   j. urinometer   instrument used to measure specific gravity of urine
3. a. asepsis   without
   b. bradycardia   slow
   c. dysuria   difficult
   d. hypertension   above, excessive
   e. hypotension   low, deficient
   f. pandemic   all
   g. polyuria   many
   h. gerontology   aged
   i. premenstrual   before
   j. tachycardia   rapid
4. a. appendectomy   surgical removal
   b. hepatitis   inflammation of
   c. electrocardiogram recording of
   d. anemia   blood
   e. tracheotomy   surgical opening
   f. hematology   study of
   g. hemiplegia   paralysis
   h. apnea   breathing
   i. otoscope   instrument to examine body opening
   j. proctoscopy   diagnostic test to examine body part
5. a. adenitis   inflammation of gland
   b. cardiopathy   disease of heart
   c. leukopenia   lack of white blood cells
   d. arthroscope   instrument to examine a joint
   e. cytomegaly   enlarged cell
6. a. glucosuria   b. gynecologist   c. phlebotomy
   d. tracheotomy   e. fibroma   f. pancytopenia
   g. bradycardia   h. hypertension   i. pneumonectomy
   j. substernal
7. a. blood clot
   b. infection due to pus-producing microorganisms
   c. inflammation of lung

d. inflammation of urinary bladder
e. inflammation of breast
8. a. abdomen   b. blood   c. gastrointestinal
   d. axillary   e. genitourinary f. vaginal
   g. shoulder

Matching
1. e   2. k   3. h   4. a   5. b
6. j   7. c   8. i   9. g   10. d

Abbreviations
1. a. walk as desired
   b. take urine specimen to laboratory as soon as possible
   c. bed rest only
   d. check dressing frequently
   e. out of bed daily
   f. elevate head of bed 45 degrees
   g. discontinue clear liquid diet
   h. soap-solution enema as needed
   i. complete blood count in morning
   j. nothing by mouth before surgery
2. a. central supply   b. eyes, ears, nose, throat
   c. physical therapy   d. intensive cardiac care unit
   e. emergency department   f. post anesthesia recovery
   g. pediatrics   h. delivery room
   i. operating room   j. laboratory
3. a. ac   b. bid   c. AM   d. TID   e. pc
   f. STAT   g. qid   h. WA   i. qh   j. noc
4. a. one half   b. milliliter   c. pound
   d. kilogram   e. liter
5. a. I   b. XII   c. VI   d. IX   e. IV

Completion
1. a. adenitis—inflammation of a gland
   b. asepsis—free from germs, infection
   c. hypertension—high blood pressure
   d. bradycardia—slow heartbeat
   e. adenoma—glandular tumor
2. tissues, organs
3. a. epithelial—secretes, absorbs, forms covering
   b. connective—connects body parts and supports body parts
   c. nervous—carries messages, regulates body functions
   d. muscle—forms walls of organs, moves body parts
4. anterior—front   inferior—below   lateral—side
   medial—middle   posterior—back   superior—above
5. a. anterior   b. posterior   c. anterior   d. posterior
   e. anterior   f. superior   g. inferior   h. superior
   i. inferior   j. medial
6. front, ventral   7. back, dorsal
8. a. right iliac region (RLQ)
   b. umbilical region (UMB region)
   c. right hypochondriac region (RUQ)
   d. left iliac region (LLQ)

Matching
1. a   2. g   3. h   4. j   5. j
6. h   7. e   8. a   9. b   10. e
11. c   12. b   13. h   14. i   15. f
16. j   17. e   18. b   19. a   20. g

UNIT 6 Classification of Disease

Vocabulary Exercise

1. diagnosis   2. antibodies   3. signs   4. congenital
5. trauma   6. neoplasm   7. therapy
8. Any change from a healthy state.
9. Cause of condition, illness, or abnormality.

Matching

1. e	2. c	3. b	4. c	5. g
6. i	7. d	8. a or h	9. a	10. c
11. c	12. b	13. a	14. a	15. c
16. a	17. b	18. b	19. a	20. a
21. a	22. a	23. b	24. b	25. b

Completion

1. a. Lack of blood clotting factors—genetic
   b. Blood disease—genetic
   c. Club feet—congenital
   d. Imperfections in upper lip and palate formation—congenital
   e. Lack of functioning kidney—congenital
2. a,b: genetic   c,d,e: congenital
3. a. Downward displacement of kidney
   b. Stones in gallbladder
   c. Stones in kidney
   d. Blood clot in brain
4. obstruction
5. a. Diabetes   b. Malnutrition   c. Edema   d. Scurvy
6. tumor, gland
7. a. Diarrhea and/or constipation
   b. Nausea and/or vomiting
   c. Blood in stools
   d. Loss of weight
   e. Anxiety
   f. Pain
8. a. Unbroken skin   b. Mucus and cilia
   c. Acidity of body secretions   d. White blood cells
   e. Inflammation, immune response
9. a. Surgery   b. Chemotherapy
   c. Radiation   d. Supportive care

Clinical Situation

1. Tell Ms. Simmons she should see a physician as soon as possible.
2. a. brain   b. cerebral—relating to the cerebrum thrombus—blood clot

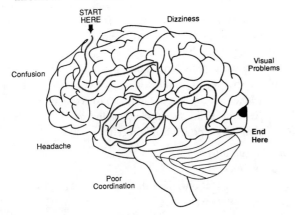

SECTION 3 BASIC HUMAN NEEDS AND COMMUNICATION

UNIT 7 Communication Skills

Vocabulary Exercise

1. symbols   2. disorientation
3. verbal communication   4. aphasia
5. shift report   6. body language
7. sign language   8. nonverbal communication
9. memo   10. communication

Completion

1. a. Describes policies and benefits for employees
   b. Contains procedures to follow in case of fire, flood, tornado, or other disasters
   c. Contains directions on how to perform all procedures
   d. Contains policies for nursing staff that pertain to the care of patients
   e. Each person knows what he or she is expected to accomplish during the shift—what his or her specific responsibilities are.
2. a. New rules and regulations   b. New procedures
   c. Health findings from recent research
   d. How to use new equipment
3. a. Sender   b. Receiver   c. Message   d. Feedback
4. a. Posture   b. Hand and body movement
   c. Activity level   d. Facial expression
   e. Overall appearance   f. Body position
5. a. Use nonthreatening words, gestures.
   b. Speak clearly and cautiously.
   c. Have patient's attention.
   d. Use pleasant tone of voice.
   e. Use appropriate body language.
      Also be alert to patient's needs, do not interrupt, reflect the patient's feelings and thoughts, ask for clarification, give only factual information, do not argue.
6. a. Name of patient   b. Room number
   c. Important information about patient
7. a. Posture   b. Hand and body movement
   c. Activity level   d. Facial expression
   e. Overall appearance   f. Body position
8. a. tone   b. loudness (volume)   c. articulate
   d. double   e. slang
9. a. anger   b. caring   c. sadness   d. happiness
10. a. see   b. hearing   c. cover   d. clearly   e. hand
11. a. objects b. lightly c. specific d. identify e. talking
12. a. one   b. substitutes   c. patronizing
    d. lengthy   e. clues
13. See text Figure 7-5d
    a. Staff Nurses   b. Nursing Assistants
    c. Nurse Manager   d. Staff Nurses
    e. Patient Care Technicians   f. Nursing Assistants
    g. Staff Nurses   h. Nursing Assistants
    i. Unit Secretaries   j. Unit Secreteries
14. See text Figure 7-3
15. To: Mr. Burke
    Date: Nov. 11
    Time: 10:00 AM

From: Father Duchene of St. Gregory's Catholic Church
Phone: 683-4972
Telephoned: (check)
Please Call: (check)
Message: Asked how Mrs. Riley was feeling.
Signed: your name

Yes or No
1. N   2. N   3. Y   4. N   5. N
6. N   7. N   8. N   9. N   10. Y

Clinical Situations
1. a. No.   b. Good morning.   c. Hurt, pain, ache, sore.
2. a. Unable to speak and/or understand written or spoken
      language; due to a stroke or brain attack.
   b. Tell him you can try again later.
   c. No.
   d. picture books, communication boards

UNIT 8 Observation, Reporting, and Documentation

Vocabulary Exercise
1. assessment   2. charting   3. process
4. graphic   5. observation   6. communication
7. Kardex   8. evaluation

Completion
1. a. Assessment   collect information about patient
   b. Planning   identify possible solutions to
                       problems, develop approaches,
                       establish goals
   c. Implementation   carry out approaches on care
   d. Evaluation   plan determine whether goals are
                       being met
2. a. Nursing diagnosis b. Approaches c. Goals, outcomes
3. the patient's problems and their etiology (causes)
4. a. actual clinical problems
   b. cause of the problem(s)
   c. risk factors for certain problems to develop
   d. wellness objectives
5. nursing care to achieve outcomes for which nurses
   are accountable.
6. other members of the interdisciplinary health care team
7. patient's medical record (chart)
8. a. Who is to carry out the approach
   b. When the approach is to be carried out
   c. How the approach is to be carried out
9. how, correctly
10. evaluation
11. the approach cannot be carried out and when the patient
    is having problems with the approach
12. a. patient's expected course of treatment
    b. expected outcomes for a DRG
13. help the patient achieve the goal

Differentiation
1. symptom   2. sign   3. symptom   4. symptom
5. symptom   6. sign   7. sign   8. sign
9. symptom   10. sign

Matching
1. c   2. d   3. b   4. b   5. a
6. a   7. d   8. a   9. a and/or d 10. a and b
11. c   12. e   13. a   14. a   15. b
16. b   17. f   18. e   19. j   20. b
21. g   22. g   23. i   24. e   25. g

Multiple Choice
1. c   2. a   3. b   4. b   5. d
6. b   7. a   8. b   9. c   10. a

Matching
1. f   2. g   3. d   4. e   5. h

Completion
1. completely   2. color   3. entry   4. sequence
5. clearly   6. spell   7. blank   8. patient
9. title   10. error

Short Answer
1. See text Figure 8-1.

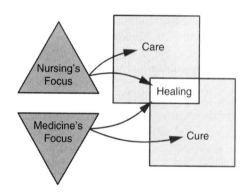

Nursing diagnosis describes the patient's response to the illness. Medical diagnosis identifies and describes the illness.

2. [Any combination of these answers is acceptable]
   - Don't be afraid of computerized charting.
   - When documenting on a specific patient, double-check to make sure you have entered the correct identification code.
   - Do not give your identification code or password to others.
   - Access only information you are authorized to obtain.
   - Document only in areas you are authorized to use.
   - Read and follow the directions for the onscreen expert reminders or error codes.
   - Know and follow facility policies for late entry and addendum documentation.
   - Stay current and attend continuing education programs to learn how to maximize the utility of computerized charting and information systems.
3. identifiable health information
4. a. Increase patient control over personal medical records
   b. Restrict the use and disclosure of patient information
   c. Make facilities accountable for protecting patient data
   d. Require facilities to implement and monitor information release policies and procedures

Clinical Situations
1. three times
2. Needs items set out, needs instruction and hand-over-hand assistance

3. Needs a shower chair, help getting into and out of shower chair, lock wheels of shower chair.
4. Communication deficits.
5. a. Paralysis on right side (right hemiplegia).
   b. Changes in circulation of blood in brain.
6. No. His hearing is not impaired; he has had brain damage that altered his ability to communicate.
7. a. Picture books   b. Gestures

UNIT 9 Meeting Basic Human Needs

Vocabulary Exercise

1. neonate—birth to one month of age; newborn infant
2. preadolescence—years between the ages of 12 and 14
3. continuum—continuous related series of events or actions
4. growth—physical changes that take place in the body during development
5. development—gradual growth
6. intimacy—feelings of closeness and familiarity
7. reflex—activity performed without conscious thought
8. sexuality—maleness or femaleness of an individual

Matching

1. a. A   b. A   c. A   d. I   e. A   f. A
2. a. 3   b. 1   c. 2   d. 4

Completion

1. tasks   2. smaller   3. 300
4. a. Independence and personal decision making
   b. Choosing a mate and establishing family life
   c. Establishing a career
   d. Optimal health
   e. Choice of friends to form support group
5. caring for both parents and children, grandchildren
6. gradual losses

Short Answer

1. Result of going through the eight stages of development.
2. Needs are on a continuum and a hierarchy in which physical needs must be met before higher-level needs become important.
3. a. Serve food at proper temperature.
   b. Avoid unpleasant odors.
   c. Remove unneeded equipment from dining area.
   d. Consider cultural preferences.
   e. Prepare patients—offer tray in pleasant manner, assist if necessary.

Clinical Situations

1. Patient is fearful—relay request to nurse.
2. Patient's self-esteem and feelings of sexuality may be affected. Remain calm and treat patient courteously. Discuss situation with nurse for guidance.
3. Patient may have unmet physical needs; check if she is hungry, thirsty, has pain or discomfort, or needs to use the bathroom. Meet needs accordingly. Offer to give backrub to help patient relax.
4. Patient wants solitude—knock on door, ask if you may enter and offer the nourishment.
5. Tell her you do not know anything about it.

6. Remain calm and professional. Say, "Please do not touch me." If behavior continues, discuss with nurse.

Relating to the Nursing Process

1. Implementation   2. Assessment
3. Assessment   4. Implementation

Unit 10 Comfort, Pain, Rest, and Sleep

Vocabulary Exercise

1. bruxism   2. sleep   3. apnea
4. narcolepsy   5. somnambulism   6. insomnia
7. REM   8. deprivation   9. rest
10. enuresis   11. hypersomnia   12. NREM
13. comfort

```
    B R U X I S M
            L         A
            E         P
  N A R C O L E P S Y N
            O         E
      I N S O M N I A
    R       N
    D E P R I V A T I O N
    M       M         R
            B         E
        E N U R E S I S
            L         T
            I
    H Y P E R S O M N I A
            M         R
                      E
              C O M F O R T
```

Short Answer

1. [Any combination of these answers is acceptable]
   - pain
   - thirst
   - illness
   - noise
   - ventilation
   - physical discomfort
   - caffeine intake
   - some foods and beverages
   - hunger
   - need to eliminate
   - exercise
   - temperature
   - light intensity
   - some medications
   - alcohol, drugs
   - lifestyle changes
   - anxiety, stress, fear, worry, emotional problems
   - changes in the environment, unfamiliar environment
   - treatments and therapies
   - staff providing routine care
2. [Any combination of these answers is acceptable]
   - verbal complaints of pain, describing the pain in the patient's exact words
   - nonverbal signs and symptoms of pain in patients who have difficulty communicating, such as facial expressions, grimacing, moaning, refusing to move, stiff, rigid, or limited movements, crying, yelling, or screaming
   - vital signs
   - skin color

- location of pain (specific site of pain on the body)
- radiation, if any (movement of pain to other areas)
- time of onset (when the pain began)
- duration (how long the pain lasts)
- frequency (how often it occurs)
- pain quality (nature and type of pain)
- pain intensity (strength and description of pain, in the patient's own words)
- aggravating and alleviating factors (things that improve or worsen the pain)
- character (properties, features, characteristics)
- variation or patterns of pain (changes in pain or cycles of pain)
- pain management history, if any (things the patient tells you about past history of pain and things that make it better or worse)
- present pain management regimen, if any, and its effectiveness (things the patient does to relieve pain, including response to comfort measures and medications)
- effect to pain upon activities of daily living, sleep, appetite, relationships, emotions, concentration, etc.
- direct observation of abnormalities at the site of the pain
- nausea or vomiting
- side effects of analgesic (pain-relieving) medications, if applicable
- response to pain medications and other forms of treatment, if applicable
- rating from pain scale, if patient has verbalized this information

3. Cultural beliefs affect the patient's outward response to pain. People from some cultures are very emotional when they are in pain. Others are very stoic. Some think that showing pain is a sign of weakness, whereas others believe that pain is a punishment from their higher power.

4. [Any combination of answers *not* noted in question 1 is acceptable]
   - pain
   - thirst
   - illness
   - noise
   - ventilation
   - physical discomfort
   - caffeine intake
   - some foods and beverages
   - hunger
   - need to eliminate
   - exercise
   - temperature
   - light intensity
   - some medications
   - alcohol, drugs
   - lifestyle changes.
   - anxiety, stress, fear, worry, emotional problems
   - changes in the environment, unfamiliar environment
   - treatments and therapies
   - staff providing routine care

5. It is a tool for communication that helps the patient accurately describe the pain.

6. The patient's self-rating of pain intensity is more accurate than anyone else's. Using a pain scale prevents subjective opinions, provides consistency between workers who are rating the pain, and eliminates some barriers to pain management.

7. The patient will wake up feeling rested and refreshed if he or she had had enough REM sleep. REM sleep restores mental function.

8. a. Pain that occurs suddenly and without warning. It is usually the result of tissue damage, caused by conditions such as injury or surgery. Acute pain decreases over time, as healing takes place.
   b. Pain that moves from the site of origin to other areas.
   c. Pain that may be caused by any one of many medical conditions. The pain lasts longer than six months, and may be intermittent or constant.
   d. Pain that occurs as a result of an amputation. The patient complains of pain in the body part that has been removed. The pain is real, not imaginary.

9. Recognize that the patient is still in severe pain. Inform the nurse right away.

True/False

1. F	2. F	3. T	4. T	5. F
6. T	7. T	8. F	9. T	10. T
11. F	12. T	13. F	14. T	15. F
16. F	17. T	18. F	19. T	20. F
21. T	22. F	23. T	24. T	

Relating to the Nursing Process

1. [Any combination of these answers is acceptable]
   - telling patients what you plan to do and how you will do it
   - providing privacy
   - assisting the patient to assume a comfortable position
   - repositioning the patient for comfort to relieve pain and muscle spasms
   - changing the angle of the bed to relieve tension on surgical sites or injured areas
   - avoiding sudden, jerking movements when moving or positioning the patient
   - performing passive range-of-motion exercises to reduce stiffness and maintain mobility
   - using pillows to support the affected body part(s)
   - providing extra pillows and blankets for comfort and support
   - straightening the bed and linen
   - giving a backrub
   - washing the patient's face and hands
   - providing a cool, damp washcloth for the patient's forehead
   - providing oral hygiene
   - providing fresh water, food, or beverages as permitted
   - playing soft music to distract the patient
   - listening to patient's concerns
   - providing emotional support
   - maintaining a comfortable environmental temperature
   - providing a quiet, dark environment
   - eliminating sources of unpleasant sights, sounds, and odors from the environment
   - waiting at least 30 minutes after the nurse administers pain medication before moving the patient, performing procedures or activities

- timing patient care to coincide with pain medication
- following the individual directions on the care plan
- applying warm or cold applications, if directed by the nurse

Developing Greater Insight

1. a. Yes. The patient's self-report of pain should be respected and accepted. Response to pain differs with individuals and in various cultures. The patient's response to pain should not be judged because of facial expression or body language.
   b. Remove the tray from the room. Provide nursing comfort measures to eliminate the pain. Tell the patient to call when she is ready to eat. Inform the nurse of the pain promptly. Check on Mrs. Hernandez after the medication is given. Offer the tray again 30 to 60 minutes after the patient has been medicated. (Follow facility policy for saving the tray on the unit and reheating it versus obtaining another tray from the dietary department.)
   c. If the tray is not available on the unit, find other items in the unit refrigerator or pantry to make a balanced meal. If they are not available on your unit, consult the nurse. He or she can ask the supervisor to get some food from dietary, or obtain food from another unit.
   d. These things make the patient uncomfortable. The discomfort causes the patient to be unable to sleep. When the room is quiet, he or she may be upset or anxious because of the discomfort.
   e. Use nursing comfort measures listed on the care plan that are most likely to work, such as applying heat or cold (if ordered), giving a backrub, repositioning the patient, changing the angle of the bed, or using pillows or props for support.

UNIT 11 Developing Cultural Sensitivity

Vocabulary Exercise

1. Stereotypes   2. Talismans   3. Ethnicity   4. Amulet
5. Sensitivity   6. Race   7. Mores

Short Answer

1. a. Caucasians   b. African Americans
   c. Hispanics   d. Asian/Pacific
   e. Native Americans f. Middle Easterners/Arabs
2. Recognizes individual within an ethnic and cultural group and provides nursing care that assures cultural as well as individual acceptance and comfort.
3. The longer a group is associated with the American culture, the less its members rely on the cultural values and traditions of the country of origin.
4. Skin color, bone structure, facial features, hair texture, blood type
5. Heritage, national origin, social customs, language
6. a. Family organization
   b. Personal space needs
   c. Communication
   d. Beliefs about health, illness, and health care practices
   e. Religions, traditions

7. a. Nature and cause of illness
   b. Types of health care practices
   c. Their relationship to a higher power
8. a. Protestantism   b. Roman Catholicism   c. Judaism
   d. Islam   e. Hinduism

True/False

1. T   2. F   3. T   4. F   5. F   6. T
7. T   8. T   9. T   10. T   11. T

Relating to the Nursing Process

1. Assessment   2. Implementation
3. Implementation   4. Implementation

Developing Greater Insight

1. a. Asian-Pacific
   b. Body has two energy forces, yin and yang
   c. Consider caring for him a duty and privilege
   d. Buddha
   e. It is disrespectful.
   f. Even though people of the same race and from the same culture may have many similar characteristics, each person is an individual with a unique personality.
2. a. See if an interpreter is available. Use body language, gestures, facial expression, pictures.
   b. Bible, medals, rosary, crucifix
   c. Holy Communion
   d. Blood, phlegm, black bile, yellow bile

SECTION 4 INFECTION AND INFECTION CONTROL

UNIT 12 Infection

Vocabulary Exercise

1. vaccine   2. yeast   3. colony   4. host
5. toxins   6. pathogens   7. antibiotics   8. hepatitis
9. carrier   10. fomites   11. bacilli

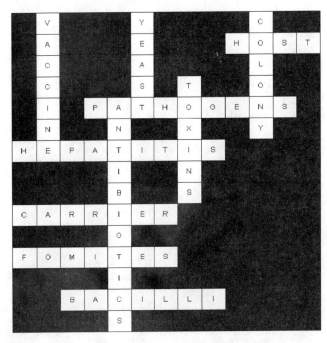

Matching

1. d	2. g	3. a	4. j	5. c
6. h	7. f	8. b	9. k	10. i
11. a	12. a	13. d	14. a	15. b
16. b	17. a	18. b	19. a	20. e

Completion

1. a. Skin   b. Tears   c. Coughing   d. Sneezing
2. a. Fever   b. Phagocytes
   c. Inflammation   d. Immune response
3. harbors a pathogen without having symptoms or being sick
4. a. Nose b. Mouth c. Vagina d. Penis e. Rectum
5. a. Nose   b. Mouth   c. Vagina   d. Penis
   e. Rectum   f. Urethra   g. Open skin or wound
6. type of pathogen
7. a. Visitors   b. Patients   c. Employees
8. a. Airborne transmission   b. Droplet transmission
   c. Contact transmission
9. a. Causative agent   b. Reservoir
   c. Portal of exit   d. Portal of entry
   e. Mode of transmission   f. Susceptible host
10. a. Malaise   b. Chills   c. Fever
    d. Muscle aches and pains   e. Cough
11. a. Hepatitis A   b. Hepatitis B   c. Hepatitis C
12. Hepatitis is readily transmitted by individuals who may have no signs and symptoms of illness. Several types of hepatitis cannot be eliminated from the body.
13. Liver
14. The liver detoxifies food and medications taken into the body. Liver failure will cause death and the only treatment for extensive damage is a transplant.
15. a. *Staphylococcus aureus*   b. enterococci

True/False

1. T	2. F	3. F	4. T	5. F
6. T	7. F	8. T	9. T	10. F
11. T	12. F	13. T	14. F	15. T
16. F	17. F	18. T	19. F	20. T
21. T	22. F	23. F	24. F	25. T
26. T	27. F	28. F	29. T	30. F
31. F	32. T	33. F	34. F	35. T
36. T	37. T			

Clinical Situations

1. a. F   b. F   c. T   d. F   e. T
   f. T   g. F   h. T   i. T
2. a. General poor health
   b. Underweight and probably malnourished
   c. Chronic illness: emphysema and congestive heart failure
3. a. adequate   b. less   c. empty
   d. front, back   e. catheter   f. urine
4. a. Susceptible host   b. Method of transmission
   c. Portal of exit   d. Source
5. infection will not occur
6. [Any combination of these answers is acceptable, as is an answer of any item that contacts secretions or excretions of the affected patient]
   - bedpans
   - soiled linens
   - environmental surfaces
   - urinals
   - laboratory specimens
   - equipment

Relating to the Nursing Process

1. Assessment   2. Implementation   3. Assessment

Developing Greater Insight

1. d   2. e   3. b   4. c   5. a
6. a. hepatitis B, influenza, measles, mumps, rubella, *Varicella zoster*
   b. [depends on vaccine]
   c. They stimulate the immune system to recognize and form antibodies to the virus, so that protective antibodies will already exist in the body when (if) exposure occurs.
   d. Yes

UNIT 13 Infection Control

Vocabulary Exercise

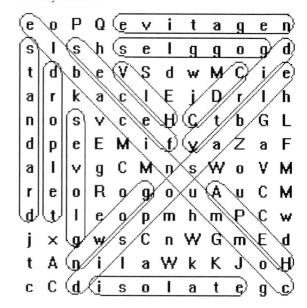

1. droplet   2. CDC   3. communicable   4. gloves
5. disposable   6. isolate   7. feces   8. goggles
9. HEPA   10. HIV   11. negative   12. dirty
13. standard   14. gown

True/False

1. T	2. F	3. F	4. F	5. F
6. F	7. T	8. T	9. F	10. F
11. F	12. F	13. T	14. F	15. T
16. T	17. F	18. F	19. T	20. F
21. F	22. F			

Completion

1. to prevent the spread of disease
2. three
3. all staff
4. prevent transmission of microorganisms
5. blood, body fluids, secretions, excretions, mucous membranes, or nonintact skin
6. nose and mouth
7. fit
8. with the outside of the gown inward
9. once

10. a. Nasal drainage   b. Saliva   c. Urine
    d. Feces   e. Blood   f. Vaginal secretions
    g. Seminal fluid   h. Vomitus   i. Wound drainage
11. cleansing, a dressing
12. They must be cleaned and disinfected.

Short Answer

1. Standard precautions
2. a. Airborne   b. Droplet   c. Contact
3. a. Droplet   b. Airborne   c. Contact
4. a. mask
   b. gown
   c. goggles or face shield
   d. gloves
   e. hazardous waste plastic bags
   f. plastic bags for soiled linen
5. a. Gown   b. Mask
   c. Goggles or face shield   d. Gloves
6. a. Handle linen as little as possible.
   b. Fold dirty linen inward.
   c. Do not shake.
   d. Do not place on floor, table, furniture.
   e. Bag soiled linen before leaving room.
   f. Keep soiled linen separate from clean linen.
   g. Transport in leakproof bag.
7. a. Should remain in room with patient.
   b. Clean and disinfect according to hospital policy.
8. Flush down toilet (except bones).
9. Biohazard bag
10. a. Autoclave   b. Gas
11. [Any of these answers is acceptable]
    • Cover the nose/mouth when coughing or sneezing.
    • Use tissues to contain respiratory secretions.
    • Dispose of tissues in the nearest waste receptacle after use.
    • Perform hand hygiene after contact with respiratory secretions and contaminated objects/materials.
12. a. ultraviolet-C , room, air duct
    b. inactivate or kill pathogens
    c. no
    d. no
13. gown, gloves, and disposable NIOSH-approved respirator
14. a face shield or goggles (eye protection)
15. yes
16. at the doorway to the patient room, or in the anteroom, if used
17. after leaving the patient's room and closing the door
18. The respirator should be discarded.

Clinical Situations

1. Put on HEPA mask.
2. Clean it in the room, put it in a biohazard bag, disinfect or sterilize before using with another patient.

Identification

1. a. Wear mask and goggles.   b. Handwashing.
   c. Gloves.   d. Gown.
   e. Proper disposal of sharps.

2. a. anteroom   b. bedroom   c. bathroom

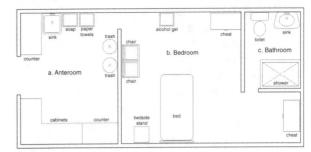

3. a. Linen against body.
   b. Hold linen away from body.
   c. Shaking linen.
   d. Do not shake linen; unfold after centering sheet.
4. a. Drawer and door open.
      Bedpan on top shelf.
      Toothbrush on bottom shelf with urinal.
   b. Place toothbrush in drawer, away from brush and comb.
      Place bedpan on bottom shelf.
      Close drawer and door.
5. Should not reach across sterile field.

Relating to the Nursing Process

1. Implementation   2. Implementation

SECTION 5 SAFETY AND MOBILITY

UNIT 14 Environmental and Nursing Assistant Safety

Vocabulary Exercise

1. incident   2. rails   3. ward
4. private   5. ergonomics   6. concurrent
7. semiprivate   8. environmental

Completion

1. all health care   2. concern
3. locked   4. 71
5. screens, curtains   6. indirect
7. shut off   8. electrical
9. ungloved hands   10. incident
11. tagged   12. checked
13. grounded   14. never
15. available to the patient   16. heat, fuel, oxygen
17. right away, supervisor   18. oils, alcohol, nail polish remover
19. upright   20. calm
21. patients   22. work-related
23. OSHA   24. MSDS

Short Answer

1. a. temperature   b. air circulation
   c. light   d. cleanliness
   e. noise control   f. walls, ceilings, floor
   g. plumbing   h. electricity
   i. equipment and furniture
2. a. fire extinguisher   b. fire hose
3. a. Pull   b. Aim   c. Squeeze   d. Sweep

4. a. Use correct body mechanics
   b. Raise beds to comfortable height
   c. Use mechanical lift
   d. Use back supports
   e. Get help
   f. Use carts for heavy objects
5. a. What precautions to take
   b. Hazard instruction for safe use
   c. Location of information, first aid measures, and how to clean up and dispose of
   d. How to read and understand labels and hazard signs
   e. Type of PPE
   f. How to manage spills
6. [Any combination of these answers is acceptable]
   - Provide support and a handle for the patient to use for turning and repositioning in bed.
   - Provide a handle for getting into and out of bed.
   - Give the patient a feeling of security.
   - Reduce the risk of falling out of bed when the patient is being transported from one location to another in bed.
   - Provide access to bed and television controls that are part of the bed rail design.
7. [Any combination of these answers is acceptable]
   - Entrapment (strangulation, suffocation, bodily injury or death when the patient or part of the patient's body become entrapped between the bars of the side rails or between the side rails and the mattress)
   - Serious injuries if the patient climbs over the rails and falls from this height
   - Skin tears, bruises, cuts, scrapes
   - Agitation, caused by a feeling of being trapped or caged in
   - Feelings of isolation or restriction
   - Sadness because of loss of independence, having to call for help
   - Actual loss of independence, such as ability to get up to use the bathroom, or retrieve an item dropped on the floor
8. [Any combination of these answers is acceptable]
   - Participate in continuing education programs to learn how to recognize and manage escalating agitation, assaultive behavior, or criminal intent.
   - Attend classes on cultural diversity that offer sensitivity training on racial and ethnic issues and differences.
   - If you are responsible for a secured area, control access to the area and keep it locked. Avoid propping locked doors and windows open. Never disable a door alarm.
   - Do not leave keys unattended. Never share security alarm codes with unauthorized persons.
   - Close shades or curtains at night.
   - Report assaults or threats of assaults to the nurse manager immediately.
   - Avoid wearing scarves, necklaces, earrings, and other jewelry that could cause injury to yourself if a patient or other individual attacks you.
   - Do not carry valuables or large sums of cash to work.
   - Avoid remote, dark areas when you are alone.

- Report lights that are burned out and locks that do not work.
- Exercise caution in elevators, stairwells, and unfamiliar areas. Immediately leave the area if you believe a hazard exists.
- Use the buddy system if personal safety may be threatened.
- If a patient or other person is acting out, or you believe you may be assaulted, do not let the person come between you and the exit.
- Keep your head up, look ahead, and be aware of your surroundings.
- If your facility has security personnel, request that they escort you in dark or potentially dangerous areas. If no security personnel are on duty, ask other staff members to accompany you.
- Park in well-lighted areas. Always lock your car when parking. Look in the car before getting in, then lock the doors. Don't roll windows down to speak with individuals approaching your car.
- Report suspicious individuals or other potential safety hazards to the proper person. Never approach a suspicious person by yourself.

9. [Any combination of these answers is acceptable]
   - Remain calm and avoid raising your voice, which may further agitate the perpetrator.
   - Speak slowly, softly, and clearly.
   - Call for help, if possible, or send someone to get help.
   - Move away from heavy or sharp objects that may be used as weapons.
   - Monitor your body language and avoid movements that could be challenging, such as placing your hands on your hips, moving toward the perpetrator, pointing your finger, or staring directly at the person. However, focus your attention on the person so you know what he or she is doing at all times.
   - Position yourself at right angles to the perpertrator. Avoid standing directly in front of him or her. Maintain a distance of 3 to 6 feet.
   - Position yourself so that an exit is accessible. Never let the perpetrator come between you and the exit.
   - Avoid making sudden movements.
   - Listen to what the person is saying. Encourage the person to talk and communicate that you care and will genuinely try to help. Acknowledge that you understand that he or she is upset. Break big problems into smaller, manageable ones.
   - Avoid arguing and defensive statements. Accept criticism in a positive way. If you sincerely feel that criticism is unwarranted, ask clarifying questions.
   - Ask the person to leave and return when more calm.
   - Ask questions to help regain control of the conversation.
   - Avoid challenging, bargaining, or making promises you cannot keep.
   - Describe the consequences of abusive behavior.
   - Avoid touching an angry person.

- If a weapon is involved, ask the person to place it in a neutral location while you continue talking. Avoid trying to disarm the person, which may put you in danger.

10.

Hidden Picture

1. crutches against wall—one without tip
2. spill on floor
3. bed wheels out, bed crank out
4. looped drainage tubing
5. drainage bag attached to side rails with drainage tubing touching floor
6. bed up to high horizontal height, side rails down
7. patient smoking while oxygen in use; no oxygen warning sign posted
8. frayed wire
9. broken wall socket
10. overloaded plug
11. excess equipment in room
12. unnecessary clutter on overbed table
13. footstool

Relating to the Nursing Process

1. Planning   2. Planning

UNIT 15 Patient Safety and Positioning

Vocabulary Exercise

1. spasms   2. orthoses   3. restraint   4. mobility
5. contracture   6. supine   7. procedure   8. splint

Completion

1. wash hands, identify the patient
2. alone
3. turning sheet
4. behind the patient's back
5. opposite side rail is up and secure
6. face
7. two hours
8. horizontal, abdomen
9. chemical, physical
10. exercised
11. falls, poisonings, thermal

True/False

1. T   2. F   3. F   4. F   5. T
6. F   7. T   8. T   9. F   10. F

Short Answer

1. Back muscles are small and easily strained.
2. It helps the patient feel more comfortable, it relieves strain and helps the body function more efficiently, it prevents deformities and complications like pressure ulcers.

3. Document behavior indicating need. Document alternative actions. Consult with family. Obtain permission from family as legal guardian. These actions all protect the patient's rights.

Name the Position

1. Prone   2. Lateral   3. Semi-Fowler's

Clinical Situations

1. a. Answer call signal immediately
   b. Check patient often
   c. Care for personal needs promptly
   d. Report mental and physical changes immediately
   e. Maintain a safe, quiet environment
   f. Provide comfortable chairs and supportive devices if needed
2. a. wrist, arm, ankle, leg   b. vest
   c. jacket   d. hand mitts
   e. geriatric chair   f. side rails, wheelchair safety belt
3. a. Get help
   b. Use turning sheet
   c. Change position frequently
4. a. Ensure that patient sits upright with head slightly flexed
   b. Feed slowly
   c. Offer liquids between solids
   d. Cut food into small pieces
   e. Place food in unaffected side of mouth
   f. Use thickeners for liquids
   g. Give oral care after feeding
   h. Know how to perform the Heimlich maneuver

UNIT 16 The Patient's Mobility: Transfer Skills

Vocabulary Exercise

1. dependent   2. full weight-   3. partial weight-
4. paralyzed   5. gait   6. pivot

Completion

1. help
2. weight
3. raised or removed
4. shoulders, hips
5. Three nursing assistants are on the far side of bed: one assistant is at head of bed to protect patient's head, neck, shoulders; one is in the middle to guide patient's trunk and hips; one is at foot of bed to guide patient's feet and legs. One nursing assistant is by side of stretcher to guide the transfer.

Corrections

1. [correct]   2. Never   3. gait belt
4. [correct]   5. strongest   6. nonslip soles
7. not acceptable 8. [correct]   9. [correct]
10. low horizontal 11. [correct]
12. the surface to which he is being transferred
13. [correct]

True/False

1. T   2. F   3. F   4. F   5. T
6. F   7. T   8. T   9. T   10. F

Clinical Situations

1. Stay with patient; do not leave patient alone.
2. Get assistance.
3. Position stretcher parallel to bed and slightly higher. Lock bed and stretcher wheels. Position one person beside stretcher and the other person on the opposite side of the bed.
4. Do not use.
5. Be available to offer assistance. Encourage use of hand rails.

Identification

[Any combination of these answers is acceptable for 1 through 4]

1. • Use strong leg muscles, do not bend from waist
   • Do not place hands under patient's armpits
   • Use transfer belt
   • front wheel improperly positioned
   • chair brakes not locked.
2. • Do not allow patient to put arms around nursing assistant's neck
   • Lock wheelchair
   • Use transfer belt
   • front wheel improperly positioned
   • chair brakes not locked.
3. • Use transfer belt
   • Lock wheelchair
   • Should have hands on transfer belt
   • front wheel improperly positioned
4. • Use transfer belt
   • Support patient's knee with nursing assistant's knee
   • Have patient place hands on bed
   • front wheel improperly positioned
   • chair brakes not locked
   • patient should not have hands on assistant's body

Relating to the Nursing Process

1. Implementation
2. Assessment
3. Implementation
4. Implementation

UNIT 17 The Patient's Mobility: Ambulation

Vocabulary Exercise

1. ambulate—to walk
2. assistive device—item that makes walking easier and safer
3. orthopedic—relating to bones and muscles
4. prosthesis—artificial body part
5. gait—the way a person walks

Completion

1. ambulation
2. heel, ball
3. swinging
4. joint
5. need
6. rails
7. affected
8. spills
9. unsafe
10. 90
11. shoes
12. arms
13. strong
14. 4
15. 90

True/False

1. F
2. T
3. T
4. F
5. F
6. T
7. F
8. F
9. T
10. T

Short Answer

1. a. stroke
   b. multiple sclerosis
   c. Huntington's disease
   d. Parkinson's disease
   e. arthritis
   f. amputation
2. a. tolerance to movement in bed, ability to move in bed
   b. ability to participate in active exercise
   c. ability to safely transfer with minimal assistance
   d. ability to stand, bear weight
   e. strength, endurance, balance
   f. clear mental status
   g. ability to walk alone, need for ambulation assistance
3. a. crutches   b. cane   c. walker
4. Crutches are cumbersome, require two strong arms and adequate balance.
5. Takes pressure off the ischia.
6. [Any combination of these answers is acceptable]
   • Make sure that the side rails are up and safety belts are fastened.
   • Push the stretcher from the head end.
   • Approach corners slowly and look before you go around them.
   • Approach swinging doors with caution. Prop the door open to propel the stretcher through the door. If this is not possible, back through swinging doors.
   • When entering an elevator, push the stop button to lock the doors open. Walk backward, pulling the head end in.
   • Stand by the patient's head while the elevator is in motion. When the elevator stops, push the stop button to lock the door open. Push the stretcher out so the feet exit the elevator first. (If the threshold is uneven, go to the foot end of the stretcher and pull it out of the elevator.) After the stretcher is safely out of the elevator, unlock the door mechanism.
   • Walk backward down ramps or inclines, looking over your shoulder to make sure that the path is clear.
   • When parking a stretcher, avoid blocking a doorway.
   • Never leave a patient unattended and unsupervised on a stretcher.

Clinical Situations

1. Do not use walker—report to proper person.
2. Help to closest chair—call for help.
3. Inform nurse, instruct—walker should be moved 8 to 12 inches and weight should be on strong leg as walker is moved forward.

Identification

1. A

Relating to the Nursing Process

1. Implementation
2. Evaluation
3. Implementation
4. Implementation

SECTION 6 MEASURING AND RECORDING VITAL SIGNS, HEIGHT, AND WEIGHT

UNIT 18 Body Temperature

Vocabulary Exercise

1. the center of the body
2. skin—outer surface of body

3. part of electronic thermometer that is inserted into body opening
4. membrane (eardrum) in ear where temperature can be taken
5. temperature, pulse, respiration, blood pressure

Completion
1. temperature
2. a. pulse   b. respirations   c. blood pressure
3. a. illness   b. environmental temperature
   c. medications   d. age
   e. infection   f. time of day
   g. exercise   h. emotions, pregnancy, menstrual cycle
4. 1 to 3 degrees   5. less   6. probe
7. cover or sheath   8. It is discarded.   9. liquid
10. one degree   11. two-tenths of a degree
12. a. Hold at eye level.
    b. Locate solid column of liquid.
    c. Read at point at which liquid ends.
13. closest line
14. a. Fahrenheit   b. Celsius
15. Wait 15 minutes.
16. a. Wipe it with a tissue.
    b. Check to be sure it is intact.
    c. Shake it down.
    d. Cover with a sheath (glass and digital thermometers), or probe cover (all other types of thermometers).
17. a. Temperature registers much more quickly
    b. Easier to take
    c. Can be used when oral temperature cannot be taken
18. a. oral   b. rectal   c. rectal   d. oral
    e. rectal   f. oral   g. rectal   h. rectal
    i. oral   j. rectal
19. a. axilla   b. groin   c. ear
20. a. 3 minutes   b. 3 minutes   c. 10 minutes
    d. few seconds   e. 20 to 60 seconds
21. a. F 98.6   b. F 100   c. C 37   d. F 101.2
    e. C 38.2   f. F 104   g. F 99.4   h. C 37.8
    i. F 98   j. C 38
22. a. electronic   b. glass oral   c. glass rectal   d. tympanic

True/False
1. T   2. F   3. T   4. F   5. F
6. T   7. F   8. T   9. F   10. T

Clinical Situations
1. Report to supervisor. Take temperature.
2. Get the sheaths; do not use probe without them.

Relating to the Nursing Process
1. Implementation   2. Assessment   3. Implementation
4. Assessment   5. Assessment

UNIT 19 Pulse and Respiration

Vocabulary Exercise
1. apical   2. cyanosis   3. pulse   4. dyspnea
5. apnea   6. tachypnea   7. rhythm   8. bradycardia

Completion
1. pressure, artery   2. arteries, skin, bone
3. carotid   4. rhythm, volume

5. dorsalis pedis
6. a. temporal   b. carotid   c. brachial
   d. radial   e. femoral   f. popliteal
   g. dorsalis pedis
7. 60, 100
8. a. illness   b. emotions
   c. age   d. exercise
   e. elevated temperature   f. sex
   g. adrenaline   h. position
   i. physical exercise   j. medications
9. high   10. second hand
11. fingertips   12. one full minute

True/False
1. F   2. F   3. T   4. T   5. F
6. T   7. F   8. T   9. F   10. F

Clinical Situations
1. Report findings to nurse.
2. Take an apical pulse.
3. 84 + 24 = 108 apical pulse (A108/84 = pulse deficit 24)
4. a. 120 − 104 = 16 (A120/R104 = 16 pulse deficit)
   b. 118 − 88 = 30 (A118/R88 = 30 pulse deficit)
   c. 92 − 50 = 42 (A92/R50 = 42 pulse deficit)
   d. 102 − 68 = 34 (A102/R68 = 34 pulse deficit)
   e. 98 − 76 = 22 (A98/R76 = 22 pulse deficit)

Relating to the Nursing Process
1. Assessment   2. Implementation   3. Assessment
4. Planning   5. Assessment

UNIT 20 Blood Pressure

Vocabulary Exercise
1. H   2. hypotension   3. depressants
4. palpated   5. brachial   6. elasticity
7. aneroid   8. sphygmomanometer   9. fasting
10. diastolic   11. stethoscope   12. stimulants

Completion
1. a. volume of blood   b. force of heartbeat
   c. condition of arteries   d. distance from heart
2. a. exercise or pain   b. eating, obesity
   c. sex of patient   d. stimulants or diseases of arteries
   e. emotional stress
3. a. rest   b. shock   c. depressants
   d. weight loss   e. fasting
4. 80% the diameter
5. a. mercury gravity   b. electronic   c. aneroid
6. hypertension   7. pulse pressure
8. paralyzed, infusion, injured   9. auscultatory gap
10. 10 mm   11. 2 mm
12. 1 to 1-1/2 inches   13. brachial artery
14. a. unable to hear it
    b. pressure higher than previous reading
    c. pressure lower than previous reading
15. one minute
16. a. stethoscope tubing   b. bell
    c. diaphragm   d. earpieces
    e. cuff   f. gauge
    g. bulb   h. pressure control valve

17. a. 90   b. 134   c. 168   d. 116
    e. 56   f. 80   g. 92   h. 68

True/False

1. F   2. F   3. T   4. T   5. F   6. T
7. T   8. T   9. T   10. F   11. T   12. F

Relating to the Nursing Process

1. Assessment   2. Planning   3. Assessment

Developing Greater Insight

1. Heart is contracting

UNIT 21 Measuring Height and Weight

Vocabulary Exercise

1. inch   2. height   3. calibrated
4. increments   5. kilogram   6. pounds
7. balance   8. scale

Completion

1. a. wheelchair   b. upright   c. bed
2. same   3. clothing   4. scale   5. empty
6. tape measure   7. paper towel   8. metric, kilograms

Reading Weights and Heights

1. 94 lb   2. 164 lb   3. 140 lb
4. 222 lb   5. 5 feet, 1 inch   6. 5 feet, 7 inches
7. 5 feet   8. 5 feet, 4 inches

True/False

1. T   2. F   3. T   4. F   5. T

Relating to the Nursing Process

1. Assessment   2. Assessment

SECTION 7 PATIENT CARE AND COMFORT MEASURES

UNIT 22 Admission, Transfer, and Discharge

Vocabulary Exercise

1. admission—procedure carried out when patient first arrives at facility
2. transfer—move patient from one nursing unit to another

3. discharge—procedures carried out when patient leaves facility
4. baseline—initial
5. assessment—evaluation

Completion

1. patient, family   2. checking the identification band
3. listed   4. meals
5. calm   6. unattended (alone)
7. comfortable, safe   8. physician's discharge order
9. observations   10. responsibility
11. documentation   12. discharge instructions
13. containing costs

Short Answer

1. a. water pitcher   b. glass   c. soap dish   d. soap
   e. basin   f. lotion   g. mouthwash
2. a. Have equipment and materials ready
   b. Be observant
   c. Document carefully and accurately
   d. Report observations
   e. Pay attention to details of each procedure
   f. Keep emotional factors in mind
   g. Be courteous
3. a. Is there a need for special equipment?
   b. What method of transportation is being used?
   c. Are there any special instructions?

Clinical Situations

1. Inform supervisor at once.
2. Return to unit; strip bed and dispose of linen.
3. Show them where to wait, let them know how long they will have to wait, tell them about the availability of coffee, answer questions about chapel activities, telephones, visiting hours, let them know when they can return.
4. Gather equipment for urine specimen, vital signs, admission kit, height and weight measurements, pad and pencil, patient's chart.

Relating to the Nursing Process

1. Implementation   2. Assessment   3. Assessment
4. Implementation   5. Implementation

UNIT 23 Bedmaking

Vocabulary Exercise

1. Stryker—special bed frame for turning patients
2. gatch—bed fitted with jointed knee and back rests that must be raised and lowered manually by means of the gatch handle
3. box pleats—special folds placed in bedding to secure blankets
4. mitered—one type of corner used to make bed
5. fanfold—procedure for folding sheet on top covers
6. side rails—metal bars on sides of beds to prevent patient from falling
7. sheet—linen used to make a bed

True/False

1. T   2. F   3. F   4. F   5. T   6. F
7. T   8. T   9. T   10. F   11. T   12. T
13. T   14. F   15. T   16. F   17. T   18. T

Identification

1. mitered
2. a. gatch bed
   b. center—raises and lowers horizontal height of bed
   c. right—raises and lowers foot of bed
   d. left—raises and lowers head of bed
3. a. low bed   b. protective floor mat
4. a. toe pleat
   b. To prevent pulling and pressure on feet to reduce the risk of skin breakdown, reduce discomfort, and reduce the risk of contractures

Short Answer

1. To conserve energy and save steps
2. Shaking sheets spreads germs
3. Open end of pillowcase facing away from door
4. To make the patient feel welcome and make it easier for the patient to get in
5. To make it easier to transfer patient from stretcher to bed
6. Provide privacy
7. Bed in lowest horizontal height and side rails up
8. Over the foot of the bed
9. After the unit is cleaned following patient discharge
10. To keep bed stationary
11. a. common   b. easier   c. confined
    d. Closed   e. out of bed   f. fanfolded

Clinical Situations

1. Lower bed before you leave.
2. Ask for assistance; be sure you are able to operate bed safely before attempting to give care.
3. A special unit that supports the body evenly, through which air is circulated, to reduce pressure.
4. Put it in the soiled linen hamper.
5. The low bed is used for patients who are confused and at risk for climbing out of a higher bed, sustaining a potentially serious injury. The patient is less likely to be injured if he or she falls from the low bed.
6. The mat on the floor is to further reduce the risk of injury if the patient falls from the bed.
7. Nursing assistants use special postural techniques called good body mechanics to prevent musculoskeletal injuries. When these techniques are used, you bend from the hips and knees, not the waist, so you are not bending over when making the bed. Squatting or kneeling on the floor mat further reduces the risk of injury. When making the bed, organize everything needed in advance, and place them within reach. Remove several pieces of linen at a time instead of all at once to further reduce the risk of injury of lifting too much weight while in an awkward position. Making one side of the bed at a time and using a fitted bottom sheet also make the job easier.
8. The electric bed is used to reduce the risk of injury to the workers from bending over to care for the patient or make the bed.
9. The height of the bed is too high for the patient to get in and out safely. The bed is lowered to prevent injury to the patient.

10. Although it would be easier to put the linen on the floor, this violates infection control principles and risks spreading infection. It is also a potential trip hazard for patients and staff.
11. The half sheet is used to help move the patient to the head of the bed and turn him or her from side to side. Pulling on the sheet is more comfortable for the patient and easier and safer for staff.
12. It is not undoing the bedmaking task. The linen is clean and tucked in tightly, which will be more comfortable for the patient. Fanfolding the linen to the foot of bed makes it easier for the patient to get in bed and covered up when he or she returns.

Relating to the Nursing Process

1. Implementation   2. Implementation
3. Implementation   4. Planning

UNIT 24 Patient Bathing

Vocabulary Exercise

1. cuticle   2. axillae   3. genitalia
4. midriff   5. pubic

Completion

1. relaxed, refreshed   2. hair, nails
3. axillae, genitals   4. 105
5. call signal   6. clean
7. towel, midriff   8. bath blanket
9. pulling the curtain   10. bedpan
11. bath blanket   12. eyes
13. inside, outside   14. breasts
15. wash basin and water   16. lotion
17. straight, fingertips   18. penis, scrotum
19. massage   20. 20
21. corns   22. massage, fingertips
23. washcloth   24. towel

Short Answer

1. a. removal of dirt and perspiration
   b. increased circulation
   c. mild form of exercise
2. a. remain with patient
   b. leave bathroom door unlocked
   c. check on patient every 5 minutes
3. a. is receiving oxygen   b. has drainage tubes
   c. is receiving an IV
4. a. Remove gloves.
   b. Reposition the patient to ensure he or she is comfortable and in good body alignment.
   c. Replace the bed covers, then remove any drapes used. Place used drapes in plastic bag to discard in trash or soiled linen.
   d. Elevate the side rails, if used, before leaving the bedside.
   e. Remove other personal protective equipment, if worn, and discard in plastic bag or according to facility policy.
   f. Wash your hands or use an alcohol-based hand cleaner.
   g. Return the bed to the lowest horizontal position.
   h. Open the privacy and window curtains.

i. Position the call signal and needed personal items within reach.
j. Wash your hands or use an alcohol-based hand cleaner.
k. Remove procedural trash and contaminated linen when you leave the room. Discard in appropriate container or location, according to facility policy.
l. Inform visitors that they may return to the room.
m. Document the procedure, your observations, and the patient's response.

5. a. Loosen gown at neck
b. Remove free arm
c. Gather gown carefully and slip sleeve down over infusion site
d. With free hand, lift IV from pole and hold at same level
e. Slip gown over IV container, do not lower container
f. Return IV container to pole

6. Wrap cloth around one hand; bring free-hanging end up over palm and tuck in the end.

7. [Any combination of these answers is acceptable]
• Faster and more economical; bath takes approximately 8 to 10 minutes
• Less fatiguing for patient
• Conserves moisture, reduces drying, and is gentler to skin than soaps
• Less friction, because the cloths are softer than regular washcloths and towels, and drying is eliminated

8. To protect self-esteem and increase circulation through exercise.
9. The nursing assistant must complete the bath for the patient.
10. oral hygiene, hair care, backrub, range-of-motion exercises
11. a. improves circulation   b. provides warmth
    c. comfort   d. cleansing
12. a. nonskid strips in tub   b. use good body mechanics
    c. check safety aids   d. encourage use of hand rails
    e. never leave patient alone f. assist in transfer activities
    g. use tub or shower chair

Clinical Situations
1. Remove plug, let water out, keep patient covered with bath towel and allow patient to rest at least 10 minutes, then assist out of tub.
2. Change water to prevent chilling.
3. Do not cut toenails, inform nurse of this need.
4. Grasp penis gently, draw foreskin back, wash and dry glans and base of penis, replace foreskin to natural position, lift scrotum, wash and dry.

Relating to the Nursing Process
1. Implementation 2. Planning   3. Implementation
4. Planning   5. Planning   6. Planning, Evaluation

UNIT 25 General Comfort Measures

Vocabulary Exercise
1. dentures   2. backrub   3. halitosis
4. oral hygiene 5. caries   6. feces

Completion
1. denture cup   2. moisture (lubrication)
3. carefully   4. patient's name and room number
5. caries   6. downward
7. lemon-glycerine swabs, sponge applicators   8. applicators
9. sitting   10. line the sink and add water
11. warm, water (or hand) 12. anticoagulants
13. taut   14. stimulates
15. bedpan or commode   16. calm, quiet
17. bedside/overbed, height 18. sheets, top
19. low   20. dishes

Short Answer
1. Prevent dental caries and halitosis.
2. Keep in labeled denture cup in patient's bedside table.
3. Increase circulation and comfort and prevent pressure ulcers.
4. Prevent scratching patients and tearing gloves.
5. Prevent cuts.
6. Apply pressure and report to nurse.
7. Separate it and comb it out.
8. The risk of cutting the patient is much higher when a disposable razor is used. Gloves are worn to protect the assistant and apply the principles of standard precautions.
9. a. unconscious   b. vomiting
   c. have high temperature d. breathing through mouth
   e. receiving oxygen   f. dying
10. a. part of cleansing bath
    b. following use of bedpan
    c. when changing dependent patient's position
    d. at bedtime
    e. whenever it could provide comfort
11. a. basin of water   b. bath towel
    c. wash cloth   d. lotion
12. To refresh the mouth and improve appetite.
13. To help patient relax and encourage restful sleep.
14. Gently speak patient's name and place hand on arm.
15. a. going to surgery
    b. having tests that prohibit eating

16. a. measuring vital signs
    b. giving backrub
    c. providing mouth and hair care
    d. assisting with toileting

Identification

1.

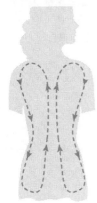

2.

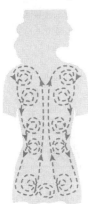

3.

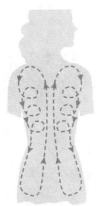

True/False

1. T   2. T   3. F   4. F   5. T
6. T   7. T   8. T   9. T   10. T

Name the Equipment

1. urinal   2. orthopedic bedpan   3. regular bedpan

Clinical Situations

1. Change position, be sure linens are dry and free of wrinkles and crumbs, notify nurse.
2. baby shampoo, detangling conditioner, and baby oil to replace oil
3. Use an orthopedic bedpan; either roll patient onto bedpan or get assistance in raising patient onto bedpan.

4. Give care to another patient and come back.
5. Allow patient to sleep if possible.
6. Carry out all ending procedure actions.

Relating to the Nursing Process

1. Implementation   2. Planning, Implementation
3. Implementation   4. Assessment
5. Assessment   6. Assessment, Evaluation

SECTION 8 PRINCIPLES OF NUTRITION AND FLUID BALANCE

UNIT 26 Nutritional Needs and Diet Modifications

Vocabulary Exercise

1. nutrition   2. cellulose   3. defecation
4. carbohydrates 5. digestion   6. protein
7. minerals   8. vitamins   9. fats

Completion

1. body, height
2. high-density (or concentrated)
3. total parenteral nutrition   4. energy
5. amino   6. cannot
7. full recovery from anesthesia is made
8. ice chips   9. defecation
10. 6 to 8   11. soft
12. diabetic   13. household
14. document the amount   15. unpleasant
16. right angle   17. therapeutic value
18. chewing, swallowing   19. swallowing
20. documented   21. dysphagia
22. thickener   23. most difficult

True/False

1. T   2. T   3. F   4. F   5. T
6. F   7. T   8. F   9. T   10. T
11. F   12. T   13. T

Short Answer

1. a. regular   b. liquid   c. soft
2. Eating should be enjoyable as well as a nutritious experience.
3. The patient must be encouraged to take more fluids.
4. a. enteral feeding   b. intravenous   c. TPN
5. a. supply heat and energy
   b. build and repair body tissue
   c. regulate body functions
6. a. proteins   b. fats   c. carbohydrates
   d. minerals   e. vitamins   f. water
7. a. meat   b. fish   c. eggs   d. poultry
8. a. corn   b. soybeans   c. peas   d. nuts
9. a. calcium   b. phosphorus c. iodine
   d. iron   e. copper   f. potassium
10. a. build teeth and bones
    b. promote growth
    c. aid normal body function
    d. strengthen resistance to disease
11. a. A   b. B complex   c. C   d. D   e. E   f. K
12. a. potato chips   b. pop (soda)   c. pickles
    d. processed foods   e. pork

13. a. one medium size   b. 1/2 cup
    c. 3 to 4 ounces   d. 2 to 3 ounces
14. Nutritional supplements are usually given to patients who have experienced weight loss and those who need additional calories to meet a medical need. Special supplements are used to treat patients with specific medical needs, such as those with renal failure, diabetes, chronic obstructive pulmonary disease, HIV, and pediatric patients.
15. Nutritional supplements must be ordered by the physician or dietitian. They are given for a specific therapeutic purpose. They are given to make up for a nutritional deficiency, strengthen the patient, or promote healing. Most facilities require documentation of nutritional supplement consumption. Nourishments are substantial food items given to patients to increase nutrient intake. These are usually regular food items, such as sandwiches or ice cream. They do not require a physician order.
16. 140, 40
17. The food cart is a clean item. The linen hamper and housekeeping cart are contaminated items. They are separated to prevent cross-contamination.
18. Serve meals promptly when carts arrive, close the door to the food cart as soon as you remove a tray, keep food covered when carrying trays in the hallway, leave trays on the food cart until you are ready to spoon-feed dependent patients.
19. A PEG tube is surgically inserted by threading the tube through the patient's mouth and into the stomach. The tube is pulled out through an incision in the patient's abdomen, with the tip remaining in the stomach. The nasogastric tube is inserted through the nose and threaded down the esophagus to the stomach, where the tip remains. Both are used for tube feeding.
20. a. are dehydrated
    b. are receiving IV infusions
    c. have recently had surgery
    d. have a urinary catheter
    e. are perspiring profusely or vomiting
    f. have specific diagnosis such as congestive heart disease or renal disease
21. a. urine   b. vomitus
    c. diarrhea   d. excessive perspiration
    e. blood   f. drainage from wound or stomach
22. All fluid taken in   23. All fluid lost
24. mL or cc   25. end of each shift

Matching
1. b   2. a   3. a   4. b   5. b   6. b

Classification
1. Group 1 Bread, cereal, rice, and pasta: cereal, rice, flour, bread, pasta
    Group 2 Milk, yogurt, and cheese: milk, cheese, ice cream, yogurt, cottage cheese
    Group 3 Meat, poultry, fish, dry beans, eggs and nuts: beef, chicken, liver, fish, bacon
    Group 4 Vegetable: peas, spinach
    Group 5 Fruit: pears, apples
    Group 6 Fats, oils, sweets: olive oil, butter, honey

Clinical Situations
1. Note how much fluid has been taken, record on I&O sheet.
2. Explain position of foods in relation to numbers on clock.
3. Encourage fluid intake each time patient contact is made.
4. Notify nurse that IV is almost empty.
5. Recognize patient's dietary restriction and provide different food.

Conversions
1. a. 16 oz × 30 = 480 mL   b. 6 oz × 30 = 180 mL
    c. 24 oz × 30 = 720 mL   d. 8 oz × 30 = 240 mL
    e. 8 oz × 30 = 240 mL

Completion
1. [activity]
2. (See graphic on next page.)
    a. active   b. 30   c. Sixty
    d. 90   e. whole   f. juices
    g. dairy   h. beans   i. lean
    j. oils   k. vegetables   l. sodium
    m. sugar   n. 6 ounces   o. 2–5 cups
    p. 2 cups   q. 3 cups   r. 5.5 ounces
3. (See table on next page.)

Relating to the Nursing Process
1. Implementation   2. Assessment   3. Assessment
4. Implementation   5. Implementation   6. Planning

SECTION 9 SPECIAL CARE PROCEDURES
UNIT 27 Warm and Cold Applications

Vocabulary Exercise
1. core   2. vasoconstrict   3. sitz
4. aquathermia   5. hypothermia   6. hemorrhage
7. vasodilate   8. warm   9. icebag
10. diathermy

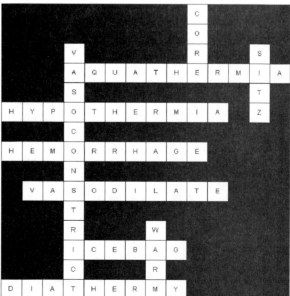

Completion
1. dry, moist
2. hot water bags, hot/wet compress, hot soak, Aquamatic K-Pad, whirlpool, sitz bath

2.

Exercise

- Adults should be physically __(a)__ for at least __(b)__ minutes most days of the week, children for 60 minutes.
- __(c)__ to __(d)__ minutes of daily physical activity may be needed to prevent weight gain or sustain weight loss.

(a) active
(b) 30
(c) 60
(d) 90

(e) whole
(f) juices
(g) dairy
(h) beans

__(j)__

- Most fat should be from fish, nuts and __(k)__ oils.
- Limit solid fats, such as butter, margarine or lard.

- Keep consumption of saturated fats, trans fats and __(l)__ low.
- Choose foods low in added __(m)__.

CATEGORY	Grains	Vegetables	Fruits	Milk	Meat and __(h)__	Recommended nutrient intakes at 12-calorie levels can be found on *mypyramid.gov*.
RECOMMENDATION	Half of all grains consumed should be __(e)__ grains.	Vary the types of vegetables you eat.	Eat a variety of fruits. Go easy on __(f)__.	Eat low-fat or fat-free __(g)__ products.	Eat __(i)__ cuts, seafood and beans. Avoid frying.	
DAILY AMOUNT *Based on a 2,000 calorie diet.*	__(n)__	__(o)__	__(p)__	__(q)__	__(r)__	

(i) lean   (j) oils   (k) vegetables   (l) sodium   (m) sugar
(n) 6 oz.   (o) 2–5 cups   (p) 2 cups   (q) 3 cups   (r) 5.5 oz.

3.

| Date | Time | Method of Adm. | Intake | | | Output | | |
| | | | Solution | Amounts Rec'd | Time | Urine Amount | Others | |
							Kind	Amount
7/16	0715	PO	water	50 mL		550 mL		
	0830	PO	tea	240 mL				
	1030	PO	cran.ju.	120 mL				
	1115	PO	water	80 mL				
	1430	PO	orange	120 mL		400 ML		
Shift Totals	1500		sherbet	610 mL		950 mL		
	1530	PO	tea	240 mL				
	1700	PO	gelatin	120 mL				
			milk	180 mL				
			soup	180 mL		375 mL		
	2130		gelatin	50 mL			vomitus	400 mL
Shift Totals	2300			770 mL		375 mL		400 mL
	2315						vomitus	200 mL
	2400						vomitus	150 mL
	0230	IV	D/W	500 mL		300 mL	vomitus	80 mL
Shift Totals	0530			500 mL		300 mL		430 mL
24 Hour Totals				1880 mL		1625 mL		830 mL vomitus

3. ice cap, ice bag, ice collar, cold/wet compress, cold soak
4. remove   5. half full
6. air   7. a doctor's written order
8. distilled water 9. one-quarter
10. standard precautions   11. 10
12. 20   13. hypothermia blanket
14. inflammation, pain   15. dilate
16. 97   17. headaches
18. heat   19. numbness, discoloration
20. air   21. away
22. strike   23. lie
24. 105   25. bath thermometer
26. asepto bulb   27. excess liquid
28. electrical outlet   29. leaks
30. covered   31. frequently
32. [Any combination of these answers is acceptable]
    • relieve pain
    • combat local infection or inflammation
    • stop bleeding
    • reduce body temperature   • reduce edema
33. [Any combination of these answers is acceptable]
    • acute inflammation
    • dermatitis
    • deep vein thrombosis
    • peripheral vascular disease
    • open wound(s)
    • recent soft tissue injuries in which swelling or bleeding would be increased by heat
    • skin sensation impairment
    • severe cognitive impairment
    • check with the nurse before using for pregnant women; patients with impaired circulation, sensory impairment, cancer, rashes, and open skin conditions; or very young and very old patients
    • hot *packs* contraindicated in paralysis or areas without sensation, acute edema or inflammation, infection, and hemophilia.
34. [Any combination of these answers is acceptable]
    • deep vein thrombosis
    • peripheral vascular disease
    • open wound(s)
    • skin sensation impairment
    • severe cognitive impairment
    • cold intolerance, cold allergy
    • rheumatoid arthritis
    • Reynaud's phenomenon
35. [Any combination of these answers is acceptable]
    • red or dark area
    • cyanosis or pale color
    • blistering
    • patient complains of numbness, tingling
    • shivering
36. a. ice bags   b. ice caps   c. ice collars
37. a. compresses   b. soaks   c. packs
38. [Any combination of these answers is acceptable]
    • changes in skin color
    • cyanosis of the lips or nail beds

• sudden changes in temperature
• marked changes in pulse, respirations, or blood pressure
• respiratory distress
• pain
• changes in sensation
• edema
• shivering and chills
• urinary output below 50 mL/hour
39. a. type of treatment   b. temperature
    c. area of application   d. length of application
    e. patient reaction
40. a. bath thermometer
    b. extra pitcher of hot water
    c. solution as ordered
    d. large rubber or plastic sheet
    e. tub or basin of proper size
    f. two bath blankets
    g. two bath towels

True/False
1. F   2. T   3. F   4. F   5. F
6. T   7. F   8. T   9. T   10. F

Clinical Situations
1. Loosen it one-quarter turn.
2. Cover ice bag (plastic or rubber should not come in contact with patient's skin).
3. Discontinue treatment.

Relating to the Nursing Process
1. Planning   2. Implementation
3. Assessment, Evaluation   4. Implementation

UNIT 28 Assisting with the Physical Examination

Vocabulary Exercise
1. lithotomy   2. percussion   3. otoscope
4. speculum   5. ophthalmoscope

Definitions
1. flat on back with knees flexed and separated
2. to cover
3. bent
4. instrument to test reflexes
5. instrument to examine eyes
6. instrument to examine ears
7. instrument to dilate body opening

Completion
1. flexed   2. back   3. left alone
4. abdomen   5. left   6. dorsal recumbent
7. lithotomy   8. knee-chest 9. sheets
10. feel   11. semi-Fowler's
12. a. supine b. semi-Fowler's c. knee-chest d. lithotomy

Short Answer
1. Prepare and clean equipment
   Drape and position patient
   Remain available throughout examination
   Assist by adjusting lights

2. Helps health care provider evaluate patient's status, establish a diagnosis, determine patient's progress and response to therapy
3. a. microscope slides and cover slips   b. cotton applicators
   c. Pap smear fixative
   d. cotton applicators
   e. cervical spatula
   f. vaginal speculum
   g. lubricant
   h. cytobrushes
   i. gloves
4. a. stethoscope—listen to body sounds
   b. otoscope—look into ear
   c. vaginal speculum—examine vagina and cervix
   d. percussion hammer—test reflexes
   e. specimen container—covered container to allow for safe transfer of specimen to lab
   f. tongue depressors—to hold tongue down while mouth and teeth are examined
   g. blood pressure cuff—to measure blood pressure
   h. gloves—perform vaginal or rectal exam
   i. tape measure—measure circumference of head, body, extremities

Clinical Situations
1. Keep calm, be reassuring, explain steps of examination
2. Place and drape patient in lithotomy position, arrange pelvic instruments, provide lighting
3. Position in high Fowler's position

True/False
1. T   2. F   3. T   4. F   5. F
6. T   7. T   8. F   9. T   10. T

Relating to the Nursing Process
1. Implementation   2. Assessment
3. Assessment, Implementation

UNIT 29 The Surgical Patient

Vocabulary Exercise
1. prosthesis 2. ambulation 3. vertigo 4. singultus
5. dangling 6. nosocomial 7. atelectasis 8. depilatory

Matching
1. e   2. h   3. j   4. i   5. k
6. g   7. f   8. c   9. b   10. a

Completion
1. a. preoperative   b. operative   c. postoperative
2. to prevent pain, relax muscles, induce forgetfulness
3. inhaled   4. vomit   5. unconscious
6. awake   7. below, lost   8. rapidly
9. [Any combination of these answers is acceptable]
   • washing, shaving operative area
   • taking, recording vital signs
   • taking care of valuables
   • removing dentures, other prostheses
   • removing nail polish, makeup, hairpins, jewelry
   • braiding long hair
   • dressing patient in hospital gown, covering hair with surgical cap or towel
   • having patient void, measuring urine
   • making room quiet and comfortable
   • putting up side rails

10. emesis basin, tissue wipes, tongue blades, vital sign equipment, pad, pencil
11. turned to one side, aspiration   12. relaxation of muscles
13. nurse   14. 2   15. pulse
16. a. clean   b. applied smoothly
    c. snug but not too tight
17. veins   18. 3 to 5, one to two hours
19. mouth care, shock   20. incisional
21. intensity, location, type   22. mobility
23. I&O   24. vital signs
25. blood pressure, weak and rapid, cool and moist
26. elevate the head, high Fowler's (or orthopnea)
27. quiet, support
28. check skin for sensitivity
29. not continue but report to nurse
30. disposable, sterile

Surgical Prep Areas
1. a. abdominal   b. anterior breast   c. posterior breast
   d. back   e. kidney   f. vaginal, rectal, perineal

Short Answer
1. a. pain receptors to receive the sensation
   b. spinal nerves to transmit sensation to spinal cord and brain
   c. areas in brain to receive and interpret sensation
2. a. about tests, medications, procedures
   b. postoperative exercises
   c. ways of decreasing postoperative discomfort
3. a. perform work efficiently
   b. be available to listen
   c. explain plans and actions before carrying out any procedure
   d. encourage patient participation in care
   e. transmit requests for spiritual support
4. a. add days to hospital stay   b. can be life-threatening
   c. increase costs
5. a. take vital signs and record
   b. take care of valuables
   c. remove and care for dentures and prostheses
   d. remove nail polish, makeup, hairpins, jewelry; tape wedding band in place
   e. dress patient in hospital gown and cap
   f. see that the patient voids, document
   g. make sure room is quiet and comfortable
6. a. elevate bed to stretcher height
   b. secure side rails in up position
   c. remove all unnecessary equipment
   d. complete surgical checklist
   e. follow facility policy regarding visitors
7. a. make a surgical bed
   b. clean top of bedside table except for needed equipment
   c. check for and obtain needed equipment
8. a. take and record vital signs
   b. check dressings
   c. check IV, rate, infusion site
   d. encourage deep breathing, moving, coughing
   e. watch for and intervene if vomiting

9. a. learn type, purpose, location of each tube
   b. check character, amount of drainage
   c. check for obstructions in tubing
   d. keep orifices clean
   e. never disconnect tubes or raise bottles above level of drainage sites
   f. never lower infusion bags below level of infusion sites
   g. do not stress tubes
   h. restrain infusion sites if necessary

10. a. Latest TPR and blood pressure charted
    b. Wrist identification band on patient
    c. Fingernail polish and makeup removed
    d. Metallic objects removed (rings may be taped)
    e. Dentures removed
    f. Other prostheses removed (such as artificial limb or eye)
    g. Bath blanket and head cap in place
    h. Bed in high position and side rails up after preop medication given
    i. Patient has voided

11. Perioperative hypothermia develops in the operating room as a result of anesthesia and some sedatives. The drugs promote heat loss by reducing the shivering response and preventing blood vessel constriction. The operating room is purposefully kept very cool, because cooler temperature reduces oxygen requirements. Open body cavities, and administration of blood and IV fluids, also contribute to temperature loss. The body cannot return the temperature to normal until the concentration of anesthetic in the brain decreases and the normal temperature-regulating responses can take over. Return to normal temperature may take 2 to 5 hours. The nursing assistant must monitor patients closely and identify and report subnormal temperatures, if present. Keep the patient warm, using warm blankets, if possible.

12. The legs must be measured with a tape measure and the measurements compared with a size chart to determine what size to use. Hosiery that does not fit increases the risk of complications, including ischemia and serious skin breakdown.

True/False

1. F   2. T   3. F   4. F   5. T   6. T
7. F   8. T   9. F   10. T   11. T

Clinical Situations

1. Clip hair with scissors before shaving.
2. Gently lower patient to floor, protecting head, and signal or call for help.
3. Remove stockings, reapply smoothly.
4. Notify nurse immediately, patient may be going into shock.
5. Notify nurse immediately, patient may be experiencing pulmonary embolus.

Relating to the Nursing Process

1. Assessment   2. Implementation
3. Planning   4. Implementation
5. Implementation   6. Assessment, Implementation

UNIT 30 Caring for the Emotionally Stressed Patient

Vocabulary Exercise

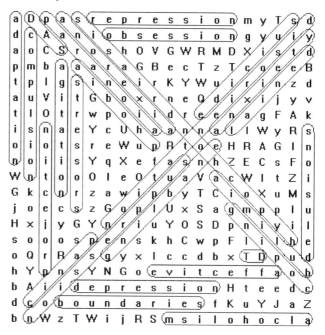

1. a. adaptation—adjustment
   b. affective—pertaining to mood
   c. agitation—mental state characterized by irregular, erratic behavior
   d. alcoholism—dependency on alcoholic beverages
   e. anorexia—eating disorder in which the patient has a disturbed body image; he or she views the body as being fat even though it may be skeletal
   f. anxiety—fear, apprehension, or sense of impending danger
   g. boundaries—unseen or unspoken limits on physical and emotional relationship with patients
   h. bulimia—a body image disorder that causes persons to binge-eat in huge amounts, then vomit (*purge*) to undo the binge
   i. compulsion—a purposeful, repetitive behavior that is done many times each day and is problematic enough to cause distress
   j. coping—managing or dealing with stress
   k. delusions—false beliefs
   l. denial—refusal to accept the truth
   m. depression—morbid sadness or melancholy
   m. disorientation—loss of recognition of time, place, or person
   o. DT—delirium tremens; part of a serious withdrawal syndrome seen in persons who stop drinking alcohol following continuous and heavy consumption
   p. enabling—shielding the patient from the consequences of his or her actions
   q. hypochondriasis—abnormal concern about one's health
   r. obsession—a frequent idea, impulse, or thought that is usually senseless

s. panic—feeling extremely fearful, as if one is in overwhelming danger

t. paranoia—state in which one has delusions of persecution or grandeur; feeling singled out as if others are blaming or watching

u. phobia—an unfounded, recurring fear that causes the person to feel panic

v. projection—denying one's own unacceptable traits and blaming them on someone or something else

w. repression—involuntarily excluding a painful or difficult experience from one's conscious memory

x. SAD—seasonal affective disorder; a depression that recurs each year at the same time. The cause is unknown, but thought to be related to lack of exposure to sunlight or having abnormal melatonin levels

y. stressors—problems that cause a person concern for his or her well-being

z. suicide—self-destruction, killing oneself

aa. suppression—consciously refusing to accept unacceptable feelings or thoughts

Completion

1. adaptation
2. stressor
3. maladaptive behaviors
4. interrelated
5. coping
6. defense
7. frustration
8. coping with stress
9. slows down
10. unfavorably
11. good
12. calm, gentle
13. motor
14. reality
15. paranoia
16. verbal
17. reliable
18. attempts
19. demanding
20. Boundaries
21. danger zone
22. Enabling

True/False

1. T	2. F	3. F	4. F	5. T
6. T	7. T	8. F	9. F	10. T
11. T	12. T	13. F	14. T	15. T
16. F	17. T	18. T	19. F	20. T
21. F	22. F	23. F	24. T	25. T
26. F	27. T	28. T	29. T	30. F
31. F	32. T	33. F	34. T	35. T
36. T	37. F	38. T	39. F	40. T
41. F	42. T			

Short Answer

1. a. hospitalization   b. illness   c. loss of spouse
    d. loss of job   e. loss of status

2. a. attributing one's own unacceptable feelings and thoughts to others
    b. blocking out painful or anxiety-producing events or feelings
    c. behaving like another who is held as an ideal
    d. using imagination to solve problems
    e. excelling in one area to make up for lack in another

3. a. learn and appreciate underlying problem
    b. establish rapport
    c. maintain open communication
    d. be consistent in manner of care

4. a. do not allow yourself to be manipulated
    b. listen with empathy
    c. help explore coping mechanisms
    d. make sure no alcohol is available
    e. follow limits that have been set

5. a. bad taste in mouth, flatulence, burning tongue
    b. preoccupation with constipation, pain in lower abdomen
    c. vague discomfort, burning on urination
    d. crying spells, apathy, backache, fatigue
    e. stiff joints, anorexia, trouble sleeping, inability to concentrate

6. a. inability to think quickly and clearly
    b. bewilderment
    c. faulty memory
    d. illusions
    e. inability to follow directions
    f. misinterpret stimuli
    g. delusions
    h. hallucinations

7. a. keep sensory aids in place
    b. speak often to patient, identifying yourself
    c. keep clock and calendar in view
    d. encourage familiar objects and refer to them
    e. post activity board
    f. call attention to color-coding in facility

8. [Any combination of these answers is acceptable]
    • family or marital problems
    • naivete
    • low self-esteem
    • loneliness, feelings of isolation
    • addiction (chemical or sexual)
    • financial problems
    • stress, burnout

9. [Any combination of these answers is acceptable]
    • protecting the patient from the natural consequences of his or her behavior
    • keeping secrets about a patient's behavior from others
    • making excuses for a patient's behavior
    • taking steps to get a patient out of personal trouble
    • blaming others for the patient's behavior
    • seeing the patient's problems as a result of something else
    • giving money to patients
    • attempting to control patients' lives and activities
    • doing things for the patient that she should do herself

Clinical Situations

1. a. report observations to nurse
    b. be consistent in approach
    c. observe closely

2. a. protect him and other patients
    b. be calm in approach
    c. assist with reality orientation
    d. maintain limits

3. a. noise   b. frustration at loss
    c. organic brain disease   d. boredom
    e. depression   f. constipation
    g. restraints   h. drug interactions

Relating to the Nursing Process

1. Implementation   2. Assessment
3. Assessment   4. Assessment, Planning, Evaluation
5. Implementation   6. Assessment
7. Implementation

UNIT 31 Caring for the Bariatric Patient

Vocabulary Exercise

1. a. advocate—a person who speaks on behalf of the patient.
   b. bariatrics—field of medicine that focuses on the treatment and control of obesity and medical conditions and diseases associated with obesity.
   c. BMI—body mass index; a mathematical calculation used to determine whether a person is at a healthy, normal weight, is overweight, or is obese.
   d. comorbidities—diseases and medical conditions that are either caused by or contributed to by morbid obesity.
   e. diabetes—chronic disease related to problems with carbohydrate metabolism; common comorbidity of obesity.
   f. (gastric) bypass—the most common procedure of the six bariatric surgical techniques that are widely accepted.
   g. hypertension—high blood pressure over 140/90; common comorbidity of obesity.
   h. hyperventilation—breathing abnormally fast and deep, resulting in excessive amounts of oxygen in the lungs and reduced carbon dioxide levels in the bloodstream.
   i. IBW—ideal body weight; a concept developed from life insurance statistics related to life span (longevity) and health.
   j. (minimally) invasive (surgery)—any surgical procedure that does not require a large incision.
   k. laparoscopic—minimally invasive surgery done through a scope or instrument inserted deep into the body through the skin.
   l. morbid (obesity)—having a BMI of 40 or higher and being 100 pounds or more over the ideal body weight.
   m. obesity—being overweight by 20 to 30% of the ideal body weight.
   n. overweight—condition in which a person weighs more than he or she should, according to standards set based on the person's height and bone (frame) size. A person who is overweight has a body weight that is greater than is considered desirable or medically advisable.
   o. panniculus—fatty apron of abdominal skin.
   p. reflux—backflow of fluid, such as when stomach juices and food flow back from the stomach into the esophagus and mouth.
   q. stenosis—narrowing of a passageway, same as a stricture.
   r. stricture—narrowing of a passageway in the body, often the result of inflammation or scar tissue.
   s. trapeze—a triangular frame that hangs on a chain from the ceiling or base support attached to the bed; used by the patient to assist with lifting and moving.

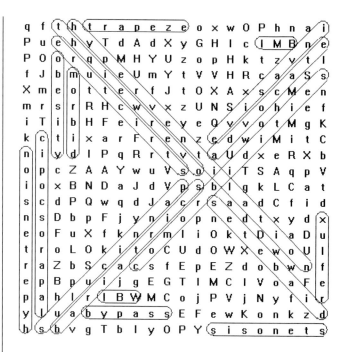

True/False

1. F	2. F	3. T	4. F	5. T
6. F	7. F	8. T	9. T	10. T
11. T	12. F	13. F	14. T	15. T
16. F	17. F	18. F	19. T	20. T
21. F	22. F	23. F	24. T	25. T

Short Answer

1. Support the upper leg on pillows.
2. The wide gait helps the patient balance and the wide girth accommodates the width of the legs.
3. The binder gives the patient a secure feeling of support and keeps the large abdomen from interfering with safe patient handling and movement.
4. Protect the patient's head.
5. a. vomiting   b. reflux   c. diarrhea
6. Postoperative care is targeted to reduce pressure and strain on both the internal and external staples.
7. The patient's stomach will hold only a few ounces, and overfilling it risks rupturing a staple and causing a leak.
8. [Any combination of these is acceptable] rhythm disturbances; pulse/heart rate above 100, hypotension; patient feels anxious, complains of anxiety or a sense of impending doom; hypoxia, decreased oxygen saturation, signs of air hunger; fever above 102°F; change in appearance or volume of gastric or wound drains; signs or symptoms of wound infections; nausea, vomiting, or diarrhea; presence of blood in emesis or stool; persistent cough
9. [Any combination of these is acceptable]
   • Vital signs according to postoperative routine
   • Abdominal binder
   • Ice packs to the incision
   • Check dressing over incision and drain hourly, or as instructed

- Use the incentive spirometer at least 10 times every hour
- Coughing and deep breathing
- Anti-embolism hosiery, circulation checks to feet every 2 to 4 hours
- Sequential compression therapy
- Up in chair with assistance one or more times
- Catheter care
- Keep patient NPO except for ice chips
- Intake and output monitoring and recording
- Monitor the pulse oximeter for alarms

Relating to the Nursing Process

1. Implementation, Assessment
2. Implementation, Assessment
3. Evaluation, Planning
4. Assessment
5. Planning, Implementation

UNIT 32 Death and Dying

Vocabulary Exercise

1. critical
2. postmortem
3. hospice
4. terminal
5. denial
6. moribund
7. anointing
8. autopsy
9. bargaining
10. rigor mortis

Completion

1. physician
2. Catholic
3. natural
4. six months or less
5. teams
6. slow
7. hearing
8. rapid, weaker
9. physician
10. nursing assistant
11. strength, comfort
12. privacy
13. journey, alone

True/False

1. F   2. F   3. F   4. T   5. T
6. T   7. F   8. F   9. T   10. T
11. F   12. T

Short Answer

1. a. denial   b. anger   c. bargaining
   d. depression   e. acceptance
2. a. control of pain
   b. coordinating all support systems
   c. providing legal and financial counseling
3. a. report pain, provide comfort measures
   b. encourage patient to actively participate in care
   c. know and be supportive of family members
   d. provide care with dignity and respect
4. a. pupils become permanently dilated
   b. heat is lost from body
   c. blood pools
   d. rigor mortis develops
   e. progressive protein breakdown
5. a. shroud   b. clean gown
   c. three or four tags   d. gauze squares for padding
   e. safety pins

6. Close doors and empty corridors of visitors and patients before transporting body to morgue.
7. Health care providers will come in contact with body fluids, which may be infectious even after death.

Clinical Situations

1. Respond to his mood, report mood change to nurse, recognize that mood swings are common.
2. Report to nurse so arrangements can be made.
3. a. remove unneeded equipment
   b. place body on back with head and shoulders on pillow
   c. close eyes
   d. replace dentures
   e. make sure room and linen are neat and clean
4. a. oxygen   b. fluid by mouth
   c. medication for discomfort   d. personal, physical care
5. durable power of attorney for health care
6. No action to resuscitate.

Relating to the Nursing Process

1. Assessment   2. Implementation
3. Assessment, Implementation   4. Implementation

SECTION 10 OTHER HEALTH CARE SETTINGS

UNIT 33 Care of the Elderly and Chronically Ill

Vocabulary Exercise

1. nocturia
2. sepsis
3. goals
4. hypothermia
5. residents
6. vitality
7. dentition
8. flatulence
9. losses
10. reminiscing
11. dementia
12. dehydration
13. reflux

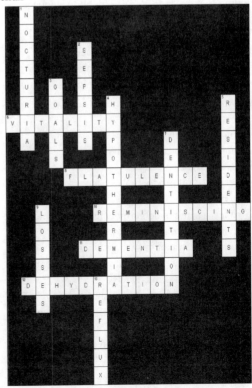

Definitions
1. federal and state-funded program to pay for medical care for individuals whose income falls below a certain level.
2. skin coloration
3. weakening
4. general care and nursing care provided to person mostly capable of self-care
5. behavior in which a person becomes more agitated and disoriented during evening hours
6. thinking and talking about the past
7. inflammation of diverticula in intestinal tract
8. sequential order
9. disorder of the brain that involves thinking, memory, judgment
10. personal care provided over an extended period of time to persons with chronic illnesses

Matching
1. d   2. j   3. b   4. g   5. i   6. a
7. h   8. e   9. k   10. c   11. f   12. f
13. e   14. d   15. c   16. b   17. b   18. e
19. c   20. b   21. a

True/False
1. F   2. F   3. F   4. T   5. F   6. F
7. T   8. T   9. T   10. F   11. T

Completion
1. humor, communicate   2. respect
3. older (or elderly), chronic   4. slower, small
5. individual   6. time clock
7. slower, accurate   8. aware
9. weight loss   10. Validation therapy
11. malnutrition   12. 30° to 45°
13. Delirium   14. sepsis
15. eloping   16. body language
17. trigger   18. 75
19. three   20. in-service
21. 24   22. helplessness
23. limitations, muscular   24. malnutrition
25. lubricate or moisturize   26. night

Short Answer
1. a. loss of fat and water
   b. thickened nails
   c. increased areas of pigmentation
   d. loss of hair color
   e. decreased oil production
2. a. to be loved
   b. to feel a sense of achievement and recognition
   c. to have a degree of economic security
   d. to have a sense of self-worth
3. a. do not obstruct open area with equipment
   b. wipe up spills immediately
   c. encourage residents to use hand rails
   d. provide adequate lighting
   e. eliminate noise and distractions
   f. do not leave resident alone in tub or shower
   g. check clothing for fit
   h. care for personal needs promptly

4. [Any combination of these answers is acceptable]
   - need help eating and drinking
   - eat less than half their meals and/or planned snacks
   - have mouth pain
   - have no dentures, or have dentures that do not fit correctly
   - have difficulty chewing or swallowing
   - have difficulty getting utensils or glasses to their mouth
   - cough or choke while eating
   - are sad, have crying spells, or withdraw from others
   - are confused, wander, or pace
   - have diabetes, lung disease, cancer, HIV, or other chronic diseases
5. [Any combination of these answers is acceptable]
   - drink less than 6 cups of liquid a day
   - have dry mouth
   - have cracked lips
   - have sunken eyes
   - have dark urine
   - need help drinking from a glass
   - have trouble swallowing liquids
   - have diarrhea, vomiting, or fever
   - are mentally confused or confusion has worsened
   - are weak or tired
   - are lethargic and have difficulty staying awake
6. The actions of a person to overwhelming stimuli that can lead to hallucinations, delusions, injury.
7. [Any combination of these answers is acceptable]
   - unfamiliar environment/relocation to a new room or new to facility
   - vascular insufficiency
   - central nervous system infection
   - trauma
   - tumors or masses, malignancies
   - chemotherapy
   - seizures
   - migraine
   - decreased cardiac output, reduced blood flow, interrupted blood flow
   - urinary retention
   - pressure ulcers
   - hypotension
   - inadequate oxygenation
   - pneumonia or other lung infection
   - systemic infections, acute and chronic
   - metabolic disorders
   - anemias
   - decreased renal function
   - endocrine system disorders
   - nutritional deficiencies, malnutrition
   - emotional stress
   - pain
   - surgery, anesthesia
   - alteration in temperature regulation—hyperthermia, hypothermia
   - dehydration, fluid and electrolyte imbalances
   - depression

- anxiety
- grief
- fatigue
- sensory/perceptual deficiencies
- sensory deprivation/isolation, confinement to a restricted area
- sensory overload
- immobility, bedrest
- exposure to toxic substances
- restraints
- medication reactions
- use of invasive equipment such as nasogastric tube or catheter
- lack of prosthetic devices, including glasses, hearing aid, dentures
- lack of items that complete body image, such as canes, purses, walkers
- loss of family contact
- loss of control over body processes

8. [Any combination of these answers is acceptable]
   - loud noise
   - uncomfortable environmental temperature
   - boredom
   - unmet physical needs
   - feeling stressed
   - pain
   - hunger
   - thirst
   - needing to use the bathroom
   - dehydration
   - illness
   - inadequate coping mechanisms
   - medications
   - unfamiliar environment

True/False

1. F   2. T   3. T   4. F   5. T
6. F   7. F   8. F   9. T

Multiple Choice

1. c   2. d   3. b   4. c   5. b   6. d

Clinical Situations

1. Recognize that she is probably frustrated, be calm, reassuring, and try to communicate with her. The resident may have an unmet physical or mental need, such as loss of control over her body or over factors in the environment that displease her. Offer her choices and give her as much control over daily routines as possible. If you identify an unmet need or approach that is effective, inform the nurse.

2. Realize that many elderly do not really remember how much fluid has been consumed. The resident may not remember how much fluid she has consumed. Another possibility is that she may have had the extra fluid at mealtime, in activities, or when snacks or juice were passed. Another assistant or the nurse may have given her fluids. Explore all possibilities before making assumptions about the resident's intake. If, after investigation, you

believe the resident's fluid intake is not adequate, notify the nurse.

3. Report and repair the tip before using.

Hidden Picture

1. a. right arm of resident hanging down over wheel of chair
   b. right leg dragging
   c. walker with no rubber tip on one leg
   d. blanket on floor
   e. second resident in geri-chair in poor alignment
   f. safety belt tied incorrectly
   g. third resident in bed with high horizontal position and side rails down
   h. overbed table too far away to reach water
   i. call bell on table, not close at hand
   j. drainage bag hanging on side rail
   k. spilled water on floor
   l. open window
   m. frayed electrical cord

Relating to the Nursing Process

1. Implementation   2. Implementation
3. Assessment   4. Implementation
5. Implementation   6. Implementation
7. Implementation

UNIT 34 The Organization of Home Care: Trends in Health Care

Vocabulary Exercise

1. Record of care given, client's response, observations, housekeeping if assigned
2. Care given at intervals
3. Record of how time was spent with client

Completion

1. part-time   2. complete, one
3. independence   4. home health care team
5. insurance group   6. records
7. hospital, skilled nursing facility 8. assistance
9. number   10. developed, nurse
11. taught   12. accuracy, calculations

Short Answer

1. a. government-sponsored   b. private agency
   c. hospital-sponsored
2. a. greater time flexibility
   b. more independence
   c. satisfaction of giving complete care
   d. part-time employment, if desired
3. a. time of arrival
   b. time of departure
   c. length of time required for specific activities
   d. travel time if working on more than one case
   e. mileage or transportation costs
4. a. be sure to have written job description
   b. carry out procedures as taught
   c. keep safety factors in mind and watch for hazards
   d. be familiar with client's rights
   e. ask for assistance with procedures you have not performed

5. a. care given   b. client's response
   c. observations   d. housekeeping tasks completed

Matching

1. b   2. e   3. c   4. a   5. b
6. c   7. c   8. d   9. a   10. d
11. a   12. d   13. c   14. b

Computations

1. a. 0815 − 0850 = 35 min
   b. 1005 − 1115 = 1 hr, 10 min
   c. 1120 − 1305 = 1 hr, 45 min
   d. 1410 − 1515 = 1 hr, 5 min
   e. 1545 − 1630 = 45 min

Clinical Situations

1. 45 minutes, 5 miles
2. Give care, be available to play games, watch TV.
3. Explain that these actions are not part of your responsibilities.

Relating to the Nursing Process

1. Implementation
2. Planning
3. Assessment

UNIT 35 The Nursing Assistant in Home Care

Vocabulary Exercise

1.

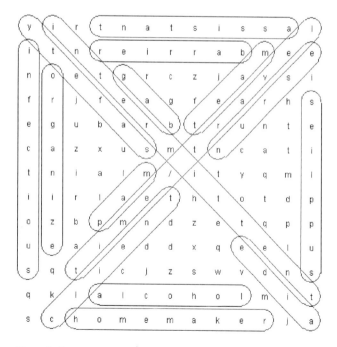

Completion

1. the care planning conference   2. purchases
3. daily   4. using, instructions
5. wipe, clothesline   6. mending
7. alone   8. give direct care
9. housekeeping service   10. household
11. honest   12. family routine

13. reusable   14. reported
15. disoriented or confused 16. germs

Short Answer

1. a. client's response to care
   b. interactions with others
   c. support services that might be needed
2. a. carry out approaches as indicated on care plan
   b. be efficient in work performance
3. a. be accurate and concise when reporting
   b. make honest appraisals
4. a. light housekeeping   b. shopping for meals
   c. preparing meals
5. a. washing windows   b. waxing floors
   c. moving heavy furniture
6. a. the home care agency   b. supervising nurse
   c. family member
   d. 911 or emergency numbers if 911 is not available
7. Wear gloves.
8. [Any combination of these answers is acceptable]
   • Be alert to conditions and people around you.
   • Inform the employer if you believe unsafe conditions exist.
   • Trust your instincts. If something doesn't feel right, it probably isn't.
   • Map out the route in advance.
   • Inform the patient of your anticipated time of arrival.
   • Lock purse in the trunk. Use a fanny pack or belt pack to carry essentials.
   • Wear scrubs or easily identifiable clothing.
   • In potentially dangerous areas, ask the agency to make joint visits with a coworker or use an escort.
   • If neighbors, relatives, or others become a safety problem, make visits when they are away from the home.
   • If a patient suggests a family member escort you, accept the offer, but never get into someone else's car.
   • Keep gas tank full.
   • Avoid parking on deserted streets or in dark areas.
   • Keep car windows up and doors locked.
   • Attend classes on personal safety and self-defense.
   • Purchase a cell phone.

True/False

1. T   2. T   3. F   4. T   5. F   6. F
7. F   8. F   9. T   10. F   11. T

Clinical Situations

1. Use extra pillows or cardboard backrest.
2. Put ice cubes in plastic bag, seal, wrap in towel, apply.
3. Use a bed tray.
4. Use a folded sheet as a lifter and get help.
5. Use a lightweight cotton blanket or spread or cotton sheet.
6. Entire bed can be put on blocks.
7. Use a shoebag attached to the bed.
8. Place pillowcase on back of chair as laundry bag.
9. Give enemas when ordered with reusable equipment; clean between uses.

10. Attach paper bag to bedframe, collect tissues, seal bag, burn if possible.
11. Report incident to supervisor, document, make no judgment.
12. a. Elevate head of bed on blocks
    b. Use plastic covered with twin sheet as bed protector
    c. Use extra pillows to change position
    d. Use cotton blanket or lightweight spread as bath blanket

Relating to the Nursing Process
1. Assessment   2. Assessment   3. Assessment, Evaluation

Unit 36 Subacute Care

Vocabulary Exercise
1. g   2. f   3. h   4. i   5. j
6. a   7. d   8. c   9. b   10. e

Completion
1. transitional   2. skilled nursing
3. 3 to 4 weeks   4. areas
5. participate   6. emotional
7. approaches   8. consistency
9. peripheral   10. hyperalimentation

Short Answer
1. Care of patients who are out of the acute phase of illness but still need highly skilled care, rehabilitation, and monitoring
2. a. homes   b. long-term care facilities
   c. assisted living facilities
3. a. work closely with nurses
   b. have extensive knowledge of patients and their conditions
   c. give care during complicated treatments and assist the nurse as directed
   d. have excellent observational skills
   e. be a contributing member of interdisciplinary care team
4. a. stroke   b. orthopedic surgery
   c. neurological disorders
5. a. medications   b. total parenteral nutrition
6. peripheral intravenous central catheter
7. a. change drip rate
   b. disconnect any tubing
   c. manipulate tubing and needle
   d. alter dressing over site
8. [Any combination of these answers is acceptable]
   • swelling of hands, feet, or face
   • changes in vital signs
   • changes in weight
   • variation in intake or output measurements
   • shortness of breath
   • complaint of pain at site of fistula or graft
9. [Any combination of these answers is acceptable]
   • catheter dislodgment   • changes in respiration
   • itching   • nausea, vomiting
   • change in mental status
10. a. changes in mental status   b. dislodged tube
    c. dyspnea or respiratory distress   d. need for suctioning

Completion
1. drip   2. full
3. tubing   4. lie
5. infiltration 6. junctions (connections)
7. leakage   8. dyspnea, cyanosis

True/False
1. T   2. F   3. F   4. T
5. T   6. F   7. T   8. T
9. T   10. F   11. T   12. T

Clinical Situations
1. a. daily weight in same clothes, same time, same scales
   b. take vital signs on arm opposite graft
   c. I&O
   d. restrict fluids
   e. special diet
2. The Kelly is used to clamp the central IV tubing close to the patient's body if the line breaks or is accidentally pulled loose. Air in the central intravenous line can cause fatal complications. Because of this, the Kelly clamp must be visible so it can be used quickly in an emergency.
3. The patient has both a pump and a spinal catheter implanted that are joined together during surgery. The medication pump incision is on the abdomen and the spinal catheter incision is on the mid-back.

Relating to the Nursing Process
1. Assessment, Evaluation   2. Assessment
3. Assessment, Evaluation

UNIT 37 Alternative, Complementary, and Integrative Approaches to Patient Care

Vocabulary Exercise
1. e   2. k   3. d   4. i   5. b   6. h
7. l   8. a   9. g   10. f   11. j   12. c

Completion
1. physician   2. osteopathy   3. yoga
4. privilege   5. herbal therapy 6. guided imagery
7. supplements   8. modalities   9. holistic
10. chelation   11. empowered   12. mind

Short Answer
1. [Any combination of these answers is acceptable]
   • Be sensitive to the patients' paths and choices.
   • Avoid passing judgment about patients' religious, spiritual, ethnic, and cultural practices and choices in health care treatment.
   • Pay attention to what the patient is saying.
   • Listen, reflect, and clarify information.
   • Avoid interpreting or defining spiritual meaning or truth to the patient.
   • Avoid imposing your beliefs on the patient.
   • Avoid pat, uncaring answers to questions.
   • Never give patients false hope.
   • Never use problem-solving techniques to analyze spiritual truths.

- Admitting you do not know an answer is all right.
- Be sensitive to patients' spiritual concerns.
- Provide privacy and support.
- Inform the nurse or social worker of the patient's concerns, as appropriate.

2. Prevent illness, enhance treatment of medical conditions, manage signs and symptoms.

3. [Any combination of these answers is acceptable]
   - toxicity
   - negative interactions with other medications and foods
   - risk of exceeding safe dosage range if combination products are used
   - interference with drugs and therapies used in treating other medical conditions
   - liver and kidney damage
   - harm to fetus in pregnancy
   - potential complications during surgery if physician does not know of alternative regimen

4. [Any combination of these answers is acceptable]
   - Alternative medical systems—Therapeutic or preventive health care practices that do not follow generally accepted methods and may not have a scientific explanation for their effectiveness. These treatments are usually based on complete systems of medical practice. Many were developed in other countries and have been used for centuries, predating conventional medical practices.
   - Mind-body therapy—Practices that employ various techniques to enhance the mind's ability to affect bodily function and symptoms (mind-over-matter principle). Many have been accepted by the medical community and are part of integrative health care practices and treatments.
   - Biological therapy—Biologically based practices using natural substances, such as vitamins, herbs, and foods. Other natural products, such as shark cartilage, are also used.
   - Body-based therapy—Practices that are based on direct body contact, including manipulation or movement of one or more parts of the body.
   - Energy therapy—The study of how living organisms interact with electromagnetic energy fields. Although some practitioners believe touch is necessary for healing, others believe they can effect healing by placing the hands within the field. Two types of energy therapy are commonly used. *Biofield therapies* work by laying hands on the body or through its energy field to transfer a healing force. The biofield may also be called an *aura*. The energy field is believed to permeate the body and extends outward for several inches. *Biomagnetic-based therapy* is a form of energy therapy in which the hands are placed in or through the energy field to apply pressure on the body.

5. In nursing, we look at and care for the whole person. We know that one weakness can affect the patient's overall

health and well-being. We anticipate and take preventive measures to support the weaknesses to strengthen the patient and prevent complications.

True/False

1. F   2. T   3. F   4. T   5. F
6. T   7. T   8. F   9. T   10. F
11. T   12. T   13. T

Vocabulary Exercise

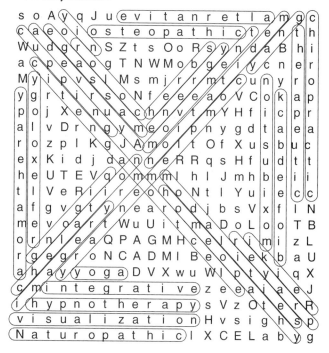

Relating to the Nursing Process

1. Planning, Implementation
2. Assessment
3. Implementation
4. Planning
5. Evaluation
6. Implementation
7. Evaluation, Assessment

SECTION 11 BODY SYSTEMS, COMMON DISORDERS, AND RELATED CARE PROCEDURES
UNIT 38 Integumentary System

Definitions

1. blue discoloration of skin due to lack of oxygen
2. scab
3. remove dead tissue
4. overweight
5. redness of skin
6. against current treatment
7. a sensitivity response to an allergen
8. changes in the tissue due to injury or disease
9. unusual paleness in the skin
10. dead tissue

Vocabulary Exercise

```
p e d i c u l o s i s q r l g c c a c w b
m a l o d o r o u s k o r h p y k o h a n
s c a b i e s g g x x d o j l k h k r o o
e s c h a r y b d e t b o v q l y r d u a
c t m d s l w w d o j e l u c a m u x b j
p o o o p z s n p g l d i p e l f r q c
m u n w b d b o u e y z x z o e a a s o c
i n r t g w f g e m q z i t s m s v l s b
t k o p u n w b e m p v j h o i d l y n e
e d u i u s o h e u p h j t o e o s v q r
s m l s t r j i t t q t a n c i u k w e l
s m q b h c a o t f v m c u d o b l v p j
m p g q d e i s n a e a b a e h v t a x g
r c b s l c a r h i i l n g x g g f y d
c r q k y d w r f m t r a j b s s s k b a
b a m b c f h c i u r t o y x a w u z i b
z d v d v b j h s n u e x c l m l k o n a
a g z q w j i u r c g x d j x p c e h i r
o k x q j j l s b l u b z i z e v p o o b
c s g k m t z u k p a p d y p v m w i b u
s b k k n n s u s y i k t v u e p m m g r
```

Anatomy Review

1. epidermis   2. dermis   3. sebaceous (oil) gland
4. hair shaf   5. sweat glands   6. artery

Completion

1. sensitivity
2. anaphylactic
3. contraindicated
4. gently, rubbing
5. prevented, cured
6. breasts, buttocks
7. first
8. covered
9. drainage, odor
10. blue-gray
11. pressure
12. infection
13. 1
14. disease, trauma, aging
15. special instruction
16. remain stationary or move in the opposite direction
17. fluid loss, pain
18. bridging
19. Elevate
20. hip
21. turned, 2 hours
22. blue, black
23. Abrasions
24. Contusions
25. ecchymosis
26. hematoma
27. Lacerations
28. senile purpura
29. Skin tears
30. pediculosis
31. Scabies
32. nodules

Short Answer

1. a. fever   b. lack of oxygen   c. dehydration
2. a. macule   b. excoriation   c. vesicle   d. scabs
3. a. elderly   b. very thin   c. obese   d. unable to move
4. a. change position at least every 2 hours
   b. wheelchair patients should raise themselves every 10 minutes
   c. proper nutrition and fluids
   d. keep skin dry and clean
   e. keep linens free from wrinkles
   f. bathe patient frequently
   g. massage around reddened areas

h. do not use lotion on broken areas
i. check areas of friction (under breasts, for example) frequently
j. check for improperly fitting braces or restraints
k. check body orifices with tubes for irritation
l. relieve pressure on susceptible areas
5. a. replace fluids and electrolytes to combat shock
   b. relieve pain and anxiety
   c. prevent contractures, deformities, infections
   d. provide emotional support and motivation
6. a. report pain
   b. maintain proper alignment
   c. use gentle positioning
   d. encourage high-protein diet
   e. give emotional support
   f. prevent infection
7. a. position patient properly
   b. use mechanical aids
   c. provide backrubs
   d. perform active/passive exercise
8. a. painful
   b. portal of entry for infectious microorganisms
   c. leads to further breakdown
9. High.
10. right side, left side, back, right side, left side
11. [Any combination of these answers is acceptable]
    • toes (if covered with bedding)
    • heels, sides of feet   • backs of knees
    • buttocks, hips   • sacrum, coccyx
    • elbows   • shoulders
    • back of ears   • back of head

Clinical Situations

1. Immerse your finger in cold water immediately or apply ice.
2. Report to nurse for special instructions; soap and lotions may be contraindicated.

Relating to the Nursing Process

1. Assessment   2. Implementation   3. Assessment
4. Implementation   5. Implementation   6. Assessment

Unit 39 Respiratory System

Vocabulary Exercise

1. dyspnea   2. expectorate   3. ventilation
4. trachea   5. cyanosis   6. pneumonia
7. alveoli   8. asthma   9. oxygen
10. larynx

Definitions

1. removing a small amount of tissue for examination
2. mucus/matter brought up from lungs
3. upper respiratory infection
4. shortness of breath
5. chronic obstructive pulmonary disease
6. tube inserted through stoma to keep it open
7. external opening of an ostomy
8. breathing stops for 10 seconds or more during sleep

Anatomy Review

1. Areas to be colored are:
   a. nose   b. pharynx   c. larynx   d. trachea
   e. bronchi   f. bronchioles   g. alveoli

Completion

1. mucus, bronchial, mucous membrane
2. persistent   3. feathers, food
4. elevation of temperature   5. alveoli
6. elasticity   7. oxygen
8. expiration   9. flow
10. Hypoxemia   11. washed, dried
12. stoma   13. laryngectomy
14. water, powder, lint, dust (or any foreign body)
15. Chest tubes   16. breathe

Short Answer

1. a. cover nose and mouth when coughing or sneezing
   b. dispose of soiled tissues in plastic or paper bag
   c. turn face away when coughing or sneezing
   d. wash hands after handling soiled tissues
2. a. dyspnea
   b. change in respiratory character
   c. presence and character of respiratory secretions
   d. any cough
3. a. assist in proper breathing techniques
   b. encourage breathing exercises
   c. position to improve ventilation
   d. assist with incentive spirometer
   e. assist with postural drainage
   f. provide care during oxygen therapy
   g. provide nutrition and fluids
   h. encourage patients to avoid crowds
   i. instruct patients to avoid going outdoors when temperature is 35 to 40 degrees or lower.
   j. discourage smoking
4. a. check gauge at each patient contact
   b. keep additional tank on hand
   c. return empty tank and replace
   d. be sure tank is secure and will not fall
5. [Any combination of these answers is acceptable]
   • immobility
   • bedrest
   • cardiac disease
   • pulmonary disease
   • postoperative patients for up to a week after surgery
   • sleep apnea
   • decreased level of consciousness
   • neuromuscular diseases
   • morbid obesity
   • kyphoscoliosis
   • trauma
6. [Any combination of these answers is acceptable]
   • tubing kinked, twisted, obstructed
   • vital signs change
   • pulse oximeter alarm sounds
   • dressing on the chest wall is loose
   • color or amount of drainage from the chest tube changes

• patient cough up blood
• patient becomes short of breath or cyanotic
• patient develops new swelling on the torso, neck, or face that "crackles" when touched
• the tube comes out of the chest wall

7. a. high Fowler's position
   b. overbed table with pillows, patient leaning forward on arms
   c. back supported by pillows
8. a. blowing against water resistance
   b. blowing a feather or ping pong ball across a table
   c. incentive spirometer
9. a. chest tapping   b. postural drainage
10. [Any combination of these answers is acceptable]
    • Avoid opening, touching, or spilling the container.
    • Flush with water if skin or clothing contacts liquid oxygen.
    • Never seal the cap or vent port on the bottle.
    • If a bottle falls or tips, evacuate the room and close the door.
    • Follow all regular oxygen safety precautions for preventing sparks and fires.

Hidden Picture

1. [Answers may be in any order, and any combination of these is acceptable]
   • electric razor on table
   • smoking cigarette
   • tank on left not chained or secured in carrier or base
   • tank on left is not capped or does not have a regulator attached (this makes it more unsafe because it is not secured)
   • tank on right not chained or secured in carrier or base
   • electric call bell
   • frayed call bell cord
   • kinked oxygen tube
   • bottle of alcohol on table (flammable)
   • no "oxygen in use" signs posted
   • candle burning on table
   (The lack of a humidifier on the oxygen tank is not an error.)

Clinical Situations

1. Report at once to nurse.
2. Provide mouth care.
3. Check with nurse to make sure oxygen can be discontinued temporarily. If so, provide patient with safety razor and discontinue flow of oxygen while patient is shaving.
4. rinse mouth with water
5. Brown, James   604
   12/30/xx   689473
   Smith   culture and sensitivity
   Sputum

Relating to the Nursing Process

1. Implementation   2. Implementation
3. Assessment   4. Implementation
5. Implementation   6. Implementation
7. Planning

Unit 40 Circulatory (Cardiovascular) System

Vocabulary Exercise
1. anemia—decrease in quality or quantity of blood
2. aorta—largest artery
3. embolus—moving blood clot
4. ischemia—loss of blood supply
5. thrombus—stationary blood clot
6. hypertrophy—increase in size
7. angina—cardiac pain
8. diuresis—temporary increase in urinary output
9. atheroma—roughened area
10. dyscrasias—abnormalities

Anatomy Review
1. tricuspid
2. bicuspid (mitral)
3. pulmonary semilunar
4. aortic semilunar
5. blue—SVC, IVC, right atrium, right ventricle, pulmonary arteries; red—pulmonary veins, aorta, left atrium, left ventricle
6. left lung
7. left atrium
8. left ventricle
9. right ventricle
10. inferior vena cava
11. right atrium
12. right lung
13. superior vena cava
14. aorta
    A. blood enters right atrium from vena cava
    B. blood goes from right ventricle to lungs
    C. blood returns to left atrium
    D. blood leaves left ventricle, travels to aorta

Completion
1. renal, pulmonary
2. peripheral
3. dyscrasias
4. arterial, venous
5. sodium
6. open
7. replaces
8. ischemic

Short Answer
1. [Any combination of these answers is acceptable]
   - keeping the feet clean and drying them well after bathing
   - checking the feet and legs daily; reporting abnormalities
   - protecting the feet from injury
   - making sure the patient is wearing properly fit footwear when out of bed
   - making sure the patient wears socks under shoes
   - not allowing the patient to ambulate barefoot or wearing only socks
   - not cutting toenails
   - not using sharp objects such as a nail file on the toes
   - making sure bed linen is not too tight on the feet; using a bed cradle, if ordered
   - checking the skin under support hose regularly; removing the hose periodically, according to the care plan
   - making sure footwear is not too tight
   - propping bedfast patients' calves on pillows so the heels are elevated from the surface of the bed, or positioning patients so the heels hang over the end of the mattress with the soles of the feet against a footboard
   - making sure the feet are supported on footrests when the patient is using the wheelchair, avoid dragging feet

2. a. skin color changes
   b. skin temperature changes
   c. changes in pulse rate or character
   d. changes in blood pressure
   e. edema
3. a. coldness   b. tingling   c. loss of sensitivity
   d. headaches   e. dizziness   f. memory lapses
4. a. brain   b. heart   c. legs
5. a. diabetes mellitus   b. lack of exercise
   c. obesity   d. heredity
   e. stress   f. diet high in fats, cholesterol
   g. smoking
6. a. exercise   b. proper diet
   c. reduction of stress   d. control of smoking and obesity
7. a. myocardial infarction   b. coronary occlusion
   c. coronary thrombosis   d. coronary embolism
8. a. signs of recurrence   b. bleeding   c. vital signs
9. a. peripheral edema   b. moist lung sounds
   c. cyanosis   d. changes in pulse rate and rhythm
10. a. low sodium diet
    b. careful monitoring of I&O
    c. daily weighing of patient
    d. measure apical heart rate
    e. assist with oxygen therapy
    f. position patient in orthopneic or high Fowler's position
    g. assist with activities of daily living

True/False
1. F   2. T   3. F   4. T
5. F   6. T   7. F   8. T
9. T   10. F   11. T

Clinical Situations
1. Try to calm the situation, because stress could precipitate an attack. Notify the nurse.
2. Remove it. The patient would be on a low-sodium diet.
3. Take the pulse apically and report findings to nurse.
4. Check I&O carefully. Check for edema. Weigh patient daily, report findings to nurse.
5. Report to nurse—may be a TIA.

Relating to the Nursing Process
1. Assessment
2. Implementation
3. Implementation
4. Implementation
5. Assessment

UNIT 41 Musculoskeletal System

Vocabulary Exercise
1. bursitis
2. cartilage
3. comminuted
4. supination
5. vertebrae
6. extension
7. adduction
8. dorsiflexion

Anatomy Review

1. bones are colored as follows
   a. femur—red   b. humerus—blue   c. ribs—brown
   d. ulna—green   e. radius—red   f. sternum—brown
   g. pelvis—blue   h. cranium—green   i. tibia—yellow

Matching

1. o   2. i   3. e   4. n   5. h
6. c   7. f   8. a   9. b   10. d
11. g   12. e   13. j   14. l   15. m
16. p

Completion

1. exercised   2. contracture   3. abduction
4. adduction   5. opposition   6. internal rotation
7. bursae   8. arthritis   9. fracture
10. compound   11. balanced

Short Answer

1. a. joints become stiff and deformed
   b. muscles atrophy and lose strength
   c. bones lose minerals
   d. general circulation slows
2. a. check for special instructions
   b. never exercise a joint to point of pain
   c. perform each exercise 3 to 5 times
   d. stop exercise if pain develops
   e. support above and below the part being exercised
3. a. joint immobilization
   b. weight control
   c. relieve pain and reduce inflammation
   d. physical therapy to maintain mobility
   e. surgery if joints are badly damaged
4. a. pins, nails   b. screws   c. bone plates
   d. cast   e. traction
5. a. CircOlectric bed   b. Stryker frame
6. a. support cast in good alignment
   b. turn patient frequently to allow air circulation to all parts of cast
   c. never use fingers to support cast
   d. observe extremities for color and temperature
   e. pad rough areas of cast to prevent friction
   f. turn patient to non-casted side
   g. always support cast
   h. supply and encourage use of trapeze
7. a. do not disturb weights
   b. keep patient in good alignment
   c. check for areas of pressure
   d. keep straps, halters, and belts smooth
8. a. straightening angle of a joint
   b. moving away from body center
   c. rolling away from center of body
   d. pointing sole of foot outward
   e. pointing sole of foot inward
   f. palms down
   g. turning wrist toward thumb side
   h. turning wrist toward little finger
   i. toes pointed down
   j. toes pointed up

9. a. odor   b. drainage
10. [Any combination of these answers is acceptable]
    • A trapeze is attached to the bed.
    • The patient is instructed to avoid pressing down on the affected foot.
    • Anti-embolism stockings are applied.
    • A fracture bedpan is used initially; an elevated toilet seat is used later.
    • The head of the bed is not elevated more than 45° without a specific order.
    • Avoid acute flexion of the hip and legs.
    • An abduction pillow may be ordered to keep the legs apart.
    • Avoid crossing the legs.
11. [Any combination of these answers is acceptable]
    • apply anti-embolism hosiery
    • do exercises to unaffected leg
    • apply sequential compression therapy
    • avoid elevating head more than 45° without specific permission
    • avoid acute hip flexion
    • use abduction pillow
    • give continuous passive motion therapy
12. a. enhances circulation, reduces risk of blood clots
    b. reduces edema
    c. promotes collagen formation to enhance healing
    d. reduces scarring
    e. decreases stiffness
    f. improves range of motion
    g. reduces risk of complications, such as contractures and adhesions
    h. helps reduce pain
13. a. untreated infections
    b. unstable fractures
    c. known or suspected blood clots (deep vein thrombosis)
    d. hemorrhage
14. a. fever   b. increasing redness or irritation
    c. increasing warmth   d. edema
    e. bleeding   f. increased or persistent pain
15. [Any combination of these answers is acceptable]
    • severe pain, especially when muscle is moved
    • pain out of proportion to injury
    • severe pain when the muscle is gently stretched
    • tenderness when the area is touched gently
    • pain on deep breathing (in some patients)
    • tingling
    • burning
    • numbness
    • feeling tight or full in the affected muscle
    • abnormal sensations in the affected area
    • weakness or inability to use the muscle
    • color of the extremity may appear pale, cyanotic, or red
    • skin of an extremity with no cast may feel warm to touch
    • fingers or toes of a casted extremity may feel cool to touch
    • edema
    • loss of the pulse in the extremity

16. a. greenstick   b. complete (simple)
    c. complete (compound)   d. comminuted
17.

Form	Tissue Affected	Possible Cause	Age Affected
Rheumatoid Arthritis	Joint tissues, especially the lining	autoimmune	any age
Osteoarthritis	Cartilage found at the bone ends	aging, trauma, obesity	older age group

18. A. Never cross affected leg over midline of body.
    B. Never internally rotate hip on affected side.

Clinical Situations

1. Report to the nurse immediately.
2. Check her position and adjust for comfort if necessary. Use nursing comfort measures listed on the care plan. Promptly inform the nurse that the patient says the pain has not been relieved.
3. Remain in the room and call for help by yelling, using the call signal, or telephone. Avoid moving the patient until the nurse gives instructions.
4. The patient will probably need to sit in a shower chair. Cover the cast with a plastic bag and secure the top well before turning the water on.
5. Do not start the CPM unit. Inform the nurse immediately.
6. Inform the nurse immediately.
7. Do not force activity; report observations and complaints to nurse.
8. When positioning extremity, avoid abduction and flexion of hips and avoid flexion of knee.

Relating to the Nursing Process

1. Implementation
2. Implementation
3. Assessment, Implementation
4. Implementation
5. Assessment
6. Implementation
7. Implementation
8. Planning

UNIT 42 Endocrine System

Vocabulary Exercise

1. glucose
2. hormone
3. morbidity
4. thyroxine
5. glycosuria
6. adrenal
7. iodine
8. glands
9. sperm

Definitions

1. basal metabolic rate
2. more than normal production of secretions
3. increase in size of organ or structure
4. proportion of deaths in population
5. excessive thirst
6. excessive muscular contraction

Anatomy Review

1. ovaries—red
2. thyroid gland—green
3. pituitary gland—blue
4. parathyroid glands—black
5. adrenal gland—brown
6. pancreas—red
7. pineal body—green
8. testes—yellow

Completion

1. hormones
2. control
3. cool
4. reduce
5. hypertrophies
6. calcium, phosphates
7. tetany
8. Cushing's syndrome
9. stress
10. American Diabetes Association, U.S. Public Health Service
11. household
12. exercise
13. hypoglycemic
14. diabetic coma (hyperglycemia)
15. hypoglycemia
16. freshly
17. inspecting
18. podiatrist or RN
19. barefoot
20. thyroid function
21. feet

Short Answer

1. Irritable, restless, nervous, tense, increased pulse rate, increased appetite, weight loss, sensitive to heat.
2. a. signs of bleeding
   b. signs of respiratory distress
   c. inability to speak
   d. greatly elevated temperature and pulse
   e. pronounced apprehension and irritability
   f. numbness, tingling, or muscle spasm
3. a. heredity   b. age
   c. obesity   d. sedentary lifestyle, lack of exercise
   e. improper diet
4. a. eye disease
   b. renal disease
   c. circulatory impairment, which may lead to gangrene and amputation
   d. poor healing
   e. cardiovascular complications
   f. hypertension
   g. diabetic coma
   h. insulin shock
5. Important role, weight reduction encouraged.
6. a. stress   b. illness   c. dehydration
   d. injury   e. forgotten medication   f. poor diet
7. a. unusual activity
   b. stress
   c. vomiting
   d. diarrhea
   e. omission of planned snack, skipping meals
   f. interaction of drugs
   g. forgotten medication   h. illness
8. [Any combination of these answers is acceptable]
   - know signs and symptoms of insulin shock and diabetic coma
   - be alert for signs and symptoms of insulin shock and diabetic coma
   - know location of easily assimilated carbohydrates
   - keep easily assimilated carbohydrates on hand
   - serve correct tray
   - do not give extra nourishment without permission
   - document food consumed
   - report uneaten food to nurse
   - give special foot care
   - test urine for acetone if instructed to do so

9. a. polyuria b. polydipsia c. polyphagia d. glycosuria
10. a. insulin-dependent diabetes mellitus
    b. non-insulin-dependent diabetes mellitus
11. a. wash daily, dry carefully
    b. report abnormalities
    c. keep area between toes dry
    d. have podiatrist give care
    e. inspect carefully
    f. use well-fitting shoes, clean socks
12.

	Diabetic Coma	Insulin Shock
Respirations	deep	shallow
Pulse	full and bounding	rapid and weak
Skin	hot, dry, and flushed	pale and moist

Clinical Situations

1. Do not awaken for AM care; keep NPO; provide bedpan if needed; maintain quiet, restful environment.
2. Report to nurse; patient may have NIDDM.
3. Report to nurse immediately.
4. Assist patient into semi-Fowler's position; support neck and shoulders.

Relating to the Nursing Process

1. Assessment
2. Implementation
3. Implementation
4. Assessment
5. Assessment
6. Assessment, Implementation

UNIT 43 Nervous System

Vocabulary Exercise

1. cochlea
2. chorea
3. nerve
4. neurotransmitter
5. hemiplegia
6. hemiparesis
7. diplegia
8. cornea
9. tremors
10. intracranial
11. axon
12. monoplegia
13. tetraplegia
14. paraplegia

Definitions

1. difficulty and slowness in carrying out voluntary muscle activities
2. small bones in middle ear
3. inability to express and understand language
4. membranes that surround brain and spinal cord
5. involuntary trembling
6. loss of voluntary muscle control
7. tingling, shock-like sensation that passes down neck and spinal column when spine is flexed
8. paralysis of all four extremities
9. jerky eye movements
10. seizure

Anatomy Review

1. movement—red
2. hearing—yellow
3. pain and other sensations—green
4. seeing—brown
5. speech and language—blue
6. spinal cord—black

Completion

1. intracranial
2. brain attack
3. brain
4. language
5. frustration
6. ministrokes
7. age
8. pressure to the affected eye
9. sharp pain
10. middle ear, fusion
11. wet
12. cold
13. monitoring
14. paralysis
15. Mental
16. overfull bladder
17. increased

Short Answer

1. a. alteration in pupil size
   b. headache
   c. vomiting
   d. loss of consciousness or sensation
   e. paralysis
   f. convulsions
2. a. speak in short, concise sentences
   b. use gestures
   c. speak often with patient to provide practice
   d. be patient and supportive of patient's attempts to communicate
3. a. position patient on side, elevate bed to semi-Fowler's height
   b. keep side rails up
   c. change position every 2 hours
   d. apply elastic hose if ordered
   e. monitor vital signs
   f. check catheter drainage
   g. maintain open airway
   h. carry out ROM exercises as ordered
4. a. fatigue that may be debilitating
   b. new joint and muscle pain
   c. new weakness in muscles affected by polio; unaffected muscles are also affected; may be more prominent on one side of the body
   d. new dyspnea and other respiratory problems
   e. severe cold intolerance
   f. muscle spasms and cramps

g. difficulty swallowing

h. difficulty falling asleep and waking frequently during the night

5. a. cold, violent shivering

   b. drug side effects

   c. blood loss

   d. respiratory problems due to muscle weakness and lung problems

   e. repositioning, need for support of body parts

   f. vomiting; fainting if the patient is upright

   g. choking on secretions

   h. transfers, ambulation

6. a. positioning

   b. range of motion and light exercise

   c. incentive spirometry

   d. conserving muscle strength, encouraging adequate rest

   e. small, frequent feedings

   f. swallowing precautions to prevent choking

   g. not washing solid foods down with liquids

   h. checking the mouth after meals; providing mouth care promptly after each meal

   i. scheduling rest and activities to preserve the patient's strength and energy

   j. preventing infection

7. a. Changes in patient before the seizure, such as an aura, confusion, or change in behavior

   b. Description of the way the seizure looked, including body parts involved

   c. Loss of bowel or bladder control, eyes rolling upward, rapid blinking, biting tongue

   d. The time the seizure started and stopped, if known

   e. Condition of the patient after the seizure

   f. Vital signs

8. [Any combination of these answers is acceptable]
   • overfull bladder
   • urinary retention
   • urinary infection
   • blocked catheter
   • overfilled urinary drainage bag
   • constipation or fecal impaction
   • hemorrhoids
   • infection or irritation in the abdomen, such as appendicitis or acute abdominal conditions
   • pressure ulcers
   • prolonged pressure by an object in the chair, shoe, sitting on wrinkled clothing, etc.
   • minor injury, such as cut, bruise, or abrasion
   • ingrown toenails
   • burns, including sunburn
   • pressure on the skin from tight or constrictive clothing
   • menstrual cramps
   • labor and delivery
   • overstimulation during sexual activity
   • fractured bones

9. a. blood pressure over 200/100

   b. severe headache

   c. red, flushed face

d. red blotches on the skin above the level of spinal injury

e. sweating above the level of spinal injury

f. stuffy nose

g. nausea

h. bradycardia

i. goose bumps below the level of injury

j. cold, clammy skin below the level of injury

10. a. prevent injury

    b. maintain open airway

11. a. regular turning

    b. proper positioning

    c. ROM exercises

12. a. lip reading

    b. sign language

13. a. momentary loss of awareness, may involve erratic behavior

    b. bilateral generalized motor movements and muscular rigidity, loss of consciousness, aura may be present

    c. continuous state of convulsions

True/False

1. T   2. T   3. F   4. T   5. T

6. F   7. T   8. T   9. F

Clinical Situations

1. Provide airway, loosen clothing, turn head to one side, move articles out of way so patient doesn't strike them, stay with patient, ring for assistance.

2. Report this to the nurse immediately.

3. Since she is in a private room, check with the nurse to see if the bed can be moved to the opposite wall or turned around. Caution her to call for help when getting up. Make sure the call signal is in reach.

4. Inform the nurse of the problem promptly. Always follow the care plan approaches for feeding. Have the patient rest before meals. Provide small, frequent feedings. When feeding, take swallowing precautions and use positions and techniques recommended by the speech language pathologist to prevent choking. Unless instructed otherwise, position the patient as upright as possible with the neck flexed slightly forward at mealtime. Avoid washing solids down with liquids. Check the mouth for food particles and provide mouth care after meals.

Relating to the Nursing Process

1. Assessment   2. Implementation

3. Implementation   4. Assessment, Implementation

5. Implementation   6. Assessment, Implementation

7. Implementation

UNIT 44 Gastrointestinal System

Vocabulary Exercise

1. cholecystectomy   2. gastrectomy

3. colostomy   4. defecation

5. colon   6. hernia

7. impaction   8. flatus

9. urgency   10. gastric

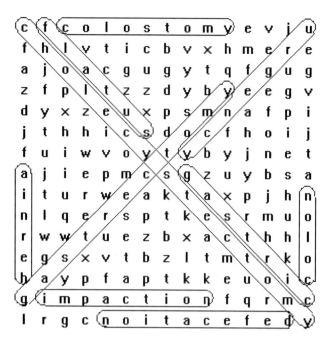

Definitions

1. hydrochloric acid
2. gallstones
3. rhythmic waves of alimentary tract
4. repair of hernia
5. severest form of constipation
6. feeding through tube
7. savory, meaty, or protein taste
8. pertaining to groin
9. tiny bumps on the tongue; tastebuds
10. tap water enema

Anatomy Review

1. esophagus—blue
2. stomach—yellow
3. small intestines—green
4. liver—red
5. gallbladder—black
6. colon—blue
7. appendix—brown
8. pancreas—blue

Completion

1. malignancies
2. accidental tube removal
3. colostomy
4. watery stools
5. low-residue
6. HCl, ulcer
7. mouth care
8. fat
9. drains
10. semi-Fowler's
11. enemas, diet
12. soap and water
13. left Sims'
14. before
15. doctor's order
16. soap-solution
17. 2 to 4 inches
18. 12 inches, anus
19. cool
20. distention
21. peristalsis
22. long as possible
23. once
24. gloves, hands
25. *H. pylori*

Short Answer

1. a. fresh blood on dressing   b. increased jaundice
   c. darkened urine
2. [Any combinations of these answers is acceptable]
   - aging
   - disease

- surgery
- diet that does not contain enough fiber, fruits, or vegetables
- medications
- lack of privacy
- bedrest
- inactivity, immobility
- inadequate exercise
- inability to chew foods properly
- loose or missing teeth
- inadequate fluid intake
- stress
- change in environment
- change in diet

3. [Any combination of these answers is acceptable]
   - complaints of constipation or inability to pass stool
   - abdominal or rectal pain
   - nausea
   - loss of appetite
   - feeling the need to have a bowel movement, but cannot
   - passing excessive flatus
   - bloating and abdominal distention
   - frequent urination
   - inability to empty the bladder
   - leaking around the catheter
   - mental confusion
   - fever
   - liquid stool or mucus seeping from the rectum

4. a. cleanse colon before X-rays
   b. before surgery
   c. before testing
   d. bowel retraining programs
   e. to relieve constipation

5. a. date and time
   b. type of enema and amount of solution
   c. character of returned solution
   d. patient reaction

Clinical Situations

1. Wait one hour before administering enema.
2. Clamp tube, encourage patient to take deep breaths, wait a few minutes.
3. Give routine postoperative care; position in semi-Fowler's; do not disturb drains; report increase of jaundice, dark urine, fresh bleeding.
4. Encourage to deep breathe, insert suppository beyond sphincter.

Relating to the Nursing Process

1. Implementation   2. Implementation   3. Implementation
4. Implementation   5. Assessment

UNIT 45 Urinary System

Vocabulary Exercise

1. dysuria—painful urination
2. hematuria—blood in urine
3. hydronephrosis—enlarged kidney
4. kidneys—organs that produce urine

5. retention—unable to eliminate urine from bladder
6. ureter—tube leading from kidney to urinary bladder
7. nephritis—inflammation of kidney
8. cystitis—inflammation of bladder
9. glomeruli—units in kidney that produce urine

Definitions

1. decreased urinary output   2. kidney stones
3. intravenous pyelogram   4. inability to secrete urine
5. tube for evacuating or injecting fluid
6. tube-like opening

Anatomy Review

1. right kidney—red   2. ureters—blue
3. bladder—green   4. urethra—yellow
5. adrenal glands—brown   6. left kidney cortex—red
7. left kidney medulla—blue   8. left kidney pelvis—yellow

Completion

1. women   2. sitz
3. encouraged   4. elevated
5. produce urine   6. obstructions
7. colic   8. hematuria
9. strained   10. forced
11. crush   12. hydronephrosis
13. balloon   14. sterile, nurse, physician
15. male   16. closed drainage system
17. sterile   18. 15
19. refrigerated   20. 120 mL
21. meatus   22. empty
23. collected

Short Answer

1. a. frequency of urination   b. hematuria
   c. dysuria   d. bladder spasm
2. a. absolute bedrest   b. low-sodium diet
   c. vital signs frequently   d. fluids may be restricted
3. Check drainage tubing to be sure there are no kinks and note amount and type of drainage.
4. a. bleeding   b. pain
   c. chilling   d. elevated temperature
   e. increased edema   f. reduced output
5. a. French (straight)   b. Foley (indwelling)
6. [Any combination of these answers is acceptable]
   • make sure tubes are in good position and unblocked
   • measure and record intake and output
   • keep end of drainage tube above urine in bag
   • do not permit drainage bag to touch floor
   • keep bag below patient's hip level
   • coil drainage tube on bed with direct drop to bag
   • do not disconnect catheter
   • Secure the catheter to the leg (or abdomen) with a catheter strap or tape.
7. a. tip of drainage tube   b. end of catheter

Clinical Situations

1. Use catheter care kit, drape patient, clean meatus, check drainage tube and collection bag, measure output and record.
2. Remove condom, clean genitalia, replace with new condom, check tubing and drainage bag, measure and record output.

3. Place graduate or paper towel on floor under bottom of drainage bag, open tubing and allow urine to flow into graduate, reclose tubing, measure and record output.
4. a. empty bag more often
   b. have straight drop of tubing from catheter
   c. tension on catheter must be minimal
   d. use proper technique when connecting and disconnecting

Relating to the Nursing Process

1. Assessment   2. Implementation
3. Implementation   4. Implementation
5. Implementation   6. Implementation
7. Implementation   8. Implementation
9. Implementation

UNIT 46 Reproductive System

Vocabulary Exercise

1. endometrium   2. rectocele   3. genitalia
4. mastectomy   5. testes   6. uterus
7. oviduct   8. vagina   9. scrotum
10. sterility   11. gonorrhea   12. vaginitis

Anatomy Review

Male tract
Pathway of sperm: testes, epididymis, ejaculatory duct, urethra—red
1. urinary bladder—yellow   2. penis—blue
3. testis—brown   4. prostate gland—green
Female tract (internal)
Pathway of egg: ovary, oviduct, uterus, vagina—red
5. uterine walls—yellow   6. right ovary— blue
7. right oviduct—green
Female tract (external)
8. labia majora—red   9. clitoris—yellow
10. urinary meatus—green   11. labia minora—blue

Completion

1. hypertrophy   2. urethra
3. retention   4. emotionally
5. Foley catheter   6. month
7. shower   8. vaginal
9. incontinence   10. fungal
11. Pap smear   12. D & C
13. salpingectomy   14. back
15. leukorrhea   16. unaware
17. placenta   18. inflammation, scarring
19. orchiectomy   20. brachytherapy
21. replication   22. immune system
23. cure

Short Answer

1. a. reproduction   b. sexual expression
   c. hormone production
2. a. do not stress or dislodge tubes
   b. note color, character, and amount of drainage
   c. report sudden increase in bright redness or clots in tubing
   d. report wet dressing
   e. be patient and understanding
   f. refer questions relating to sexual function and urinary incontinence to nurse

g. provide emotional support

h. wear personal protective equipment and apply the principles of standard precautions

i. assist with elimination as needed

j. keep patient clean and dry

3. So hormones will still be produced.

4. a. monthly on last day of period

b. one selected day each month after menopause

c. routinely and faithfully

d. with fingertips

e. using rolling motion

f. be sure to include axillae

5. a. at least once each month

b. during warm shower

c. with soapy fingers

d. palpating testes between fingers and thumb

6. a. hemorrhoids   b. constipation

7. Slowing of pelvic blood supply can result in clot formation.

8. a. painless lump or mass   b. nipple discharge

c. retraction of nipple   d. scaly skin around nipple

e. dimpling of skin   f. enlarged lymph nodes

Clinical Situations

1. Refer questions to nurse.

2. Explain that a lumpectomy removes only the lump and a small amount of breast tissue.

3. Refer concerns to nurse.

Relating to the Nursing Process

1. Assessmen   2. Assessment   3. Assessment

4. Implementation   5. Assessment

SECTION 12 EXPANDED ROLE OF THE NURSING ASSISTANT

UNIT 47 Caring for the Patient with Cancer

Vocabulary Exercise

1.

```
                              B
      P A L L I A T I V E
                    M       N
                    M       I
                    U       G
        M A L I G N A N T
                    O       R   B
            M E T A S T A S I S
                    H       D   O
      C A R C I N O G E N     I   P
                    R       A   S
                    A       T   Y
  C H E M O T H E R A P Y   I
  A             Y       O
  N                     N
  C
  E
  R
```

Completion

1. cell growth

2. oxygen, nutrients

3. benign

4. metastasize

5. malignant

6. carcinogen

7. one or more

8. monthly

9. testicular, monthly

10. biopsy

11. Chemotherapy

12. eat, drink, chew gum

13. handling

14. Radiation therapy

15. Immunotherapy

16. severe

Short Answer

1. [Any combination of these answers is acceptable]

- age
- lifestyle and habits
- family history, genetics
- environmental pollution
- harmful substances in the environment
- chemicals
- radiation
- prolonged sun exposure
- infections and some viruses

2. a. no more than 30% of total calories from fat

b. total cholesterol from diet should not exceed 300 mg a day

c. at least 55% of total calories from complex carbohydrates

d. salt from all food sources should not exceed 1 teaspoon a day

3. a. not smoking

b. limiting intake of alcoholic beverages

c. following the food guide pyramid and eating a healthy diet

d. regular exercise

e. maintaining a healthy weight

f. avoiding sun exposure, particularly between 10:00 AM and 3:00 PM

g. get genetic testing and counseling if at risk for familial cancers

4. C = Change in bowel or bladder habits

A = A sore that does not heal

U = Unusual bleeding or discharge

T = Thickening or lump in the breast, testicles, or any part of the body

I = Indigestion or difficulty swallowing

O = Obvious change in a wart, mole, or skin condition

N = Nagging cough or hoarseness

5. a. alopecia, or hair loss

b. nausea and vomiting

c. anorexia, loss of appetite

d. anemia

e. fatigue

f. low white blood cell count, increased risk of infection

g. fewer platelets, increased risk of bleeding

h. destruction of the mucous membranes of the mouth, causing burning, pain, redness, and breakdown inside the mouth

6. [Any combination of these answers is acceptable]

- fever over 101°F
- chilling
- swelling, redness, irritation inside the mouth

- rectal pain or tenderness
- change in bowel or bladder habits
- pain or burning on urination
- redness, swelling, open area, or pain on the skin
- cough or shortness of breath
- decreased level of consciousness
- decreased urine output
- warm, flushed, dry skin

7. a. fatigue   b. nausea, vomiting
   c. diarrhea   d. skin redness, irritation, peeling
   e. change in taste   f. irritation of mucous membranes
   g. cough   h. shortness of breath
8. a. Do not remain in the patient's room any longer than necessary.
   b. Stay at least three feet away from the patient unless direct care is being given.
   c. Inform the nurse if an implant comes out of a body cavity (if so, do not touch it).
   d. Find out if special precautions are necessary for handling soiled linens, tissues, or dressings.
   e. Inform the nurse if you are pregnant or suspect you may be pregnant.
9. a. fever or chills
   b. pulse over 100, respirations over 24
   c. cyanosis
   d. shortness of breath
   e. restless, apprehensive
   f. diarrhea, nausea, or vomiting
   g. complaints of itching
10. [Any combination of these answers is acceptable]
    - spend as much time as possible with the patient if he or she wants to talk
    - encourage/allow the patient to talk about feelings and fears
    - develop proficiency at providing physical care and assistance with ADLs
    - anticipate patients' needs before they ask
    - respect the patient's beliefs and wishes
    - provide emotional support
    - respect the patient's privacy if he or she wants to be alone
    - make the patient feel respected and valued as a person
    - avoid giving the patient false hope

True/False
1. T   2. T   3. F   4. F   5. T
6. T   7. T   8. T   9. F   10. T
11. F   12. T   13. T   14. F   15. F
16. T   17. T   18. T   19. T   20. F
21. T   22. T   23. F   24. F   25. F

Relating to the Nursing Process
1. Evaluation, Assessment   2. Planning   3. Assessment
4. Evaluation   5. Implementation

UNIT 48 Rehabilitation and Restorative Services

Vocabulary Exercise
1. handicap   2. physiatrist   3. adaptive devices
4. restorative care   5. disability

Completion
1. optimum level of performance   2. disability
3. rehabilitation   4. problems, care
5. strength   6. influence
7. self-care deficit   8. disease or injury
9. retraining   10. same approach

Short Answer
1. a. increase in physical abilities
   b. preventing complications
   c. maintenance of current abilities
   d. adaptation to specific limitations
   e. increased quality of life
2. a. bathing   b. hair and nail care
   c. dressing and undressing   d. eating
   e. toileting   f. mobility
   g. oral care
3. a. adapt to present circumstances
   b. learn to direct others who give the care
   c. use adaptive devices to increase independence
4. a. physical therapist   b. occupational therapist
   c. speech therapist   d. psychologist
   e. social worker
5. a. procedures to prevent complications
   b. mobility skills
   c. personal care
   d. bowel and bladder training programs
   e. maintaining nutritional status
   f. programs to increase patient independence
6. a. treatment begins as soon as possible
   b. stress the patient's ability, not disability
   c. activity strengthens and inactivity weakens
   d. treat the whole person
7. a. decreased strength   b. lack of endurance
   c. limited range of motion   d. depression
   e. disorientation
   f. perceptual deficit
8. a. inability to organize a task
   b. lack of judgment
   c. inability to identify common objects
   d. inability to use common objects
   e. inability to initiate a task
   f. inability to sequence a task
9. a. setup   b. verbal cues
   c. hand-over-hand technique   d. demonstration
10. An environment in which caregivers are consistent, that promotes maintenance or improvement, is arranged to maximize independence and self-esteem, and addresses the importance of quality of life.

Clinical Situations
1. Keep directions simple but not childish.
2. Avoid distractions; do ADLs in private.
3. Be patient and encouraging; realize that progress may be uneven and inconsistent.
4. Know reason for self-care deficit; read care plan and follow carefully for consistency.
5. Use adaptive devices correctly and consistently.
6. Collect needed items, prepare bath, help patient with bath.

7. Use verbal cues with each action.
8. Use gestures to simulate brushing the teeth (demonstration) while simultaneously using verbal cues. If this is ineffective, progress to hand-over-hand technique.
9. Remember that mental and physical activity are essential to patient well-being.
10. a. restoration   b. rehabilitation, restoration
    c. rehabilitation   d. rehabilitation
    e. restoration   f. rehabilitation
    g. restoration

Relating to the Nursing Process
1. Implementation   2. Implementation
3. planning   4. Assessment

UNIT 49 Obstetrical Patients and Neonates

Vocabulary Exercise
1. lochia   2. neonate   3. fetal
4. episiotomy   5. umbilical   6. placenta
7. efface   8. amniotic

Definitions
1. transabdominal perforation of amniotic sac to obtain sample
2. vaginal discharge after childbirth
3. after birth
4. milk production
5. incision in perineum to avoid laceration
6. newborn
7. top of uterus
8. afterbirth
9. to open up or enlarge
10. fluid that surrounds the growing fetus in the uterus

Completion
1. obstetrical   2. 1, 3
3. morning sickness, amenorrhea, darkening of area around the nipples
4. umbilical cord   5. placenta
6. bonding   7. fetoscopy
8. uterine contractions, cervix   9. thins
10. fetal monitor   11. identified
12. cesarean   13. head
14. bleeding   15. back, hand
16. back   17. before, after, diaper
18. each time diaper is changed   19. blood
20. his or her own   21. massage
22. 6 to 8   23. hemorrhage
24. returning to normal (contracting)   25. retention
26. gloves, inward, paper towel   27. toilet
28. circular, nipple   29. infant, one, five
30. good   31. temperature
32. length   33. 7 to 10
34. doura

Short Answer
1. The nine-month period is divided into three separate three-month periods, each called a trimester.
2. a. complaints of persistent headache
   b. elevated blood pressure, vaginal bleeding
   c. complaints of dizziness
   d. swelling of hands and feet
3. a. epidural   b. regional caudal block
   c. pudendal block
4. a. allows mother to be awake and to participate
   b. encourages a person to act as coach for mother
   c. necessitates little if any pain control medication
5. [Any combination of these answers is acceptable]
   • supporting the mother
   • comforting the mother
   • enhancing communication between the mother and the medical professionals
   • remaining with patient during labor and delivery
   • helping family adjust to new member
6. a. check vital signs   b. check perineum
   c. check vaginal flow   d. check surgical dressing
7. a. ice packs   b. sitz bath   c. anesthetic sprays
8. a. provides antibodies   b. has a mild laxative effect
9. a. heart rate   b. respiratory effort
   c. muscle tone   d. reflex irritability
   e. color of skin
10. a. wash hands and nipples before feeding
    b. during shower, wash breasts with circular motion from nipples outward
    c. apply lotion to nipples between feedings
    d. use breast pads if leaking
    e. wear well-fitting support bra
11. a. grasp ankles, lifting legs and buttocks with one hand
    b. slide the other hand under the buttocks to shoulders and neck to support head

Clinical Situations
1. Instruct her to squeeze her buttocks together and hold them in this position until seated upright.
2. Mother and baby are cared for in a single unit.
3. a. provide clean gown and linen
   b. check level and firmness of uterus
   c. check vital signs
   d. check perineum
   e. check flow and discharge

Identification
1. a. umbilical cord   b. placenta
   c. uterus   d. fetal membranes
   e. rectum   f. cervix
   g. vagina   h. bladder

Relating to the Nursing Process
1. Assessment   2. Implementation
3. Assessment   4. Assessment, Implementation
5. Implementation   6. Assessment

UNIT 50 Pediatric Patients

Vocabulary Exercise
a. fantasies   b. foster   c. siblings
d. regress   e. infant   f. deviate
g. school-age   h. adolescent   i. pediatric
j. autonomous   k. developmental

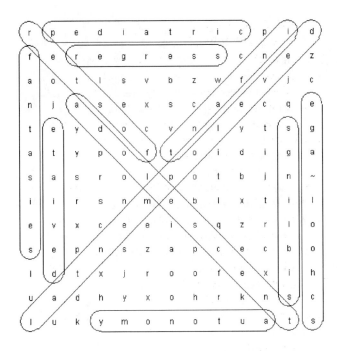

Completion

1. a. by age   b. by condition
2. The parent(s), legal guardian(s).
3. a. child's likes and dislikes
   b. normal times for common activities
   c. nickname
   d. routines
4. It allows primary caregiver to participate in care. Parent and child both benefit.
5. a. double birth length   b. triple birth weight
6. Development of motor skills, rolling over, sitting up, crawling, and walking.
7. Learning to trust.
8. By feeding, holding, touching, talking to infant, and keeping infant warm and dry.
9. 6 or 7 months of age
10. a. mirrors   b. mobiles   c. rattles
11. So that she can sleep after eating.
12. Weigh self; hold toddler and weigh both; subtract your weight.
13. a. crying   b. fever   c. infection
14. Before.
15. Use a pacifier.
16. The words the child uses for elimination.
17. That body parts will be injured or changed.
18. Use time references such as naptime or mealtime.
19. Allow to assist in own care.
20. As authority figures.
21. The adolescent's friends.
22. Straighten the ear canal prior to inserting the thermometer.
23. Attach a self-adhesive urine collection bag.
24. [Any combination of these factors is acceptable]
    - type 2 diabetes
    - sleep apnea
    - hypertension

- skin disorders
- weight-related orthopedic problems
- gallstones
- depression
- risk factors for atherosclerosis and other cardiac problems

25. Interrupted sleep inhibits the ability to learn; school performance is not as good as that of children with no sleep problem. Sleep disorders are believed to reduce cognitive function, which may permanently damage the growing child. Children with sleep disorders have lower scores on IQ tests and do not perform as well on tests measuring verbal skills and word usage than children with no sleep disorder.
26. Overweight and obese children are often teased and tormented by their peers. Many suffer from low self-esteem.
27. body image.

True/False

1. T   2. F   3. F   4. F   5. T
6. T   7. F   8. F   9. T   10. T
11. F   12. T   13. F   14. T   15. T
16. T   17. F   18. F   19. T   20. F
21. F   22. T

Clinical Situations

1. Understand that regression is common; the child needs comfort.
2. Ignore as long as she cannot hurt herself or others; set firm and consistent limits.
3. Allow him to read or listen to music with headphones.

Relating to Nursing Process

1. Assessment   2. Implementation
3. Implementation   4. Implementation
5. Planning

UNIT 51 Special Advanced Procedures

Vocabulary Exercise

1. appliance—bag used with colostomy or ileostomy to collect drainage from stoma
2. ileostomy—surgical opening into small bowel
3. ostomy—surgical opening
4. port—opening
5. stoma—artificial, surgical opening
6. colostomy—surgical opening into colon

Completion

1. infection   2. stool specimen   3. urination
4. port   5. 30 minutes   6. alcohol
7. nurse   8. liquid, digestive   9. irritating
10. solvent   11. legal   12. not be
13. wear gloves   14. tongue blade   15. gently (carefully)

Short Answer

1. a. all invasive procedures
   b. procedures in which the skin is broken, such as injections, and inserting intravenous needles or catheters
   c. procedures in which body cavities are entered, such as catheterization and tracheal suctioning

d. changing surgical dressings

e. changing dressings on central intravenous catheters

f. procedures involving patients with severe destruction of the skin, such as burns and trauma

2. a. tube clamp   b. completed label
   c. emesis basin   d. 10-mL syringe
   e. specimen cup and lid   f. 21- or 22-gauge needle
   g. alcohol sponges   h. gloves
   i. plastic bag

3. a. keep area clean and dry
   b. use colostomy bag to collect drainage
   c. perform routine stoma care

4. a. basic preparation
   b. experience
   c. special advanced training in skills
   d. state regulations

5. Urine in bag has accumulated over a long period of time.

6. With alcohol.

7. a. leakage   b. odor   c. irritation

8. Location of the ostomy.

True/False

1. T   2. F   3. F   4. T   5. T
6. F   7. T   8. F   9. F   10. F
11. F   12. T   13. T   14. T   15. F
16. T   17. T   18. F   19. F   20. F
21. T

Clinical Situations

1. Remove feces with toilet paper, gently wash with soap and warm water.
2. There may be too much barrier cream; wipe some off.
3. Use a commercial guide.
4. Skin care to prevent irritation, proper fitting of appliance ring to prevent leakage.

Relating to the Nursing Process

1. Implementation   2. Assessment   3. Assessment

SECTION 13 RESPONSE TO BASIC EMERGENCIES

UNIT 52 Response to Basic Emergencies

Vocabulary Exercise

1. trauma   2. arrest   3. fainting
4. incident   5. emergency   6. heart attack
7. shock   8. elevate   9. CPR
10. hemorrhage

Completion

1. danger   2. American Red Cross
3. American Heart Association   4. skill, knowledge
5. emotions   6. evaluate
7. call, quiet   8. 911
9. the tongue, jaw   10. brain
11. 30, 2   12. urgent care
13. unit   14. abdominal
15. see   16. shock
17. lying   18. cardiac arrest

19. pattern   20. harming
21. confused, disoriented   22. wood

Short Answer

1. a. keep calm   b. use a quiet voice
   c. keep onlookers away   d. proceed in methodical way

2. a. name of caller
   b. location
   c. description of scene
   d. information about types of injuries
   e. type of help needed

3. a. immediate care for victim
   b. care needed if medical help is delayed

4. Most hospitals have a core group of personnel who work in more than one facility; also, personnel periodically change jobs. In some types of codes, all health care workers must respond. In others, workers on all units must implement specific safety measures when a code is called. The margin for error is great. Having standardized code words makes them easier to remember and eliminates confusion.

5. a. ring emergency alarm
   b. use signal cord or phone
   c. ask another patient to signal
   d. call out for assistance

6. a. look for chest movement
   b. listen and feel for flow of air by putting your ear near victim's nose and mouth

7. a. degree of consciousness   b. airway
   c. heart rate   d. bleeding
   e. signs of shock

8. Victim clasps throat with neck extended, unable to speak, high-pitched sounds on inhalation.

9. a. identify bleeding area
   b. apply continuous direct pressure
   c. increase pressure and padding if necessary
   d. raise and support wounded area above heart level
   e. apply pressure over pressure point
   f. keep person comfortably warm and quiet

10. a. pale, cool, moist skin   b. complaints of weakness
    c. rapid pulse   d. irregular tachypnea
    e. restlessness and anxiety

11. a. crushing chest pain radiating up jaw and down arm
    b. face pale or grayish, perspiring
    c. absence of breathing
    d. loss of consciousness
    e. cardiac arrest

Clinical Situations

1. Get person away from danger of explosion.
2. Turn off source of electricity before touching victim.
3. Stand behind victim, position hands for abdominal thrusts, and carry out Heimlich maneuver.

Relating to the Nursing Process

1. Assessment   2. Assessment, Implementation
3. Implementation   4. Implementation
5. Implementation

SECTION 14 MOVING FORWARD
UNIT 53 Employment Opportunities and Career Growth

Vocabulary Exercise
1. résumé—a short account of one's career and qualifications, prepared by an applicant for a position
2. networking—communication between individuals with a common interest or goal
3. interview—meeting with a prospective employer
4. reference—statements about your abilities and characteristics by someone who knows you

Completion
1. assets, limitations
2. solutions
3. employment
4. responsibilities
5. networking
6. résumé
7. permission
8. relatives
9. neat, clean
10. time
11. knowledgeable
12. pleasant (positive)

Short Answer
1. a. facilities in your area
   b. the type of work you desire
   c. shifts that have openings
   d. the person to contact for information or interview
2. [Any combination of these answers is acceptable]
   - age
   - number of children
   - sex
   - weight
   - marital status
   - religion
   - height

Practical Applications
1. Make a list, which might include doctors' offices, blood banks, clinics, hospices, long-term care facilities, hospitals, rehabilitation centers.
2. Phone book, classified ads, facility where you had clinical experiences, talking with friends.

3. a. prepare several copies
   b. keep a copy for yourself
   c. type the résumé
   d. carry a copy with you when you seek employment
   e. use résumé as ready reference
   f. update résumé regularly
4. a. preparation
   b. participation in interview
   c. write a thank-you note
5. a. arrive on time
   b. perform as taught
   c. be flexible
   d. follow rules of ethical and legal conduct
   e. be open and ready to learn and grow
6. a. read nursing journals
   b. enroll in general education courses
   c. participate in staff development programs
   d. enroll in minicourses on health subjects
   e. read books relating to health issues
   f. research programs leading to advancement

True/False
1. T   2. T   3. T   4. F   5. T
6. T   7. T   8. T   9. T   10. T

Résumé Writing
1. areas to be covered:
   a. name, address, telephone number
   b. educational background
   c. work history
   d. other related experiences
   e. references
   f. personal information about interest and activities
2–3. [Application and letter of resignation will be unique for each student.]

PROCEDURE EVALUATION   Student _____

STUDENT PERFORMANCE RECORD

Your teacher will evaluate each procedure you learn and perform, but it will be helpful if you also keep a record so you will know which experiences you still must master.

PROCEDURE		Satisfactory	Marginal	Unsatisfactory
UNIT 13 Infection Control				
Procedure 1	Handwashing			
Procedure 2	Putting on a Mask			
Procedure 3	Putting on a Gown			
Procedure 4	Putting on Gloves			
Procedure 5	Removing Contaminated Gloves			
Procedure 6	Removing Contaminated Gloves, Mask, and Gown			
Procedure 7	Serving a Meal in an Isolation Unit			
Procedure 8	Measuring Vital Signs in an Isolation Unit			
Procedure 9	Transferring Nondisposable Equipment Outside of Isolation Unit			
Procedure 10	Specimen Collection from Patient in an Isolation Unit			
Procedure 11	Caring for Linens in an Isolation Unit			
Procedure 12	Transporting Patient to and from the Isolation Unit			
Procedure 13	Opening a Sterile Package			
UNIT 15 Patient Safety and Positioning				
Procedure 14	Turning the Patient Toward You			
Procedure 15	Turning the Patient Away from You			
Procedure 16	Moving a Patient to the Head of the Bed			
Procedure 17	Logrolling the Patient			

PROCEDURE	Satisfactory	Marginal	Unsatisfactory
UNIT 16 The Patient's Mobility: Transfer Skills			
Procedure 18 Applying a Transfer Belt			
Procedure 19 Transferring the Patient from Bed to Chair—One Assistant			
Procedure 20 Transferring the Patient from Bed to Chair—Two Assistants			
Procedure 21 Sliding-Board Transfer from Bed to Wheelchair			
Procedure 22 Transferring the Patient from Chair to Bed—One Assistant			
Procedure 23 Transferring the Patient from Chair to Bed—Two Assistants			
Procedure 24 Independent Transfer, Standby Assist			
Procedure 25 Transferring the Patient from Bed to Stretcher			
Procedure 26 Transferring the Patient from Stretcher to Bed			
Procedure 27 Transferring the Patient with a Mechanical Lift			
Procedure 28 Transferring the Patient onto and off the Toilet			
UNIT 17 The Patient's Mobility: Ambulation			
Procedure 29 Assisting the Patient to Walk with a Cane and Three-Point Gait			
Procedure 30 Assisting the Patient to Walk with a Walker and Three-Point Gait			
Procedure 31 Assisting the Falling Patient			
UNIT 18 Body Temperature			
Procedure 32 Measuring Temperature Using a Sheath-Covered Thermometer			
Procedure 33 Measuring an Oral Temperature (Electronic Thermometer)			
Procedure 34 Measuring a Rectal Temperature (Electronic Thermometer)			
Procedure 35 Measuring an Axillary Temperature (Electronic Thermometer)			
Procedure 36 Measuring a Tympanic Temperature			

PROCEDURE	Satisfactory	Marginal	Unsatisfactory
UNIT 19 Pulse and Respiration			
Procedure 37 Counting the Radial Pulse			
Procedure 38 Counting the Apical-Radial Pulse			
Procedure 39 Counting Respirations			
UNIT 20 Blood Pressure			
Procedure 40 Taking Blood Pressure			
Procedure 41 Taking Blood Pressure with an Electronic Blood Pressure Apparatus			
UNIT 21 Measuring Height and Weight			
Procedure 42 Weighing and Measuring the Patient Using an Upright Scale			
Procedure 43 Weighing the Patient on a Chair Scale			
Procedure 44 Measuring Weight with an Electronic Wheelchair Scale			
Procedure 45 Measuring and Weighing the Patient in Bed			
UNIT 22 Admission, Transfer, and Discharge			
Procedure 46 Admitting the Patient			
Procedure 47 Transferring the Patient			
Procedure 48 Discharging the Patient			
UNIT 23 Bedmaking			
Procedure 49 Making a Closed Bed			
Procedure 50 Opening the Closed Bed			
Procedure 51 Making an Occupied Bed			
Procedure 52 Making the Surgical Bed			
UNIT 24 Patient Bathing			
Procedure 53 Assisting with the Tub Bath or Shower			
Procedure 54 Bed Bath			

PROCEDURE		Satisfactory	Marginal	Unsatisfactory
Procedure 55	Changing the Patient's Gown			
Procedure 56	Waterless Bed Bath			
Procedure 57	Partial Bath			
Procedure 58	Female Perineal Care			
Procedure 59	Male Perineal Care			
Procedure 60	Hand and Fingernail Care			
Procedure 61	Bed Shampoo			
Procedure 62	Dressing and Undressing the Patient			

UNIT 25 General Comfort Measures

Procedure 63	Assisting with Routine Oral Hygiene			
Procedure 64	Assisting with Special Oral Hygiene			
Procedure 65	Assisting the Patient to Floss Teeth and Brush Teeth			
Procedure 66	Caring for Dentures			
Procedure 67	Backrub			
Procedure 68	Shaving a Male Patient			
Procedure 69	Daily Hair Care			
Procedure 70	Giving and Receiving the Bedpan			
Procedure 71	Giving and Receiving the Urinal			
Procedure 72	Assisting with Use of the Bedside Commode			

UNIT 26 Nutritional Needs and Diet Modifications

Procedure 73	Assisting the Patient Who Can Feed Self			
Procedure 74	Feeding the Dependent Patient			

UNIT 27 Warm and Cold Applications

Procedure 75	Applying an Ice Bag			
Procedure 76	Applying a Disposable Cold Pack			
Procedure 77	Applying an Aquamatic K-Pad			
Procedure 78	Giving a Sitz Bath			
Procedure 79	Assisting with Application of a Hypothermia Blanket			

PROCEDURE		Satisfactory	Marginal	Unsatisfactory
UNIT 29 The Surgical Patient				
Procedure 80	Assisting the Patient to Deep Breathe and Cough			
Procedure 81	Performing Postoperative Leg Exercises			
Procedure 82	Applying Elasticized Stockings			
Procedure 83	Applying Elastic Bandage			
Procedure 84	Applying Pneumatic Compression Hosiery			
Procedure 85	Assisting the Patient to Dangle			
UNIT 32 Death and Dying				
Procedure 86	Giving Postmortem Care			
UNIT 36 Subacute Care				
Procedure 87	Checking Capillary Refill			
Procedure 88	Using a Pulse Oximeter			
UNIT 39 Respiratory System				
Procedure 89	Collecting a Sputum Specimen			
UNIT 41 Musculoskeletal System				
Procedure 90	Procedure for Continuous Passive Motion			
Procedure 91	Performing Range-of-Motion Exercises (Passive)			
UNIT 42 Endocrine System				
Procedure 92	Obtaining a Fingerstick Blood Sugar			
UNIT 43 Nervous System				
Procedure 93	Caring for the Eye Socket and Artificial Eye			
Procedure 94	Applying Warm or Cool Eye Compresses			
UNIT 44 Gastrointestinal System				
Procedure 95	Collecting a Stool Specimen			
Procedure 96	Giving a Soap-Solution Enema			

PROCEDURE		Satisfactory	Marginal	Unsatisfactory
Procedure 97	Giving a Commercially Prepared Enema			
Procedure 98	Inserting a Rectal Suppository			

UNIT 45 Urinary System

Procedure 99	Collecting a Routine Urine Specimen			
Procedure 100	Collecting a Clean-Catch Urine Specimen			
Procedure 101	Collecting a 24-Hour Urine Specimen			
Procedure 102	Routine Drainage Check			
Procedure 103	Giving Indwelling Catheter Care			
Procedure 104	Emptying a Urinary Drainage Unit			
Procedure 105	Disconnecting the Catheter			
Procedure 106	Applying a Condom for Urinary Drainage			
Procedure 107	Connecting a Catheter to a Leg Bag			
Procedure 108	Emptying a Leg Bag			

UNIT 46 Reproductive System

Procedure 109	Giving a Nonsterile Vaginal Douche			

UNIT 49 Obstetrical Patients and Neonates

Procedure 110	Changing a Diaper			
Procedure 111	Bathing an Infant			

UNIT 50 Pediatric Patients

Procedure 112	Admitting a Pediatric Patient			
Procedure 113	Weighing the Pediatric Patient			
Procedure 114	Changing Crib Linens			
Procedure 115	Changing Crib Linens (Infant in Crib)			
Procedure 116	Measuring Temperature			
Procedure 117	Determining Heart Rate (Pulse)			
Procedure 118	Counting Respiratory Rate			
Procedure 119	Measuring Blood Pressure			
Procedure 120	Bottle-Feeding an Infant			

PROCEDURE		Satisfactory	Marginal	Unsatisfactory
Procedure 121	Burping an Infant			
Procedure 122	Collecting a Urine Specimen from an Infant			

UNIT 51 Special Advanced Procedures

Procedure 123	Testing for Occult Blood Using Hemoccult and Developer			
Procedure 124	Collecting a Urine Specimen Through a Drainage Port			
Procedure 125	Removing an Indwelling Catheter			
Procedure 126	Giving Routine Stoma Care (Colostomy)			
Procedure 127	Routine Care of an Ileostomy (with Patient in Bed)			
Procedure 128	Setting Up a Sterile Field Using a Sterile Drape			
Procedure 129	Adding an Item to a Sterile Field			
Procedure 130	Adding Liquids to a Sterile Field			
Procedure 131	Applying and Removing Sterile Gloves			
Procedure 132	Using Transfer Forceps			

UNIT 52 Response to Basic Emergencies

Procedure 133	Head-Tilt, Chin-Lift Maneuver			
Procedure 134	Jaw-Thrust Maneuver			
Procedure 135	Mask-to-Mouth Ventilation			
Procedure 136	Positioning the Patient in the Recovery Position			
Procedure 137	Heimlich Maneuver—Abdominal Thrusts			
Procedure 138	Assisting the Adult Who Has an Obstructed Airway and Becomes Unconscious			
Procedure 139	Obstructed Airway: Infant			
Procedure 140	Child with Foreign Body Airway Obstruction			

TRANSPARENCY MASTER 1   **ALPHABET**

CAPITAL LETTERS

small letters

NUMERALS

NURSING ORGANIZATIONAL CHART

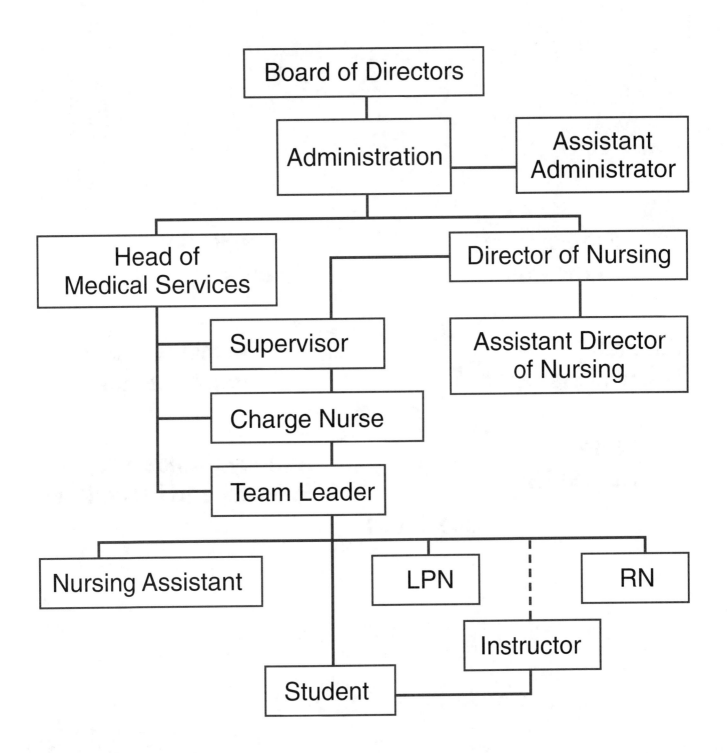

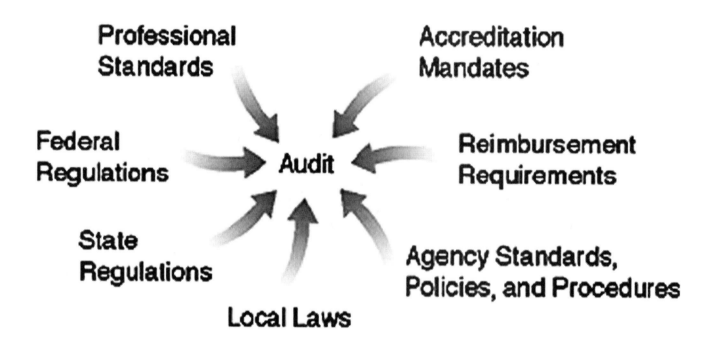

TRANSPARENCY MASTER 4

PLANES OF THE BODY

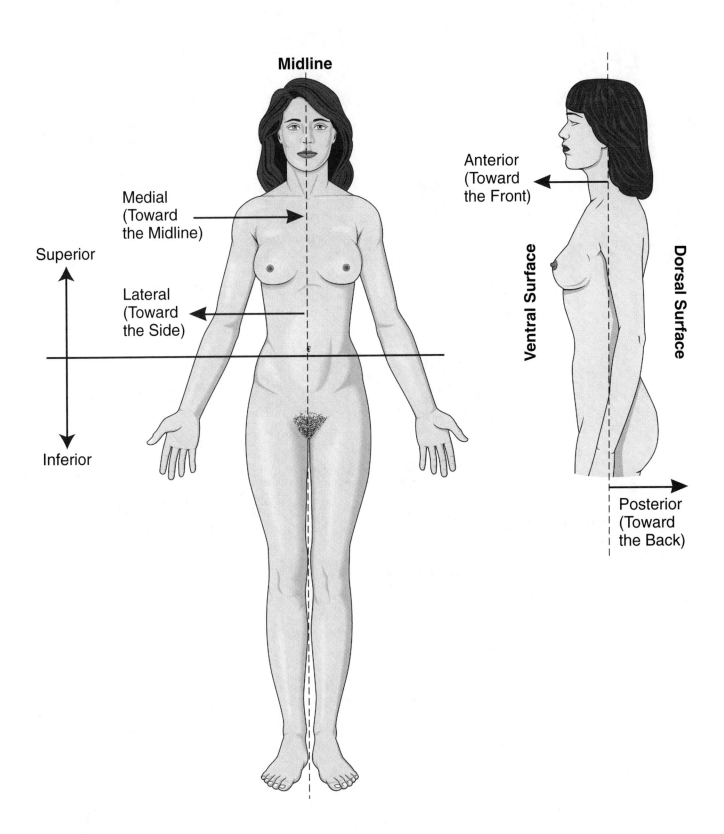

Midline

Medial
(Toward
the Midline)

Superior

Lateral
(Toward
the Side)

Inferior

Anterior
(Toward
the Front)

Ventral Surface

Dorsal Surface

Posterior
(Toward
the Back)

TRANSPARENCY MASTER 5   **LATERAL VIEW OF BODY CAVITIES**

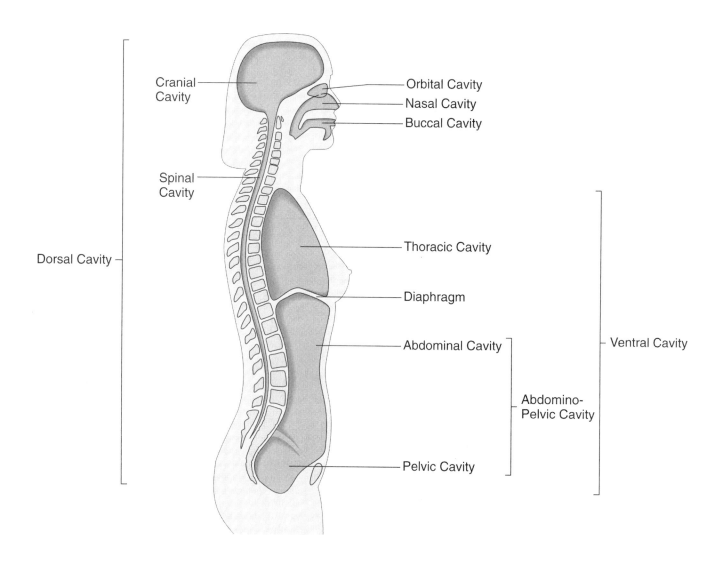

Cranial Cavity

Orbital Cavity

Nasal Cavity

Buccal Cavity

Spinal Cavity

Dorsal Cavity

Thoracic Cavity

Diaphragm

Abdominal Cavity

Ventral Cavity

Abdomino-Pelvic Cavity

Pelvic Cavity

ABDOMINAL QUADRANTS

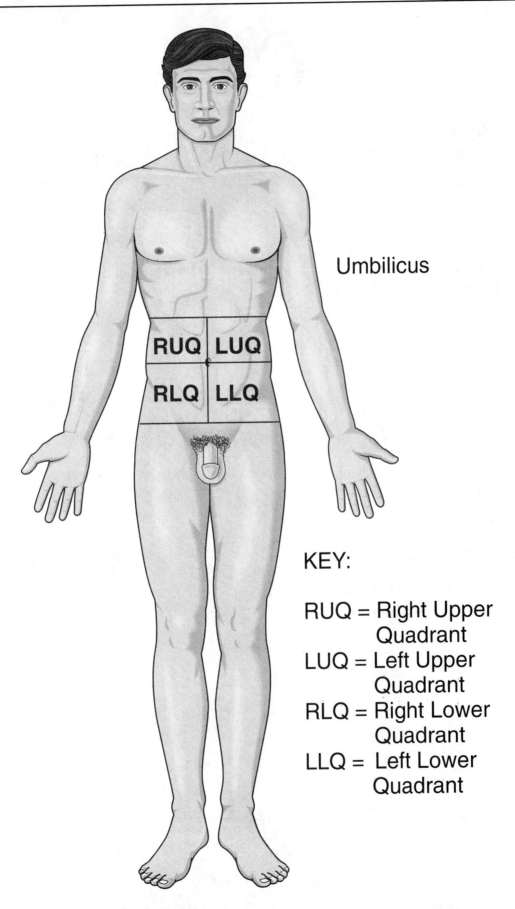

Umbilicus

RUQ | LUQ

RLQ | LLQ

KEY:

RUQ = Right Upper
          Quadrant
LUQ = Left Upper
          Quadrant
RLQ = Right Lower
          Quadrant
LLQ = Left Lower
          Quadrant

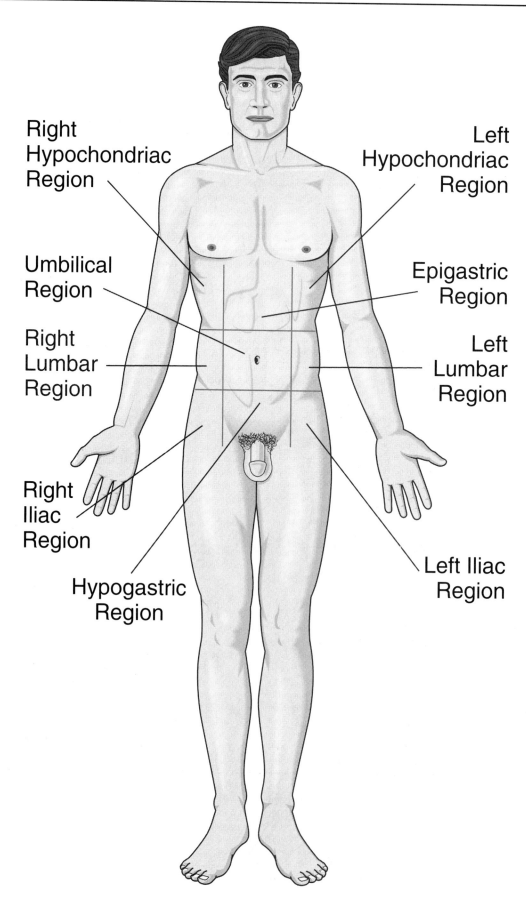

Right Hypochondriac Region

Left Hypochondriac Region

Umbilical Region

Epigastric Region

Right Lumbar Region

Left Lumbar Region

Right Iliac Region

Left Iliac Region

Hypogastric Region

TRANSPARENCY MASTER 8   **SYSTEMS OF THE BODY**

System	Function	Structures
Cardiovascular, lymph	Transports materials around the body; carries oxygen and nutrients to the cells and carries waste products away; part of the immune system that provides protective cells and chemicals to fight current infections and protect against future infections	Heart, arteries, capillaries, veins, spleen, lymph nodes, lymphatic vessels, blood,
Endocrine	Produces hormones that regulate body processes	Pituitary gland, thyroid gland, parathyroid glands, thymus gland, adrenal glands, testes, ovaries, pineal body, islets of Langerhans in pancreas
Gastrointestinal (Digestive)	Digests, transports food, absorbs nutrients, and eliminates wastes	Mouth, esophagus, pharynx, stomach, small intestine, large intestine, salivary glands, teeth, tongue, liver, gallbladder, pancreas
Integumentary	Protects the body from injury and against infection, regulates body temperature, eliminates some wastes	Skin, hair, nails, sweat and oil glands
Skeletal	Supports and protects body parts, produces blood cells, acts as levers in movement	Bones, joints
Muscular	Protects organs by forming body walls, forms walls of some organs, assists in movement by changing position of bones at joints	*Smooth* muscles—form walls of organs *Skeletal* muscles—attached to bones *Cardiac* muscles—form wall of heart
Nervous	Coordinates body functions	Brain, spinal cord, spinal nerves, cranial nerves, special sense organs such as eyes and ears
Reproductive	Reproduces the species, fulfills sexual needs, develops sexual identity	*Male:* Testes, epididymis, urethra, seminal vesicles, ejaculatory duct, prostate gland, bulbourethral glands, penis, spermatic cord *Female:* Breasts, ovaries, oviducts, uterus, vagina, Bartholin glands, vulva
Respiratory	Brings in oxygen and eliminates carbon dioxide	Sinuses, nose, pharynx, larynx, trachea, bronchi, lungs
Urinary	Manages fluids and electrolytes of body, eliminates liquid wastes	Kidneys, ureters, urinary bladder, urethra

TRANSPARENCY MASTER 9   **CROSS-SECTION OF THE SKIN**

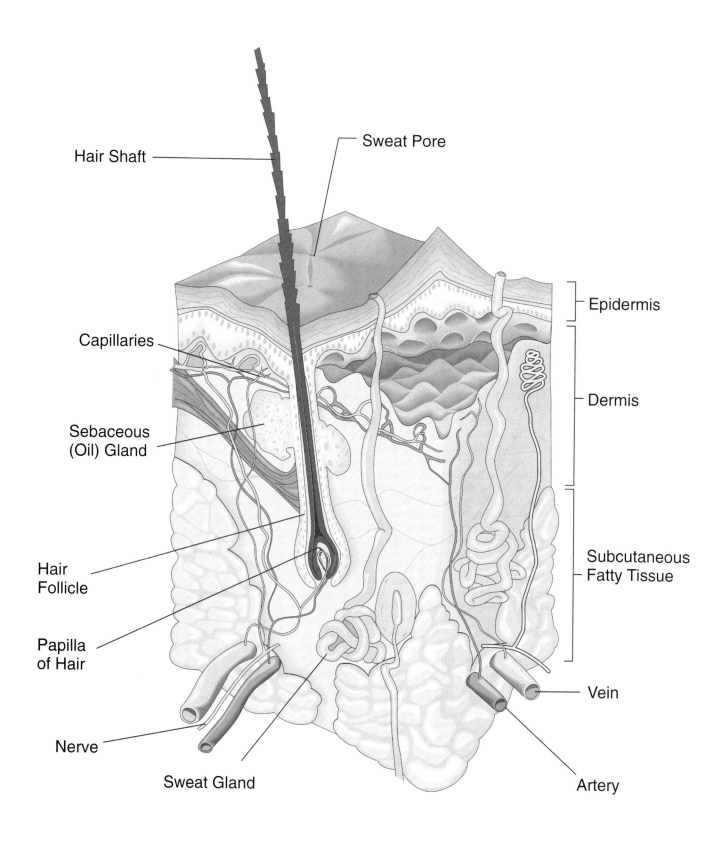

Hair Shaft

Sweat Pore

Epidermis

Capillaries

Dermis

Sebaceous
(Oil) Gland

Hair
Follicle

Subcutaneous
Fatty Tissue

Papilla
of Hair

Vein

Nerve

Sweat Gland

Artery

TRANSPARENCY MASTER 10A

ANTERIOR VIEW OF THE SKELETAL SYSTEM

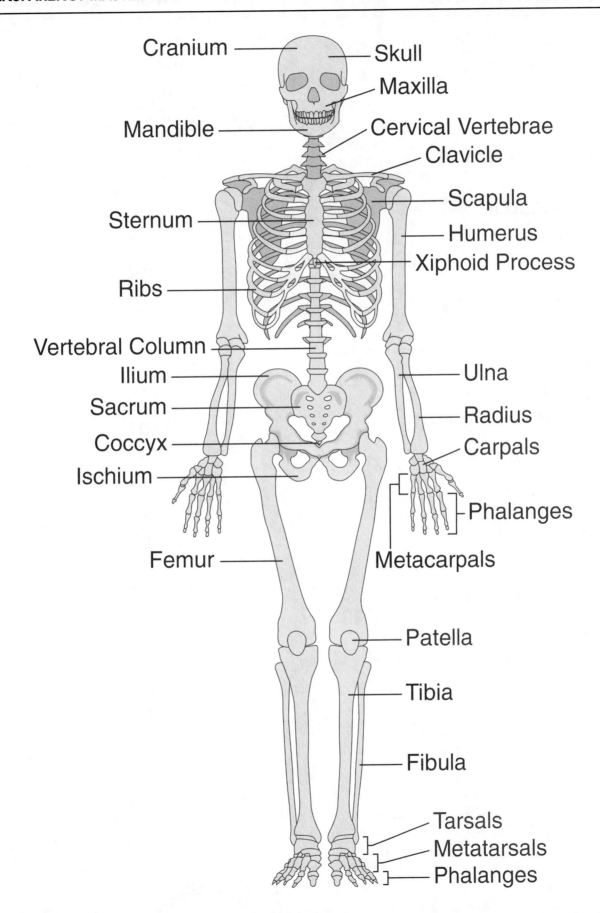

Cranium — Skull
Maxilla
Mandible — Cervical Vertebrae
Clavicle
Scapula
Sternum — Humerus
Xiphoid Process
Ribs
Vertebral Column
Ilium — Ulna
Sacrum — Radius
Coccyx — Carpals
Ischium
Phalanges
Metacarpals
Femur
Patella
Tibia
Fibula
Tarsals
Metatarsals
Phalanges

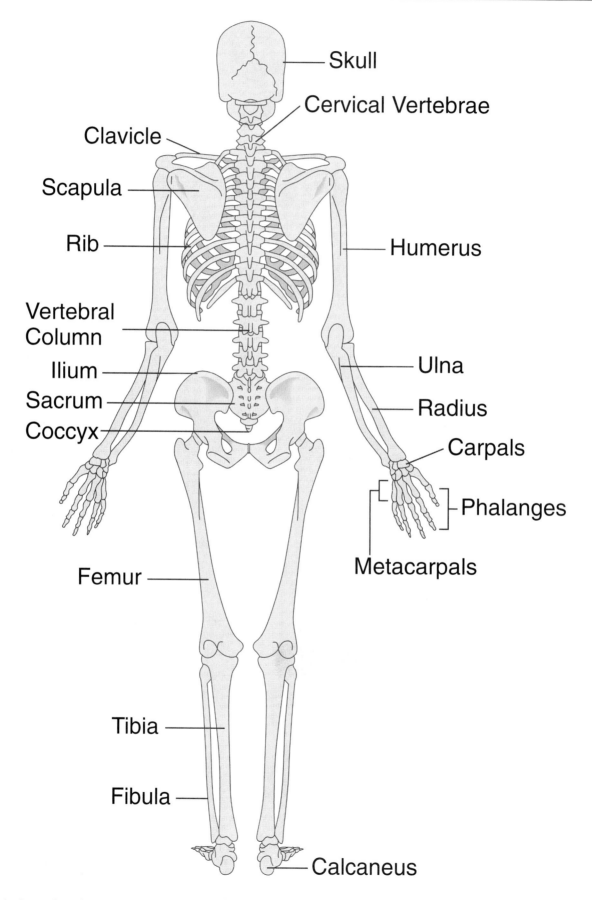

Skull

Cervical Vertebrae

Clavicle

Scapula

Rib

Humerus

Vertebral Column

Ulna

Ilium

Sacrum

Radius

Coccyx

Carpals

Phalanges

Metacarpals

Femur

Tibia

Fibula

Calcaneus

TRANSPARENCY MASTER 11A   **EXTERNAL VIEW OF THE HEART**

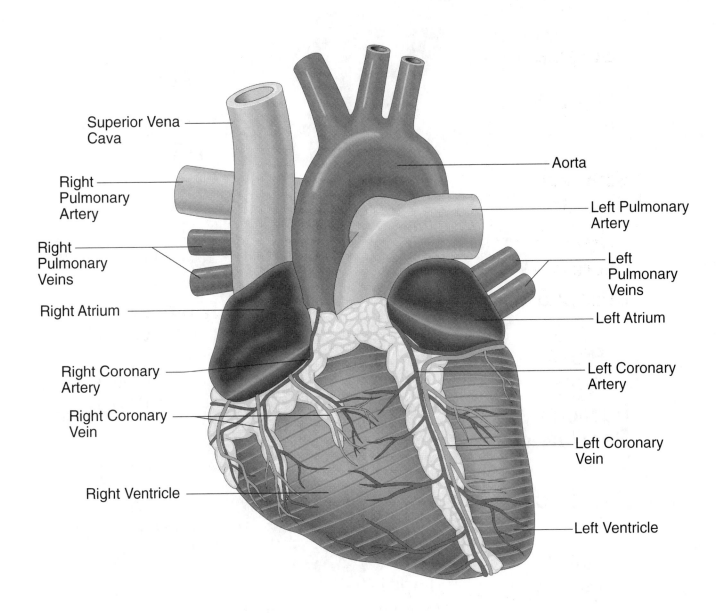

Superior Vena
Cava

Right
Pulmonary
Artery

Right
Pulmonary
Veins

Right Atrium

Right Coronary
Artery

Right Coronary
Vein

Right Ventricle

Aorta

Left Pulmonary
Artery

Left
Pulmonary
Veins

Left Atrium

Left Coronary
Artery

Left Coronary
Vein

Left Ventricle

TRANSPARENCY MASTER 11B

INTERNAL STRUCTURES OF THE HEART AND
BLOOD FLOW THROUGH THE HEART

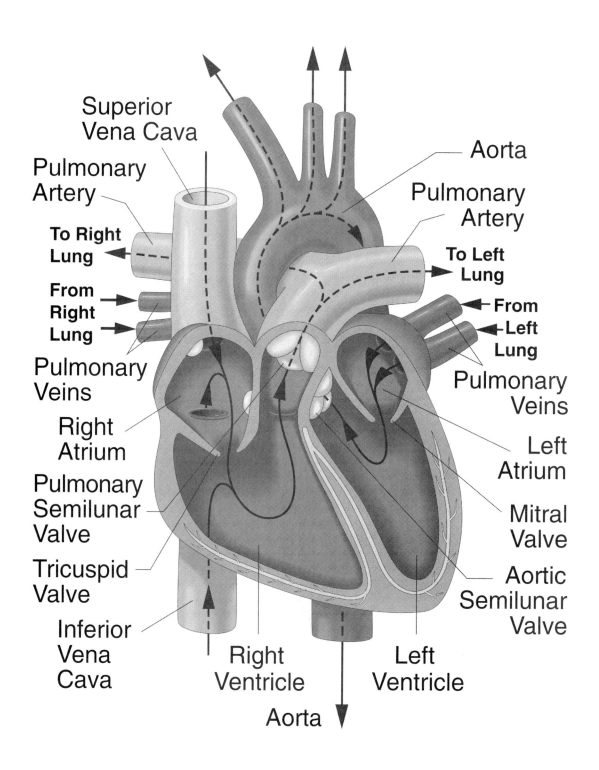

Superior
Vena Cava

Pulmonary
Artery

To Right
Lung

From
Right
Lung

Pulmonary
Veins

Right
Atrium

Pulmonary
Semilunar
Valve

Tricuspid
Valve

Inferior
Vena
Cava

Right
Ventricle

Aorta

Aorta

Pulmonary
Artery

To Left
Lung

From
Left
Lung

Pulmonary
Veins

Left
Atrium

Mitral
Valve

Aortic
Semilunar
Valve

Left
Ventricle

RESPIRATORY SYSTEM

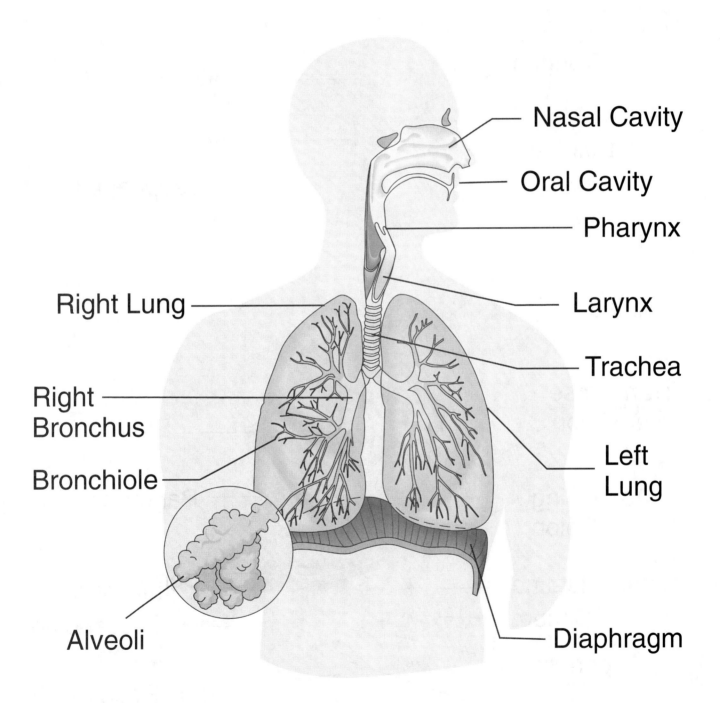

Nasal Cavity

Oral Cavity

Pharynx

Right Lung

Larynx

Trachea

Right
Bronchus

Bronchiole

Left
Lung

Alveoli

Diaphragm

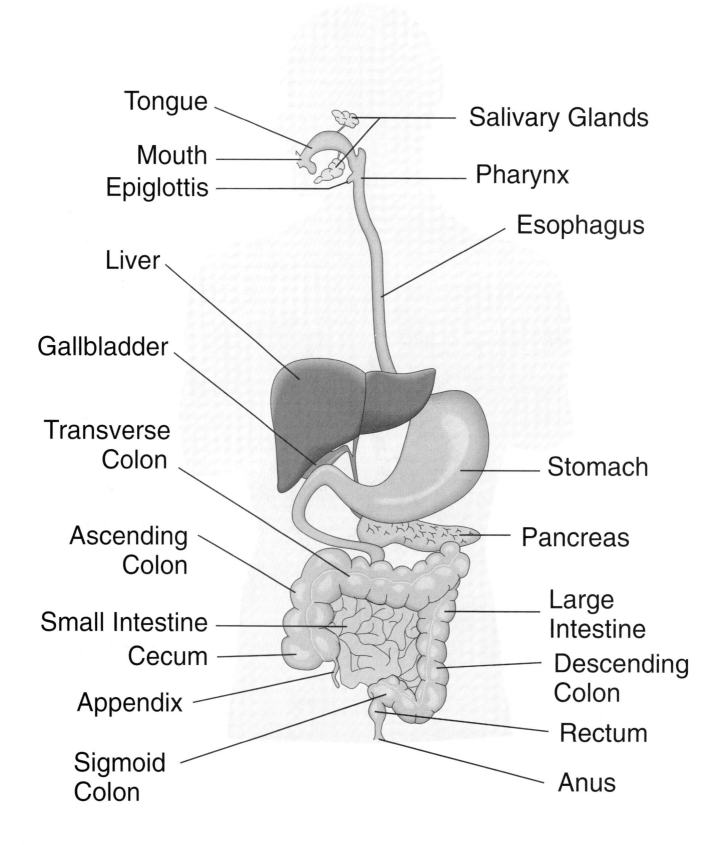

Tongue

Mouth

Epiglottis

Liver

Gallbladder

Transverse
Colon

Ascending
Colon

Small Intestine

Cecum

Appendix

Sigmoid
Colon

Salivary Glands

Pharynx

Esophagus

Stomach

Pancreas

Large
Intestine

Descending
Colon

Rectum

Anus

TRANSPARENCY MASTER 14   **URINARY SYSTEM**

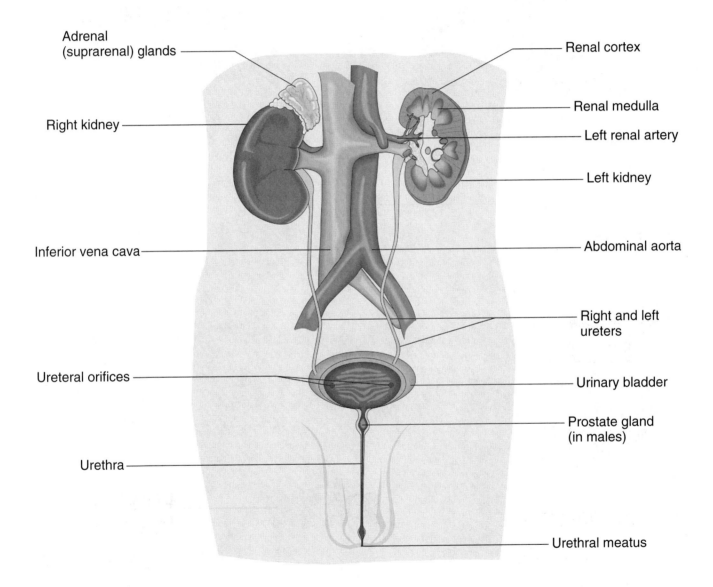

Adrenal (suprarenal) glands

Right kidney

Inferior vena cava

Ureteral orifices

Urethra

Renal cortex

Renal medulla

Left renal artery

Left kidney

Abdominal aorta

Right and left ureters

Urinary bladder

Prostate gland (in males)

Urethral meatus

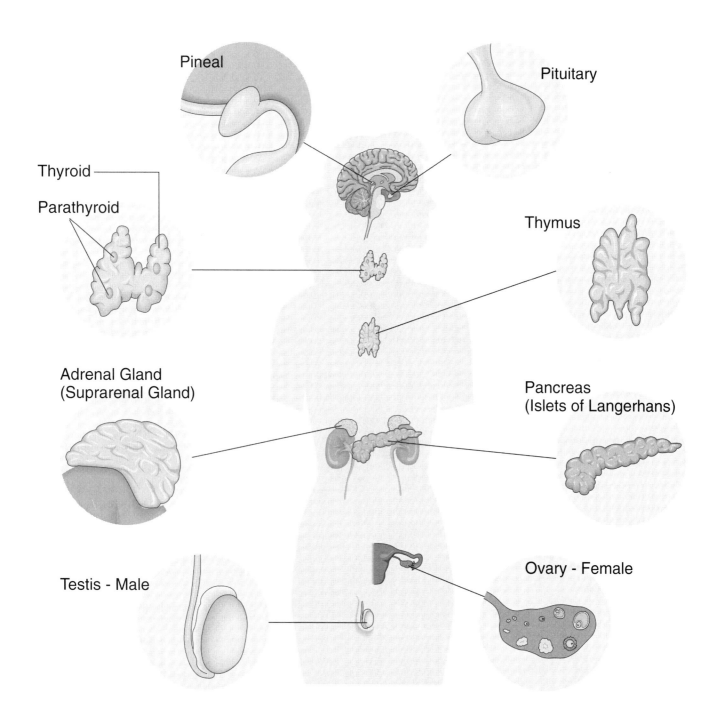

Pineal

Pituitary

Thyroid

Parathyroid

Thymus

Adrenal Gland
(Suprarenal Gland)

Pancreas
(Islets of Langerhans)

Testis - Male

Ovary - Female

TRANSPARENCY MASTER 16   **MALE REPRODUCTIVE SYSTEM**

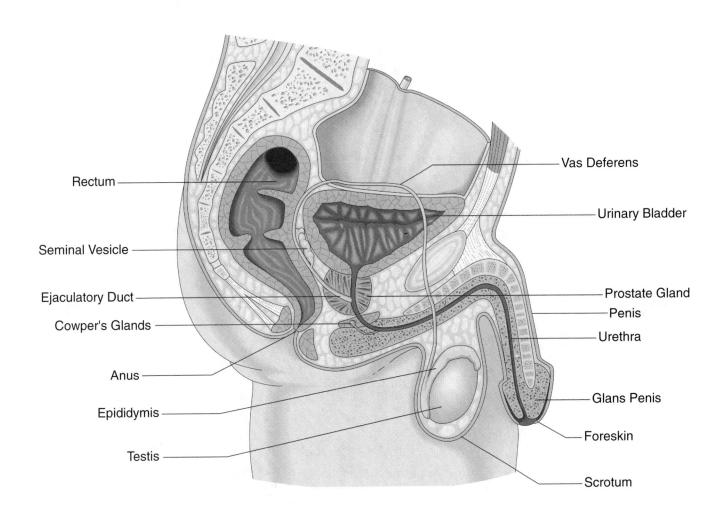

Rectum

Seminal Vesicle

Ejaculatory Duct

Cowper's Glands

Anus

Epididymis

Testis

Vas Deferens

Urinary Bladder

Prostate Gland

Penis

Urethra

Glans Penis

Foreskin

Scrotum

TRANSPARENCY MASTER 17   **FEMALE REPRODUCTIVE SYSTEM**

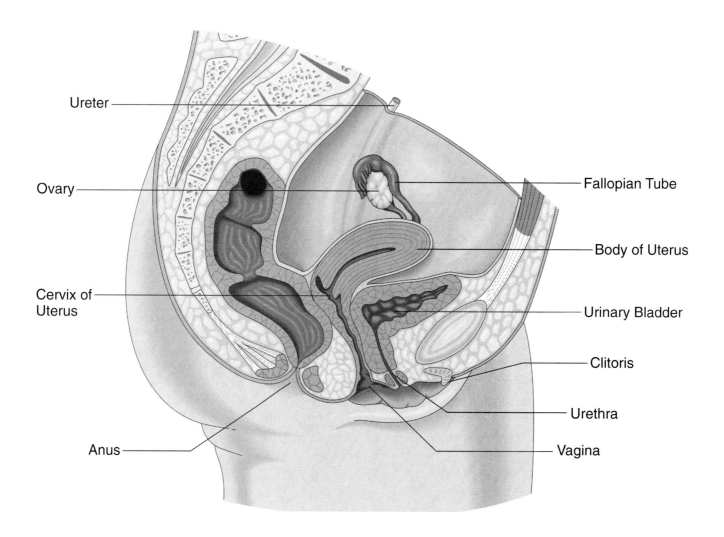

Ureter

Ovary

Cervix of
Uterus

Anus

Fallopian Tube

Body of Uterus

Urinary Bladder

Clitoris

Urethra

Vagina

TRANSPARENCY MASTER 18

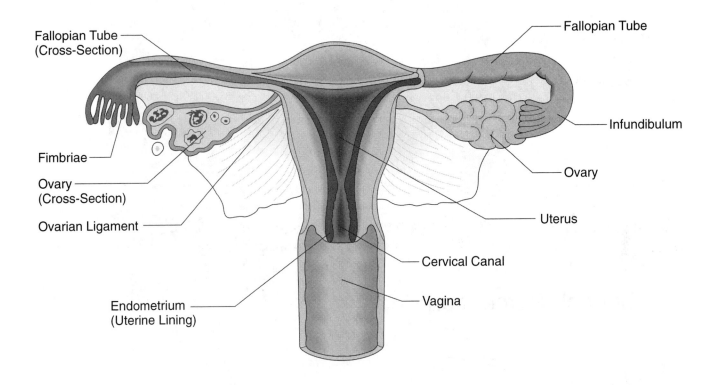

Fallopian Tube
(Cross-Section)

Fimbriae

Ovary
(Cross-Section)

Ovarian Ligament

Endometrium
(Uterine Lining)

Fallopian Tube

Infundibulum

Ovary

Uterus

Cervical Canal

Vagina

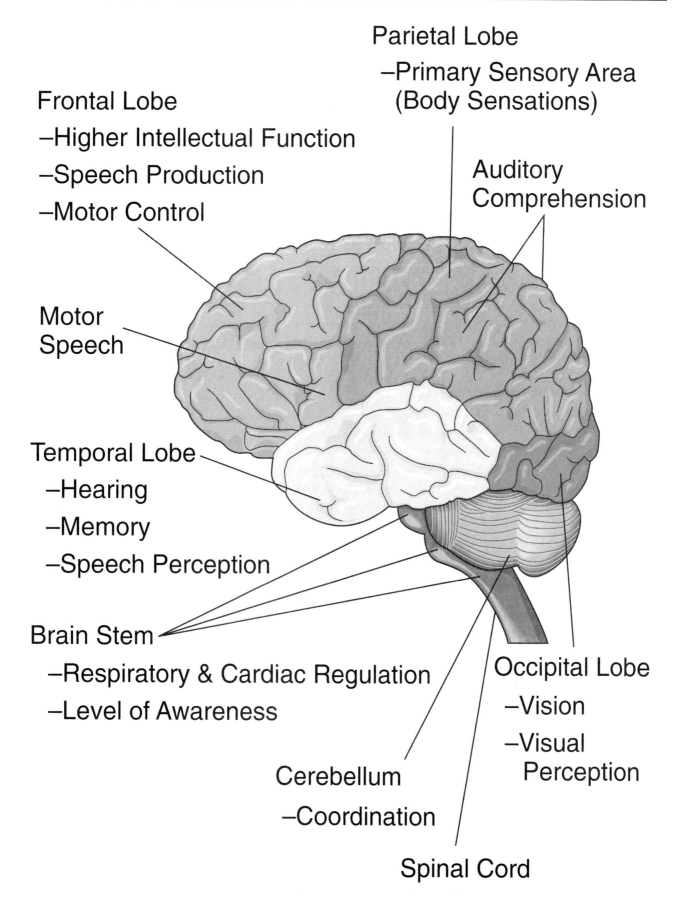

Parietal Lobe
–Primary Sensory Area
(Body Sensations)

Frontal Lobe
–Higher Intellectual Function
–Speech Production
–Motor Control

Auditory
Comprehension

Motor
Speech

Temporal Lobe
–Hearing
–Memory
–Speech Perception

Brain Stem
–Respiratory & Cardiac Regulation
–Level of Awareness

Occipital Lobe
–Vision
–Visual
Perception

Cerebellum
–Coordination

Spinal Cord

TRANSPARENCY MASTER 20A

MAJOR VEINS OF THE BODY

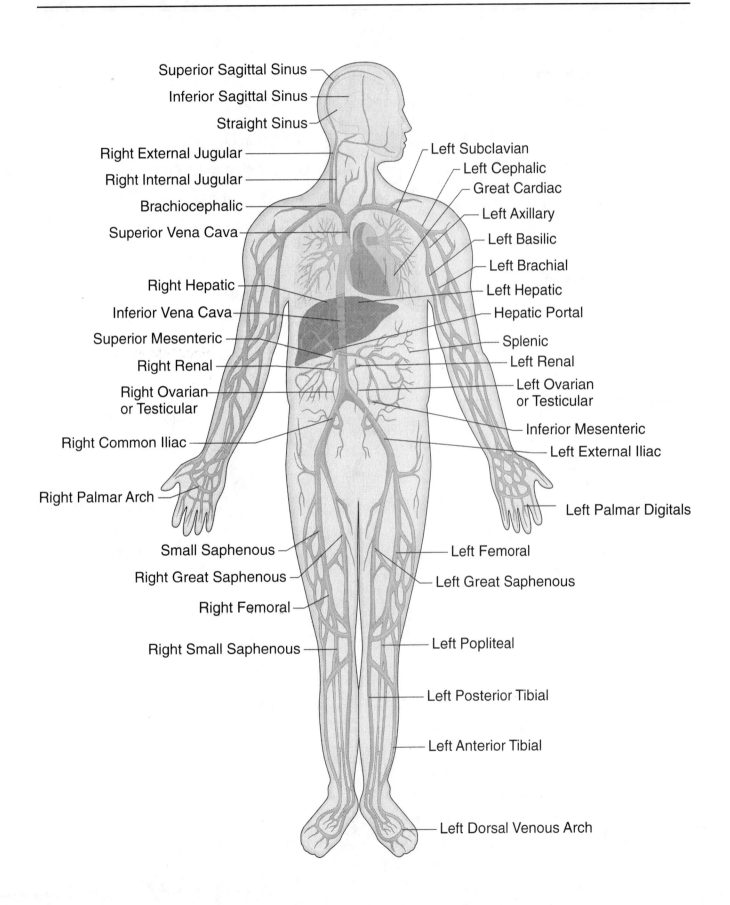

Superior Sagittal Sinus

Inferior Sagittal Sinus

Straight Sinus

Right External Jugular

Right Internal Jugular

Brachiocephalic

Superior Vena Cava

Right Hepatic

Inferior Vena Cava

Superior Mesenteric

Right Renal

Right Ovarian
or Testicular

Right Common Iliac

Right Palmar Arch

Small Saphenous

Right Great Saphenous

Right Femoral

Right Small Saphenous

Left Subclavian

Left Cephalic

Great Cardiac

Left Axillary

Left Basilic

Left Brachial

Left Hepatic

Hepatic Portal

Splenic

Left Renal

Left Ovarian
or Testicular

Inferior Mesenteric

Left External Iliac

Left Palmar Digitals

Left Femoral

Left Great Saphenous

Left Popliteal

Left Posterior Tibial

Left Anterior Tibial

Left Dorsal Venous Arch

TRANSPARENCY MASTER 20B

MAJOR ARTERIES OF THE BODY

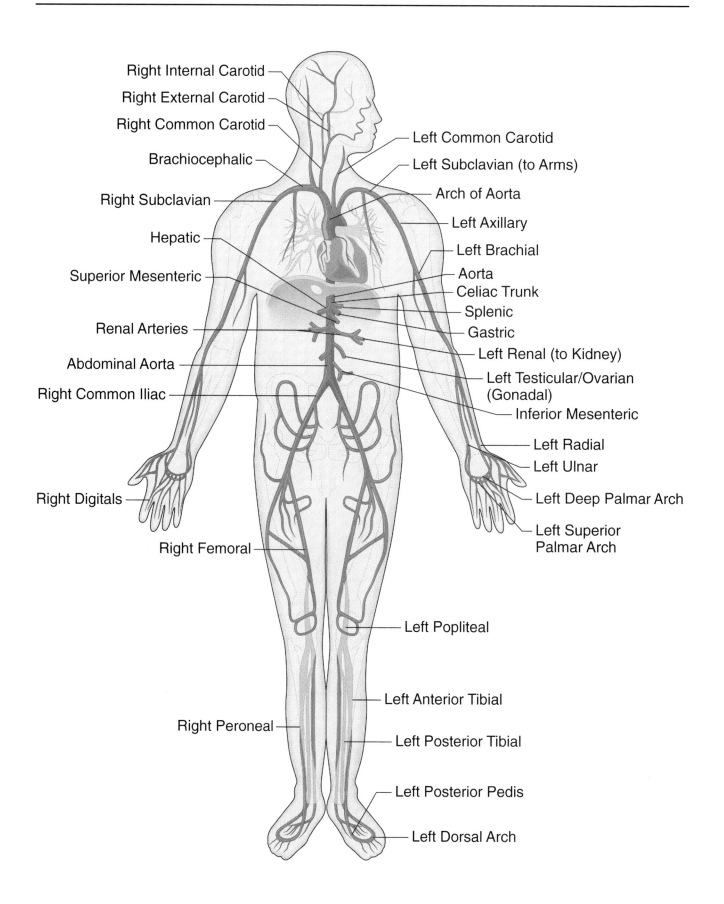

Right Internal Carotid

Right External Carotid

Right Common Carotid

Brachiocephalic

Right Subclavian

Hepatic

Superior Mesenteric

Renal Arteries

Abdominal Aorta

Right Common Iliac

Right Digitals

Right Femoral

Right Peroneal

Left Common Carotid

Left Subclavian (to Arms)

Arch of Aorta

Left Axillary

Left Brachial

Aorta

Celiac Trunk

Splenic

Gastric

Left Renal (to Kidney)

Left Testicular/Ovarian (Gonadal)

Inferior Mesenteric

Left Radial

Left Ulnar

Left Deep Palmar Arch

Left Superior Palmar Arch

Left Popliteal

Left Anterior Tibial

Left Posterior Tibial

Left Posterior Pedis

Left Dorsal Arch

TRANSPARENCY MASTER 21A   MAJOR MUSCLES OF THE BODY—ANTERIOR VIEW

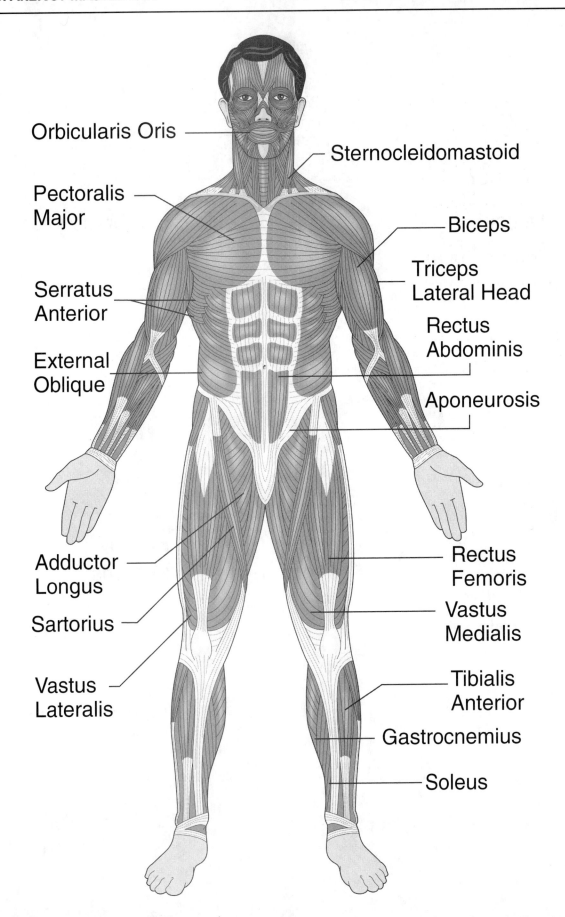

Orbicularis Oris

Sternocleidomastoid

Pectoralis Major

Biceps

Triceps Lateral Head

Serratus Anterior

Rectus Abdominis

External Oblique

Aponeurosis

Adductor Longus

Rectus Femoris

Sartorius

Vastus Medialis

Vastus Lateralis

Tibialis Anterior

Gastrocnemius

Soleus

TRANSPARENCY MASTER 21B   MAJOR MUSCLES OF THE BODY—POSTERIOR VIEW

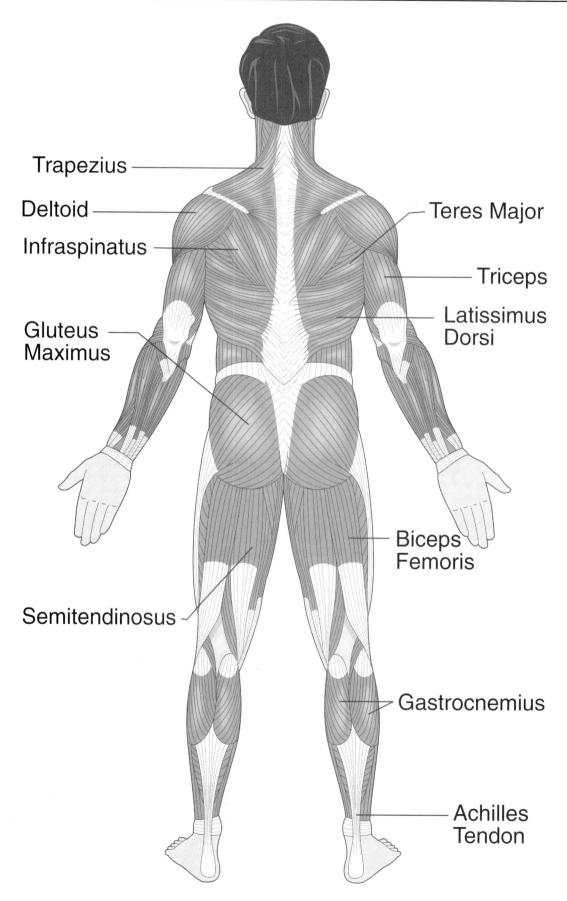

Trapezius

Deltoid

Infraspinatus

Gluteus
Maximus

Semitendinosus

Teres Major

Triceps

Latissimus
Dorsi

Biceps
Femoris

Gastrocnemius

Achilles
Tendon

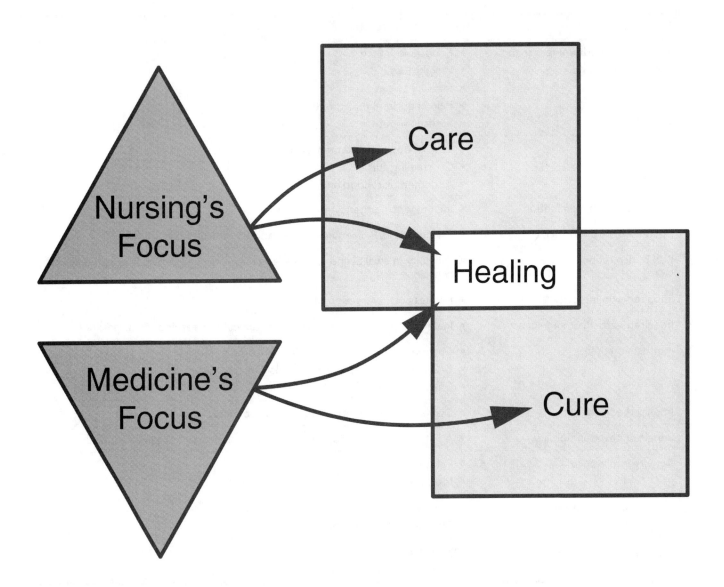

TRANSPARENCY MASTER 23   **NURSING DIAGNOSIS AND RELATED OBSERVATIONS**

Diagnosis	Observations to Make
Imbalanced nutrition; less than body requirements	• Food/fluid intake • Weight loss • Inability to eat • Pain in abdomen or mouth • Sores in mouth
Constipation	• Lack of bowel movement or hard, dry stools • C/O feeling full • Abdomen distended and firm
Impaired urinary elimination	• Incontinence, urgency, painful urination
Decreased cardiac output	• Changes in B/P, irregular pulse, fatigue, difficulty breathing
Risk of aspiration	• Difficulty in swallowing, depressed cough and gag reflex, reduced level of consciousness
Impaired skin integrity	• Redness or destruction of skin
Impaired verbal communication	• Inability or difficulty with speaking, difficulty breathing, disorientation
Ineffective coping	• Change in usual communication patterns • C/O inability to cope or meet basic needs • Change in behavior
Impaired adjustment	• Disbelief, anger, inability to solve problems
Impaired physical mobility	• Ability to move in bed, range of motion, balance, coordination, endurance
Activity intolerance	• Fatigue, weakness, shortness of breath • Irregular pulse
Disturbed sleep pattern	• C/O not sleeping • Changes in behavior or speech
Anxiety	• Shakiness, quivering voice, increased movements • Poor eye contact, helplessness

TRANSPARENCY MASTER 24A   **ACTIVITIES OF DAILY LIVING FLOW CHART, PG. 1**

DATE		1	2	3	4	5	6	7	8	9	10	11	12	13	14	15	16	17	18	19	20	21	22	23	24	25	26	27	28	29	30	31
Blood Pressure Sys/Dia																																
Temperature																																
Pulse																																
Respirations																																
Weight																																
DIET % CONSUMED	Breakfast																															
	Nourishment																															
	Lunch																															
	Nourishment																															
	Dinner																															
	Nourishment																															
INTAKE cc's	7-3																															
	3-11																															
	11-7																															
	Total																															
OUTPUT cc's	7-3																															
	3-11																															
	11-7																															
	Total																															
BATH CODE: A - Assist I - Indep. D - Dep.	7-3																															
	3-11																															
	11-7																															
PERSONAL CARE A - Assist I - Indep. D - Dep.	Oral Hygiene																															
	Shampoo																															
	Shave																															
	Nail Care																															
	Skin Care																															
AMBULATION # of feet	7-3																															
	3-11																															
	11-7																															
BED RAILS UP Y - Yes N - No	7-3																															
	3-11																															
	11-7																															

LAST NAME	FIRST NAME	INITIAL	ATTENDING PHYSICIAN	ROOM NO.	PATIENT NO.

ACTIVITIES OF DAILY LIVING FLOW CHART

TRANSPARENCY MASTER 24B   **ACTIVITIES OF DAILY LIVING FLOW CHART, PG. 2**

DATE		1	2	3	4	5	6	7	8	9	10	11	12	13	14	15	16	17	18	19	20	21	22	23	24	25	26	27	28	29	30	31
UP IN CHAIR A - Assist I - Indep. D - Dep.	7-3																															
	3-11																															
	11-7																															
ROM Exercises A - Active P - Passive	7-3																															
	3-11																															
POSITION changed A - Assist I - Indep. D - Dep.	7-3																															
	3-11																															
	11-7																															
BLADDER ACTION C - Continent I - Incontinent F - Foley # x's	7-3																															
	3-11																															
	11-7																															
BOWEL ACTION C - Continent I - Incontinent # x's	7-3																															
	3-11																															
	11-7																															
CONSISTENCY L - Liquid S - Soft formed H - Hard formed	7-3																															
	3-11																															
	11-7																															
PERI CARE A - Assist I - Indep. D - Dep.	7-3																															
	3-11																															
	11-7																															
RESTRAINT P - Pelvic W - Waist B - Belt G - Geri Chair Check q 1/2 Hr. Release q 2 hrs.	7-3																															
	3-11																															
	11-7																															
Nursing Assistant Initials	A.M.																															
	P.M.																															
	NOC.																															
Licensed Nurse Initials	A.M.																															
	P.M.																															
	NOC.																															

Nursing Assistant Initials and Signature

_____ _____   _____ _____   _____ _____

_____ _____   _____ _____   _____ _____

Licensed Nurse Initials and Signature

_____ _____   _____ _____   _____ _____

_____ _____   _____ _____   _____ _____

LAST NAME	FIRST NAME	INITIAL	ATTENDING PHYSICIAN	ROOM NO.	PATIENT NO.

TRANSPARENCY MASTER 25A   **24-HOUR TIME (MILITARY TIME)**

The 24-Hour Clock

Standard Clock	24-Hour Clock	Standard Clock	24-Hour Clock
12:00 midnight	2400 or 0000	12:00 noon	1200
1:00 a.m.	0100	1:00 p.m.	1300
2:00 a.m.	0200	2:00 p.m.	1400
3:00 a.m.	0300	3:00 p.m.	1500
4:00 a.m.	0400	4:00 p.m.	1600
5:00 a.m.	0500	5:00 p.m.	1700
6:00 a.m.	0600	6:00 p.m.	1800
7:00 a.m.	0700	7:00 p.m.	1900
8:00 a.m.	0800	8:00 p.m.	2000
9:00 a.m.	0900	9:00 p.m.	2100
10:00 a.m.	1000	10:00 p.m.	2200
11:00 a.m.	1100	11:00 p.m.	2300

Entries in the chart are made in chronological order, by date and time. Some facilities use the 24-hour clock to document the time. When this system is used, indicating times by noting A.M. or P.M. is not necessary.

TRANSPARENCY MASTER 25B   **24-HOUR CLOCK (MILITARY TIME)**

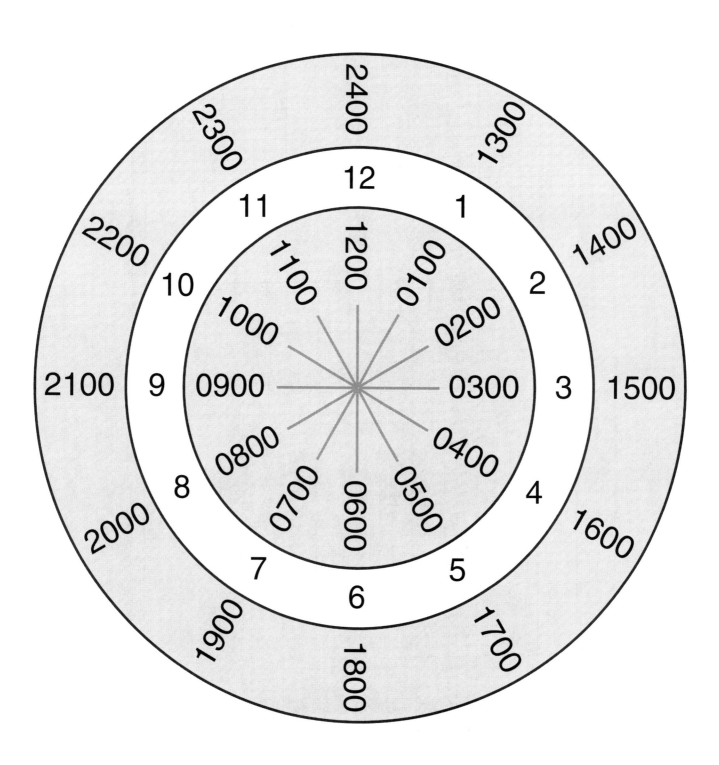

TRANSPARENCY MASTER 26A

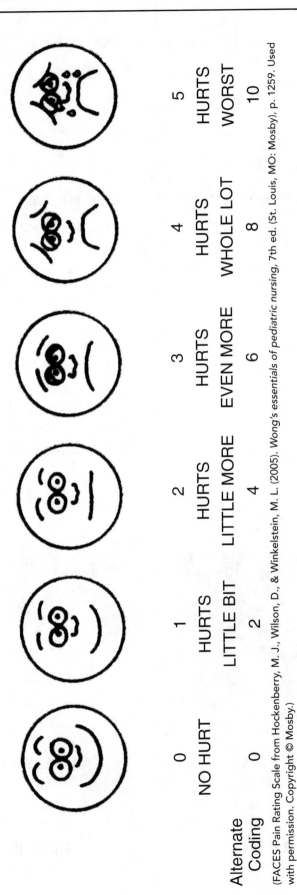

	0	1	2	3	4	5
	NO HURT	HURTS LITTLE BIT	HURTS LITTLE MORE	HURTS EVEN MORE	HURTS WHOLE LOT	HURTS WORST
Alternate Coding	0	2	4	6	8	10

(FACES Pain Rating Scale from Hockenberry, M. J., Wilson, D., & Winkelstein, M. L. (2005). *Wong's essentials of pediatric nursing*, 7th ed. (St. Louis, MO: Mosby). p. 1259. Used with permission. Copyright © Mosby.)

TRANSPARENCY MASTER 26B   **NUMERIC AND VERBAL PAIN SCALES**

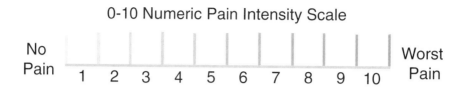

0-10 Numeric Pain Intensity Scale

No Pain | 1 2 3 4 5 6 7 8 9 10 | Worst Pain

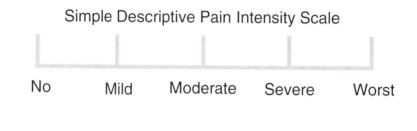

Simple Descriptive Pain Intensity Scale

No   Mild   Moderate   Severe   Worst

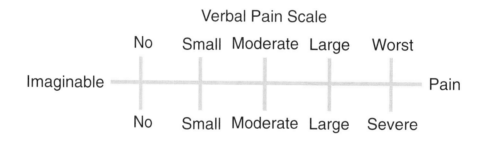

Verbal Pain Scale

No   Small Moderate Large   Worst

Imaginable ———————————————————— Pain

No   Small Moderate Large   Severe

Word Scale #1

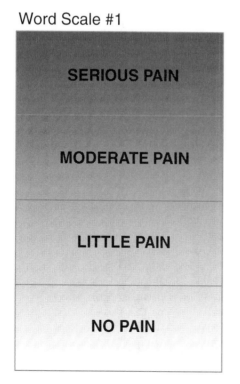

SERIOUS PAIN

MODERATE PAIN

LITTLE PAIN

NO PAIN

Word Scale #2

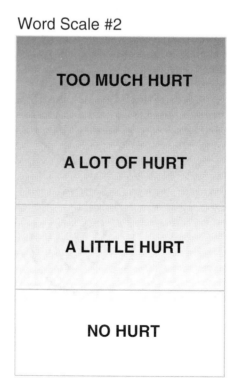

TOO MUCH HURT

A LOT OF HURT

A LITTLE HURT

NO HURT

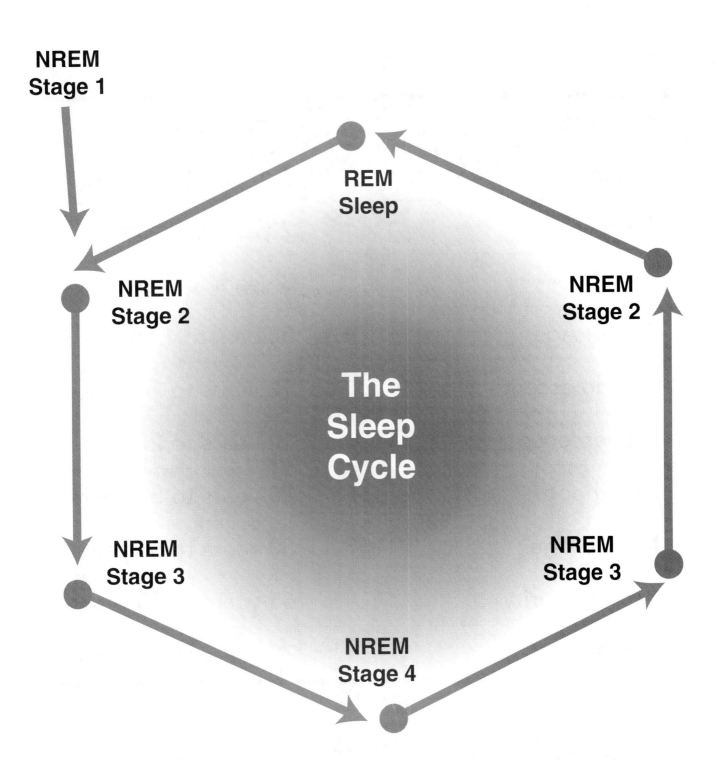

TRANSPARENCY MASTER 28   STAGES OF GROWTH AND DEVELOPMENT

Neonate	Birth to 1 month
Infancy	1 month to 2 years
Toddler	2 years to 3 years
Preschool	3 years to 5 years
School Age	5 years to 12 years
Preadolescent	12 years to 14 years
Adolescence	14 years to 20 years
Adulthood	20 years to 50 years
Middle Age	50 years to 65 years
Later Maturity	65 years to 75 years
Old Age	75 years and beyond

TRANSPARENCY MASTER 29 TASKS OF PERSONALITY DEVELOPMENT

Physical Stage	Year of Occurrence	Tasks to Be Mastered
Oral-sensory	Birth–1 year (infant)	To learn to trust (Trust)
Muscular-anal	1–3 years (toddler)	To recognize self as a being independent from mother (Autonomy)
Locomotor	3–5 years (preschool years)	To recognize self as a family member (Initiative)
Latency	6–11 years (school-age years)	To demonstrate physical and mental skills/abilities (Industry)
Adolescence	12–18 years	To develop a sense of individuality as a sexual human being (Identity)
Young Adulthood	19–35 years	To establish intimate personal relationships with a mate (Intimacy)
Adulthood	35–50 years	To live a satisfying and productive life
Maturity	50+ years	To review life's events and examine how they have influenced the development of a unique individual (Ego integrity)

Self-Actualization
Obtain full potential,
Confident, Self-secure

Esteem
Self-respect,
Has approval of others

Love and Affection
Feel sense of belonging,
Can give and receive friendship and love

Safety and Security
Free from fear and anxiety,
Feel secure in the environment

Physiological Needs
Food, Water, Oxygen, Elimination of waste,
Protection from temperature extremes, Sleep

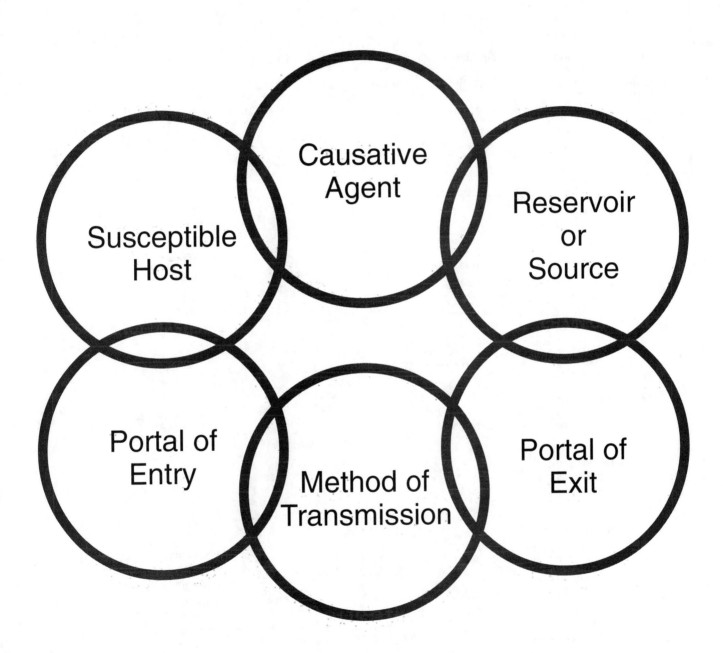

TRANSPARENCY MASTER 31B   **BREAKING THE CHAIN OF INFECTION**

Elements in the Chain of Infection

Causative Agent	Source or Reservoir	Portal of Exit	Mode of Transmission	Portal of Entry	Susceptible Host
Bacteria	People	Blood	Direct contact	Mucous membranes	Chronic diseases
Fungi	Medicine	Moist body fluid	Indirect contact	Nonintact skin	Immuno-suppression
Viruses	Food	Droplets	Airborne	Urinary tract	Surgery
Parasites	Water	Secretions	Droplet	GI tract	Diabetes
	Equipment	Excretions	Fomites	Respiratory tract	Elderly patients
		Skin	Common vehicle	Blood	Burns
			Vectors	Body fluid	Cardiopulmonary disease

Elements of the chain of infection

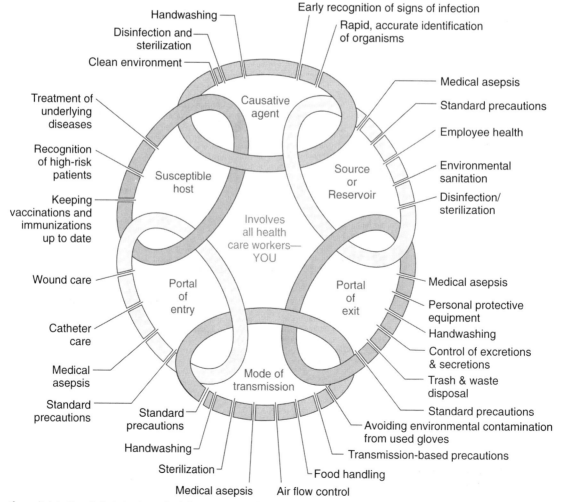

If one link in the chain is broken, the infection cannot be spread to others.

TRANSPARENCY MASTER 32

DANGER ZONE: YOUR HANDS

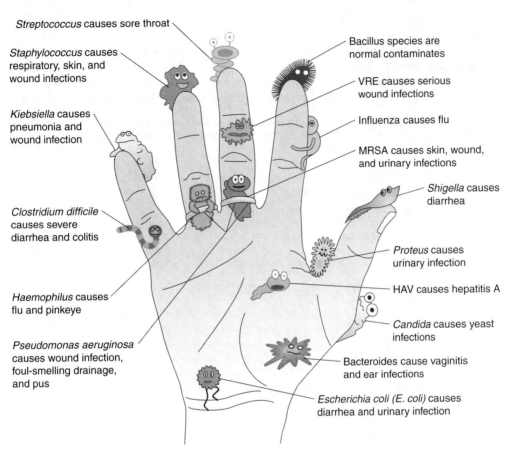

Streptococcus causes sore throat

Staphylococcus causes respiratory, skin, and wound infections

Klebsiella causes pneumonia and wound infection

Clostridium difficile causes severe diarrhea and colitis

Haemophilus causes flu and pinkeye

Pseudomonas aeruginosa causes wound infection, foul-smelling drainage, and pus

Bacillus species are normal contaminates

VRE causes serious wound infections

Influenza causes flu

MRSA causes skin, wound, and urinary infections

Shigella causes diarrhea

Proteus causes urinary infection

HAV causes hepatitis A

Candida causes yeast infections

Bacteroides cause vaginitis and ear infections

Escherichia coli (E. coli) causes diarrhea and urinary infection

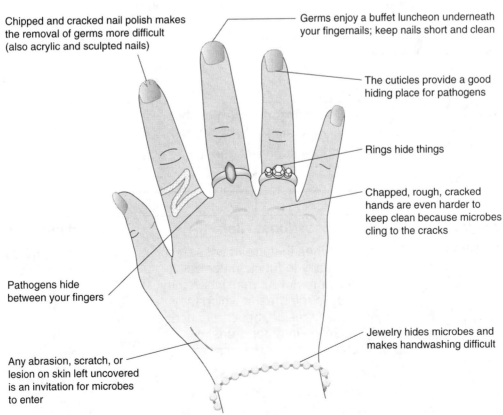

Chipped and cracked nail polish makes the removal of germs more difficult (also acrylic and sculpted nails)

Pathogens hide between your fingers

Any abrasion, scratch, or lesion on skin left uncovered is an invitation for microbes to enter

Germs enjoy a buffet luncheon underneath your fingernails; keep nails short and clean

The cuticles provide a good hiding place for pathogens

Rings hide things

Chapped, rough, cracked hands are even harder to keep clean because microbes cling to the cracks

Jewelry hides microbes and makes handwashing difficult

Modes of Transmission of Microbes	
Airborne	Tiny microbes are carried by moisture or dust particles in air and are inhaled
Droplet	Droplets spread within approximately three feet (no personal contact). Droplets are larger and heavier than airborne microbes, so they cannot travel as far. Droplet nuclei are inhaled: • Coughing • Laughing • Sneezing • Singing • Talking
Contact	Direct contact of health care provider with patient: • Touching • Rubbing • Toileting (urine and feces) • Blood, body fluid, mucous membranes, • Bathing or nonintact skin • Secretions or excretions from patient Indirect contact of health care provider with objects used by patients: • Clothing • Dressings • Bed linens • Diagnostic equipment • Personal belongings • Permanent or disposable • Personal care equipment health care equipment • Instruments and supplies used in • Environmental surfaces such as treatments counters, faucets, and doorknobs
Common Vehicle	Spread to many people through contact with items such as: • Food • Medication • Water • Contaminated blood products
Vector-Borne	Intermediate hosts such as: • Flies • Rats • Fleas • Mice • Ticks • Roaches

Examples of various methods of microbe transmission

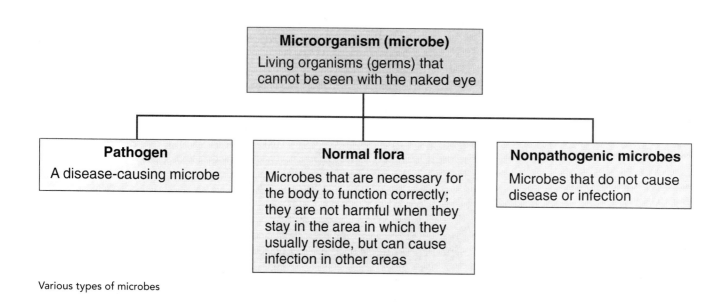

Various types of microbes

TRANSPARENCY MASTER 33B **MODES OF TRANSMISSION OF PATHOGENS**

Airborne Transmission

- Pathogens carried by moisture or dust particles in air, can be carried long distances

Droplet Transmission

Droplet Spread Within Approximately 3 Feet (No Personal Contact) of Infected Person by:

- Coughing
- Sneezing
- Talking
- Laughing
- Singing

Contact Transmission

Direct Contact with Infected Person:

- Touching
- Sexual contact
- Blood
- Body fluids (drainage, urine, feces, sputum, saliva, vomitus)

Indirect Contact with Infected Person:

- Clothing
- Dressings
- Equipment used in care and treatment
- Bed linens
- Personal belongings
- Specimen containers
- Instruments used in treatment
- Food
- Water

Note that pathogens can also be carried by insects and animals (vectors) and passed to humans.

TRANSPARENCY MASTER 34   **STANDARD PRECAUTIONS FOR INFECTION CONTROL**

Wash Hands (Plain soap)
Wash after touching **blood, body fluids, secretions, excretions**, and **contaminated items**.
Wash immediately **after gloves are removed** and **between patient contacts**.
Avoid transfer of microorganisms to other patients or environments.

Wear Gloves
Wear when touching **blood, body fluids, secretions, excretions**, and **contaminated items**.
Put on **clean** gloves just **before touching mucous membranes** and **nonintact skin**.
Change gloves between tasks and procedures on the same patient after contact with material that may contain high concentrations of microorganisms. Remove gloves promptly after use, before touching noncontaminated items and environmental surfaces, and before going to another patient, and wash hands immediately to avoid transfer of microorganisms to other patients or environments.

Wear Mask and Eye Protection or Face Shield
Protect mucous membranes of the eyes, nose, and mouth during procedures and patient care activities that are likely to generate **splashes** or **sprays** of **blood, body fluids, secretions**, or **excretions**.

Wear Gown
Protect skin and prevent soiling of clothing during procedures that are likely to generate **splashes** or **sprays** of **blood, body fluids, secretions**, or **excretions**. Remove a soiled gown as promptly as possible and wash hands to avoid transfer of microorganisms to other patients or environments.

Patient-Care Equipment
Handle used patient care equipment soiled with **blood, body fluids, secretions**, or **excretions** in a manner that prevents skin and mucous membrane exposures, contamination of clothing, and transfer of microorganisms to other patients and environments. Ensure that reusable equipment is not used for the care of another patient until it has been appropriately cleaned and reprocessed and single-use items are properly discarded.

Environmental Control
Follow hospital procedures for routine care, cleaning, and disinfection of environmental surfaces, beds, bedrails, bedside equipment, and other frequently touched surfaces.

Linens
Handle, transport, and process used linens soiled with **blood, body fluids, secretions**, or **excretions** in a manner that prevents exposures and contamination of clothing, and avoids transfer of microorganisms to other patients and environments.

Occupational Health and Bloodborne Pathogens
Prevent injuries when using needles, scalpels, and other sharp instruments or devices; when handling sharp instruments after procedures; when cleaning used instruments; and when disposing of used needles.

Never recap used needles using both hands or any other technique that involves directing the point of a needle toward any part of the body; rather, use either a one-handed "scoop" technique or a mechanical device designed for holding the needle sheath.

Do not remove used needles from disposable syringes by hand, and do not bend, break, or otherwise manipulate used needles by hand. Place used disposable syringes and needles, scalpel blades, and other sharp items in puncture-resistant sharps containers located as close as practical to the area in which the items were used, and place reusable syringes and needles in a puncture-resistant container for transport to the reprocessing area.

Use **resuscitation devices** as an alternative to mouth-to-mouth resuscitation.

Patient Placement
Use a **private room** for a patient who contaminates the environment or who does not (or cannot be expected to) assist in maintaining appropriate hygiene or environmental control. Consult Infection Control if a private room is not available.

(Courtesy of BREVIS Corporation, Salt Lake City, UT)

Head Lice
(Pediculus humanus capitis)

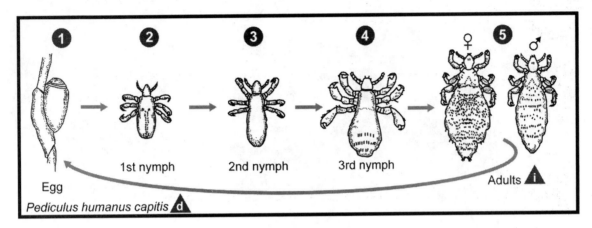

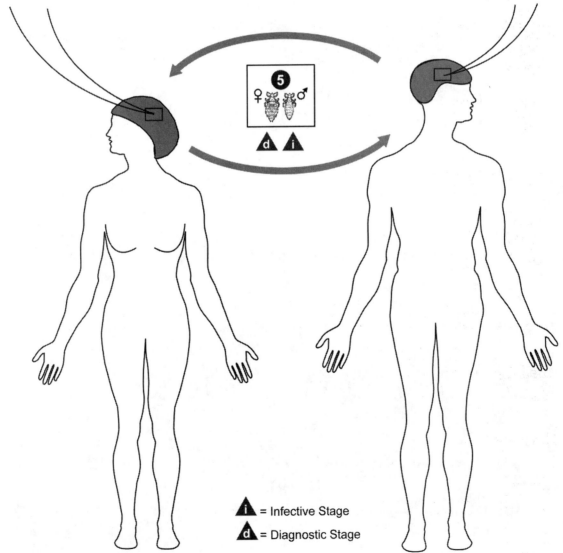

i = Infective Stage

d = Diagnostic Stage

(Courtesy of Centers for Disease Control and Prevention)

TRANSPARENCY MASTER 36   **COMPARISON OF LICE**

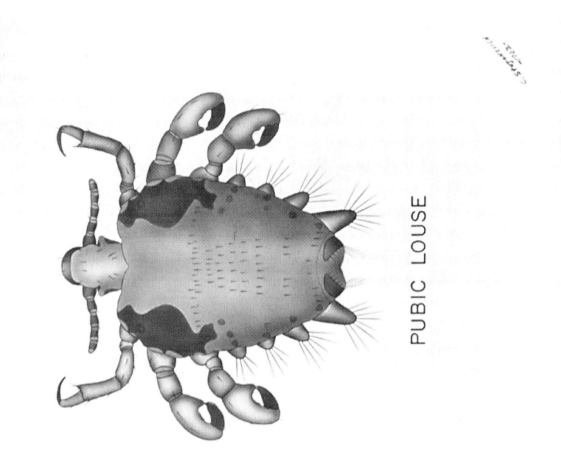

PUBIC LOUSE

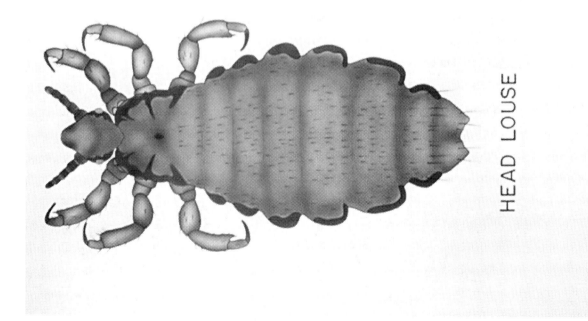

HEAD LOUSE

(Courtesy of Centers for Disease Control and Prevention)

TRANSPARENCY MASTER 37   **LIFE CYCLE OF SCABIES MITE**

Scabies
(Sarcoptes scabei)

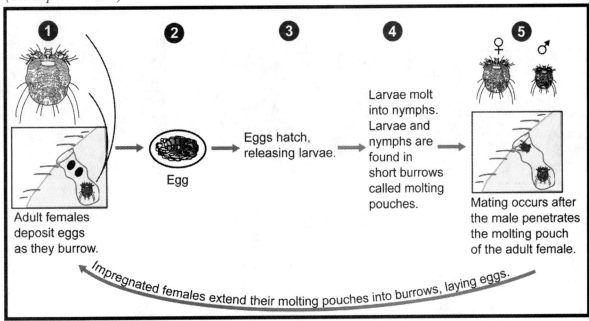

① Adult females deposit eggs as they burrow.

② Egg

Eggs hatch, releasing larvae.

④ Larvae molt into nymphs. Larvae and nymphs are found in short burrows called molting pouches.

⑤ ♀ ♂

Mating occurs after the male penetrates the molting pouch of the adult female.

Impregnated females extend their molting pouches into burrows, laying eggs.

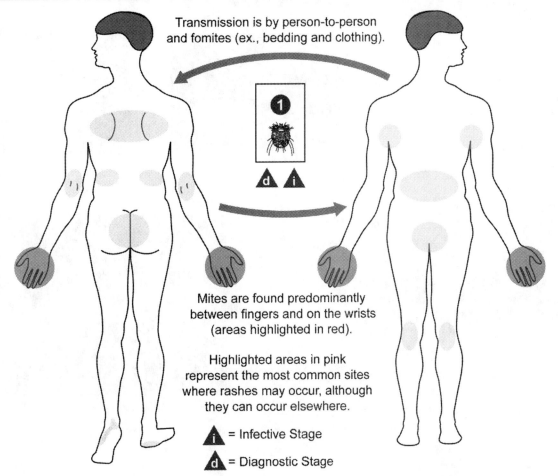

Transmission is by person-to-person and fomites (ex., bedding and clothing).

Mites are found predominantly between fingers and on the wrists (areas highlighted in red).

Highlighted areas in pink represent the most common sites where rashes may occur, although they can occur elsewhere.

▲i = Infective Stage

▲d = Diagnostic Stage

(Courtesy of Centers for Disease Control and Prevention)

TRANSPARENCY MASTER 38

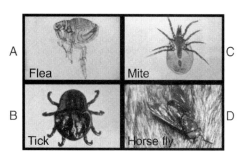

A Flea
B Tick
C Mite
D Horse fly

Brown-banded cockroach

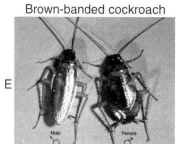

E

Male ♀   Female ♂

German cockroach
(most common type in United States)

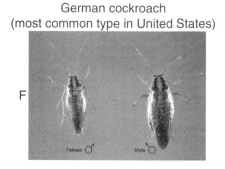

F

Female ♂   Male ♀

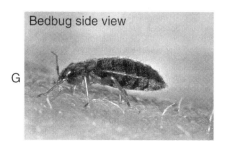

G Bedbug side view

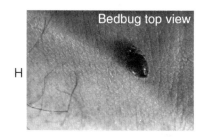

H Bedbug top view

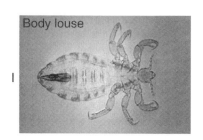

I Body louse

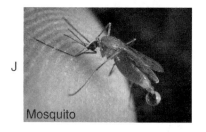

J Mosquito

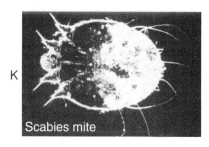

K Scabies mite

Brown recluse spider

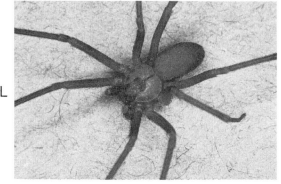

L

(Courtesy of Centers for Disease Control and Prevention)

Black widow spider

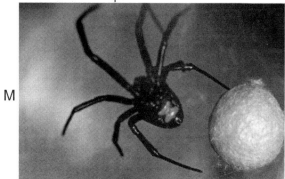

M

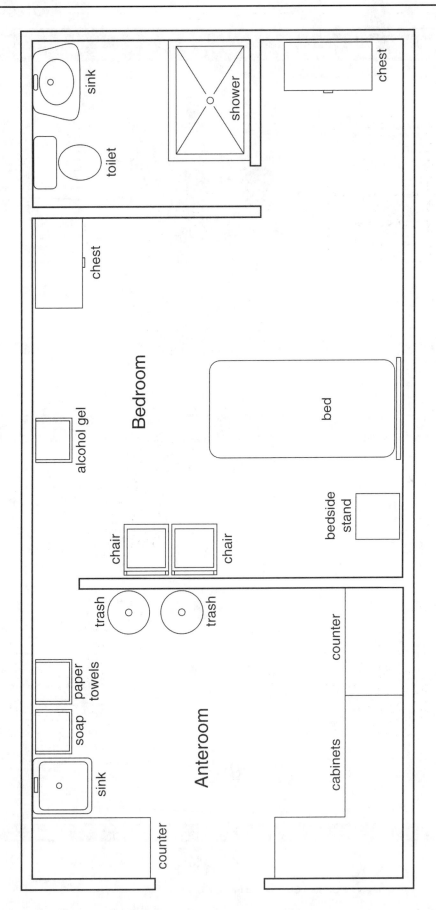

TRANSPARENCY MASTER 40

APPLYING AND REMOVING PERSONAL PROTECTIVE EQUIPMENT

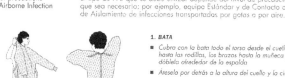

SEQUENCE FOR DONNING PERSONAL PROTECTIVE EQUIPMENT (PPE)

The type of PPE used will vary based on the level of precautions required; e.g., Standard and Contact, Droplet or Airborne Infection Isolation.

1. GOWN
- Fully cover torso from neck to knees, arms to end of wrists, and wrap around the back
- Fasten in back of neck and waist

2. MASK OR RESPIRATOR
- Secure ties or elastic bands at middle of head and neck
- Fit flexible band to nose bridge
- Fit snug to face and below chin
- Fit-check respirator

3. GOGGLES OR FACE SHIELD
- Place over face and eyes and adjust to fit

4. GLOVES
- Extend to cover wrist of isolation gown

USE SAFE WORK PRACTICES TO PROTECT YOURSELF AND LIMIT THE SPREAD OF CONTAMINATION

- Keep hands away from face
- Limit surfaces touched
- Change gloves when torn or heavily contaminated
- Perform hand hygiene

SECUENCIA PARA PONERSE EL EQUIPO DE PROTECCIÓN PERSONAL (PPE)

El tipo de PPE que se debe utilizar depende del nivel de precaución que sea necesario; por ejemplo, equipo Estándar y de Contacto o de Aislamiento de infecciones transportadas por gotas o por aire.

1. BATA
- Cubra con la bata todo el torso desde el cuello hasta las rodillas, los brazos hasta la muñeca y dóblela alrededor de la espalda
- Átesela por detrás a la altura del cuello y la cintura

2. MÁSCARA O RESPIRADOR
- Asegúrese los cordones o la banda elástica en la mitad de la cabeza y en el cuello
- Ajústese la banda flexible en el puente de la nariz
- Acomódesela en la cara y por debajo del mentón
- Verifique el ajuste del respirador

3. GAFAS PROTECTORAS O CARETAS
- Colóquesela sobre la cara y los ojos y ajústela

4. GUANTES
- Extienda los guantes para que cubran la parte del puño en la bata de aislamiento

---

UTILICE PRÁCTICAS DE TRABAJO SEGURAS PARA PROTEGERSE USTED MISMO Y LIMITAR LA PROPAGACIÓN DE LA CONTAMINACIÓN

- Mantenga las manos alejadas de la cara
- Limite el contacto con superficies
- Cambie los guantes si se rompen o están demasiado contaminados
- Realice la higiene de las manos

SEQUENCE FOR REMOVING PERSONAL PROTECTIVE EQUIPMENT (PPE)

Except for respirator, remove PPE at doorway or in anteroom. Remove respirator after leaving patient room and closing door.

1. GLOVES
- Outside of gloves is contaminated!
- Grasp outside of glove with opposite gloved hand, peel off
- Hold removed glove in gloved hand
- Slide fingers of ungloved hand under remaining glove at wrist
- Peel glove off over first glove
- Discard gloves in waste container

2. GOGGLES OR FACE SHIELD
- Outside of goggles or face shield is contaminated!
- To remove, handle by head band or ear pieces
- Place in designated receptacle for reprocessing or in waste container

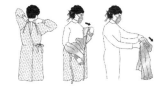

3. GOWN
- Gown front and sleeves are contaminated!
- Unfasten ties
- Pull away from neck and shoulders, touching inside of gown only
- Turn gown inside out
- Fold or roll into a bundle and discard

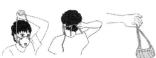

4. MASK OR RESPIRATOR
- Front of mask/respirator is contaminated — DO NOT TOUCH!
- Grasp bottom, then top ties or elastics and remove
- Discard in waste container

SECUENCIA PARA QUITARSE EL EQUIPO DE PROTECCIÓN PERSONAL (PPE)

Con la excepción del respirador, quítese el PPE en la entrada de la puerta o en la antesala. Quítese el respirador después de salir de la habitación del paciente y de cerrar la puerta.

1. GUANTES
- ¡El exterior de los guantes está contaminado!
- Agarre la parte exterior del guante con la mano opuesta en la que todavía tiene puesto el guante y quíteselo
- Sostenga el guante que se quitó con la mano enguantada
- Deslice los dedos de la mano sin guante por debajo del otro guante que no se ha quitado todavía a la altura de la muñeca
- Quítese el guante de manera que acabe cubriendo el primer guante
- Arroje los guantes en el recipiente de deshechos

2. GAFAS PROTECTORAS O CARETA
- ¡El exterior de las gafas protectoras o de la careta está contaminado!
- Para quitárselas, tómelos por la parte de la banda de la cabeza o de las piezas de las orejas
- Colóquelas en el recipiente designado para reprocesar materiales o de materiales de deshecho

3. BATA
- ¡La parte delantera de la bata y las mangas están contaminadas!
- Desate los cordones
- Tocando solamente el interior de la bata, pásela por encima del cuello y de los hombros
- Voltee la bata al revés
- Dóblela o enróllela y deséchela

4. MÁSCARA O RESPIRADOR
- La parte delantera de la máscara o respirador está contaminada — ¡NO LA TOQUE!
- Primero agarre la parte de abajo, luego los cordones o banda elástica de arriba y por último quítese la máscara o respirador
- Arrójela en el recipiente de deshechos

PERFORM HAND HYGIENE IMMEDIATELY AFTER REMOVING ALL PPE

EFECTÚE LA HIGIENE DE LAS MANOS INMEDIATAMENTE DESPUÉS DE QUITARSE CUALQUIER EQUIPO DE PROTECCIÓN PERSONAL

(Courtesy of Centers for Disease Control and Prevention)

TRANSPARENCY MASTER 41 **SELECTING PPE FOR PATIENT CARE**

Examples of Personal Protective Equipment in Basic Patient Care

Resident Care Task	Gloves	Gown	Goggles/ Face Sheild	Surgical Mask
Controlling bleeding when blood is squirting	Yes	Yes	Yes	Yes
Wiping a wheelchair, shower chair, or bathtub with disinfectant solution	Yes	No	No	No
Emptying a catheter bag	Yes	Yes, if facility policy	Yes, if facility policy	Yes, if facility policy
Serving a meal tray	No	No	No	No
Giving a backrub to a patient who has intact skin	No	No	No	No
Brushing a patient's teeth	Yes	No	No	No
Helping the dentist with a procedure	Yes	Yes, if facility policy	Yes	Yes
Cleaning a patient and changing the bed after an episode of diarrhea	Yes	Yes	No	No
Changing a bed in which the linen is not visibly soiled	No, or follow facility policy. If gloves are worn for removing soiled linen, remove and wash hands before handling clean linen	No	No	No
Taking an oral temperature with a glass thermometer (gloves are not necessary with an electronic thermometer)	Yes	No	No	No
Taking a rectal temperature	Yes	No	No	No
Taking blood pressure	No	No	No	No
Cleaning soiled utensils, such as bedpans	Yes	Yes, if splashing is likely	Yes, if splashing is likely	Yes, if splashing is likely
Shaving a patient with a disposable razor	Yes, because of the high risk of this procedure for contact with blood	No	No	No
Giving eye care	Yes	No	No	No
Giving special mouth care to an unconscious patient	Yes	No, unless coughing is likely	No, unless coughing is likely	No, unless coughing is likely
Washing the patient's genital area	Yes	No	No	No
Washing the patient's arms and legs when the skin is not broken	No	No	No	No

There are exceptions to every rule. Use this chart as a general guideline only. You are responsible for selecting the correct apparel for each procedure.

TRANSPARENCY MASTER 42   MATERIAL SAFETY DATA SHEET

Material Safety Data Sheet

PRODUCT CODE NUMBERS:
MSC5300

SECTION 1

ISSUE DATE: 9-21-96
IDENTITY: **Exuderm Hydrocolloid Ultra Dressing**

MARKETED OR DISTRIBUTED BY:
Medline Industries, Inc.
One Medline Place
Mundelein, IL 60060
1.800.MEDLINE

Emergency Telephone Number:
Contact Your Regional Poison Control Center

SECTION 2 - HAZARDOUS INGREDIENTS/IDENTITY INFORMATION

HAZARDOUS COMPONENTS (SPECIFIC CHEMICAL IDENTITY, COMMON NAME(S)	CAS#	OSHA PEL	ACGIH TLV	OTHER LIMITS RECOMMENDED	% (OPTIONAL)
None					

SECTION 3 - PHYSICAL/CHEMICAL CHARACTERISTICS

BOILING POINT: N/A	SP GRAVITY (WATER=1): N/A
VAPOR PRESSURE (MM HG): N/A	MELTING POINT: N/A
VAPOR DENSITY (AIR=1): N/A	EVAPORATION RATE (BUTYL ACETATE=1): N/A
SOLUBILITY IN WATER: N/A	
APPEARANCE AND ODOR: Light caramel in color and no odor	

SECTION 4 - FIRE AND EXPLOSION HAZARD DATA

FLASH POINT (METHOD USED): N/A

FLAMMABLE LIMITS: N/A	LEL: N/A	UEL: N/A

EXTINGUISHING MEDIA: Water, dry chemical or foam
SPECIAL FIRE FIGHTING PROCEDURES: None
UNUSUAL FIRE AND EXPLOSIVE HAZARDS: None

SECTION 5 - REACTIVITY DATA

STABILITY: Stable
CONDITIONS TO AVOID: Avoid overheating and freezing.
INCOMPATIBILITY (MATERIALS TO AVOID): N/A
HAZARDOUS DECOMPOSITION OR BYPRODUCTS: N/A
HAZARDOUS POLYMERIZATION: Will not Occur
CONDITIONS TO AVOID: N/A

SECTION 6 - HEALTH HAZARD DATA

ROUTE(S) OF ENTRY:

INHALATION: N/A	SKIN: N/A	INGESTION: N/A

HEALTH HAZARDS (ACUTE AND CHRONIC): None

CARCINOGENICITY? N/A	NTP? N/A	IARC? N/A	OSHA REGULATED? N/A

SIGNS AND SYMPTOMS OF EXPOSURE: May cause moderate irritation in eyes
MEDICAL CONDITIONS GENERALLY AGGRAVATED BY EXPOSURE: N/A
EMERGENCY AND FIRST AID PROCEDURES: Eye contact: Flush.
Excessive Ingestion: Induce vomiting and consult physician.

SECTION 7 - SPILL, LEAK, AND WASTE DISPOSAL PROCEDURES

STEPS TO BE TAKEN IN CASE MATERIAL IS RELEASED OR SPILLED: N/A
WASTE DISPOSAL METHOD: In accordance with all local, state and federal regulations.
PRECAUTIONS TO BE TAKEN IN HANDLING AND STORING: N/A
OTHER PRECAUTIONS: N/A

SECTION 8 - CONTROL MEASURES

RESPIRATORY PROTECTION (SPECIFY TYPE): N/A

VENTILATION:	LOCAL EXHAUST: N.A.	SPECIAL: N/A
	MECHANICAL (GENERAL): N/A	OTHER: N/A

PROTECTIVE GLOVES: N/A	EYE PROTECTION: N/A

SPECIAL CLOTHING: N/A
WORK/HYGIENIC PRACTICES: None

SECTION 9 - SPECIAL PRECAUTIONS

None

SECTION 10 - ADDITIONAL INFORMATION

Exuderm Hydrocolloid Dressing has passed all testing required for medical devices as outlined in the FDA Biocompatibility Guidelines for short-term devices in contact with breached or compromised skin.

The information provided in this Material Safety Data Sheet has been obtained from sources believed to be reliable.

Medline Industries, Inc. provides no warranties, either expressed or implied and assumes no responsibility for the accuracy or completeness of the data contained herein.

ISSUE DATE: 9-21-96
Revised: 10/31/01   Updated telephone information

(Courtesy of Medline Industries, Inc.; (800) MEDLINE)

TRANSPARENCY MASTER 43

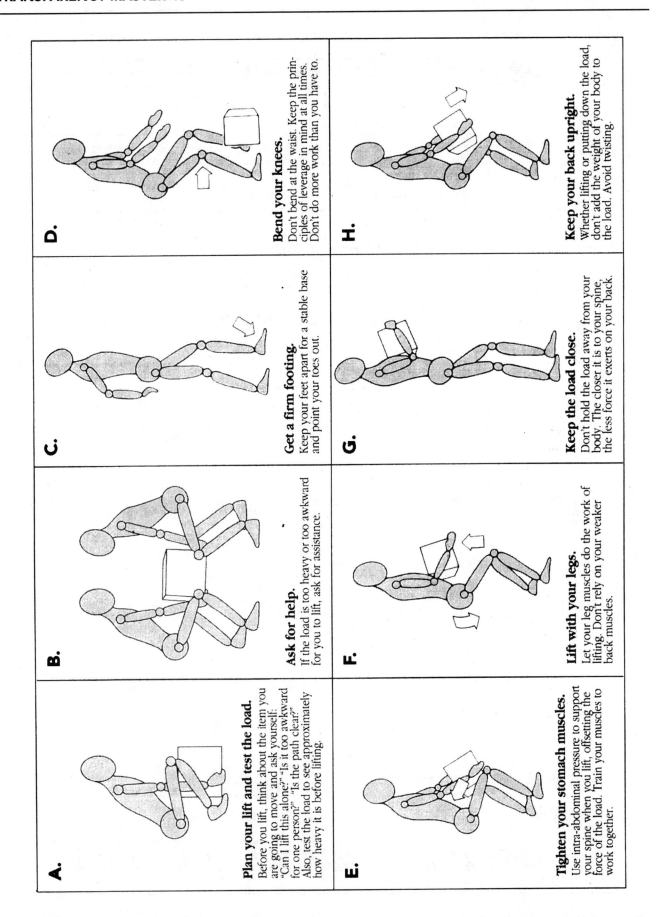

A.

Plan your lift and test the load.
Before you lift, think about the item you are going to move and ask yourself: "Can I lift this alone?" "Is it too awkward for one person?" "Is the path clear?" Also, test the load to see approximately how heavy it is before lifting.

B.

Ask for help.
If the load is too heavy or too awkward for you to lift, ask for assistance.

C.

Get a firm footing.
Keep your feet apart for a stable base and point your toes out.

D.

Bend your knees.
Don't bend at the waist. Keep the principles of leverage in mind at all times. Don't do more work than you have to.

E.

Tighten your stomach muscles.
Use intra-abdominal pressure to support your spine when you lift, offsetting the force of the load. Train your muscles to work together.

F.

Lift with your legs.
Let your leg muscles do the work of lifting. Don't rely on your weaker back muscles.

G.

Keep the load close.
Don't hold the load away from your body. The closer it is to your spine, the less force it exerts on your back.

H.

Keep your back upright.
Whether lifting or putting down the load, don't add the weight of your body to the load. Avoid twisting.

TRANSPARENCY MASTER 44   **SAMPLE GLASS THERMOMETER SCALES**

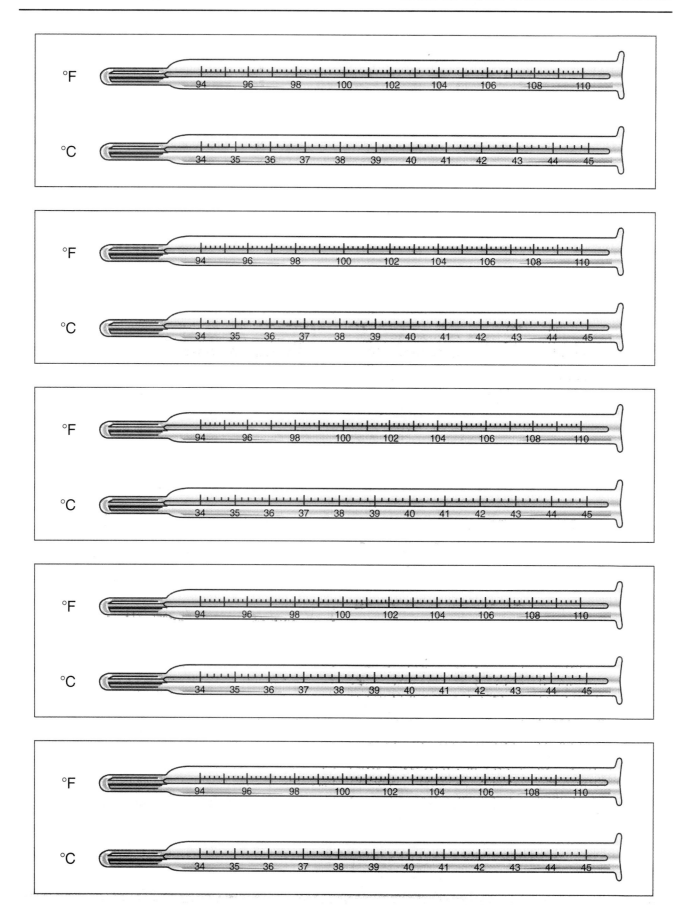

TRANSPARENCY MASTER 45   **PULSE SITES**

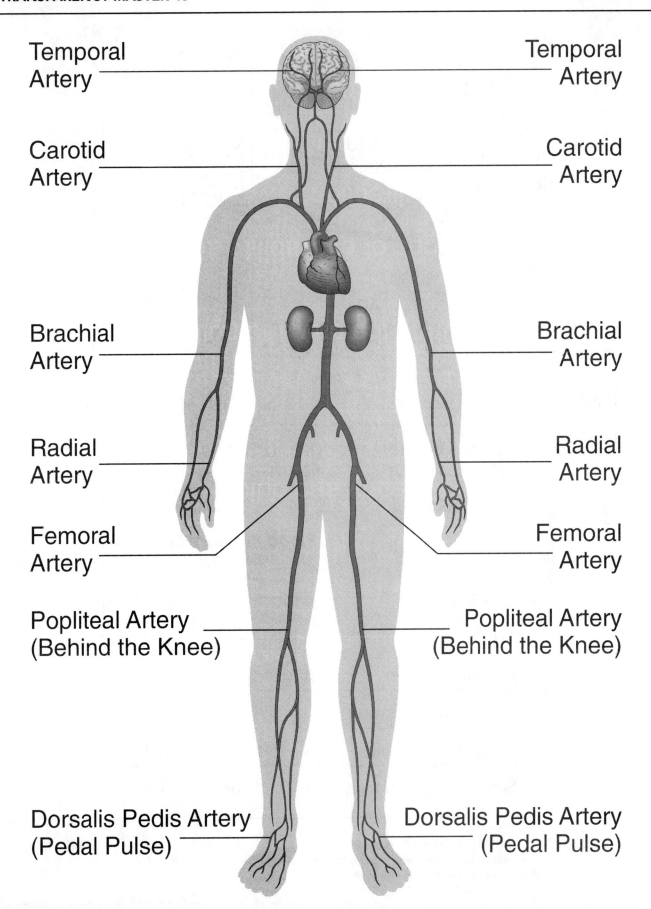

Temporal
Artery

Carotid
Artery

Brachial
Artery

Radial
Artery

Femoral
Artery

Popliteal Artery
(Behind the Knee)

Dorsalis Pedis Artery
(Pedal Pulse)

Temporal
Artery

Carotid
Artery

Brachial
Artery

Radial
Artery

Femoral
Artery

Popliteal Artery
(Behind the Knee)

Dorsalis Pedis Artery
(Pedal Pulse)

TRANSPARENCY MASTER 46   **UNDERSTANDING BLOOD PRESSURE**

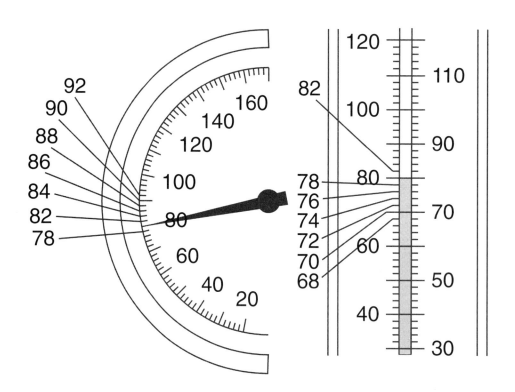

National Heart, Lung, and Blood Institute Blood Pressure Definitions 2003			
	Blood Pressure Level (mm Hg)		
Category	**Systolic**	*****	**Diastolic**
Normal	< 120	and	< 80
Prehypertension	120–139	or	< 80
High Blood Pressure			
Stage I Hypertension	140–159	or	90–99
Stage II Hypertension	≥ 160	or	≥ 100

< means less than
≥ means greater than or equal to

Source: National Heart, Lung, and Blood Institute, National Institutes of Health. 2003. For additional information, see http://www.nhlbi.nih.gov/hbp/index.html

TRANSPARENCY MASTER 47

SPHYGMOMANOMETER SCALES

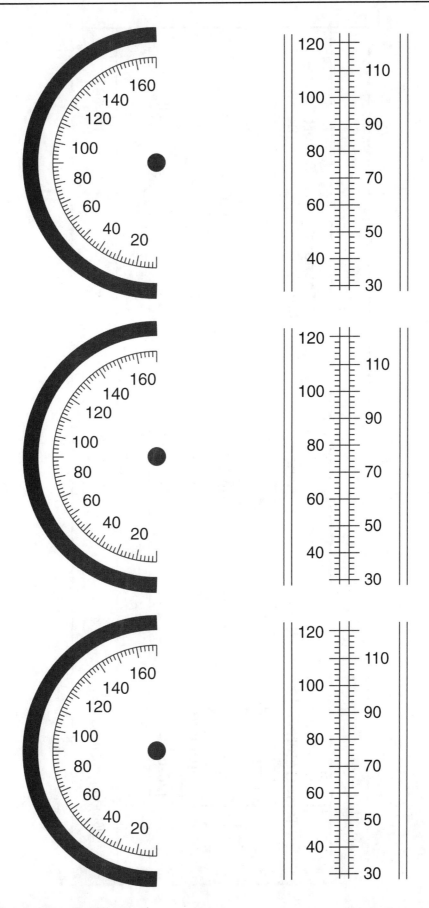

TRANSPARENCY MASTER 48   REPORTING ABNORMAL VITAL SIGNS

Normal Vital Sign Ranges for Adults

Temperature	Normal	Range	Report Changes Above	Report Changes Below
Axillary temperature	97.6°F	96.6–98.6°F	99°F	96°F
Oral temperature	98.6°F	97.6–99.6°F	100°F	97°F
Rectal temperature	99.6°F	98.6–100.6°F	101°F	98°F
Pulse	76	60–100	100	60
Respiration	16	14–20	20	12
Blood pressure	120/80	100/60–140/90	140/90	100/60

These values are guidelines only. Your instructor will inform you if reporting values are different in your facility.

TRANSPARENCY MASTER 49   **DETERMINING THE WEIGHT**

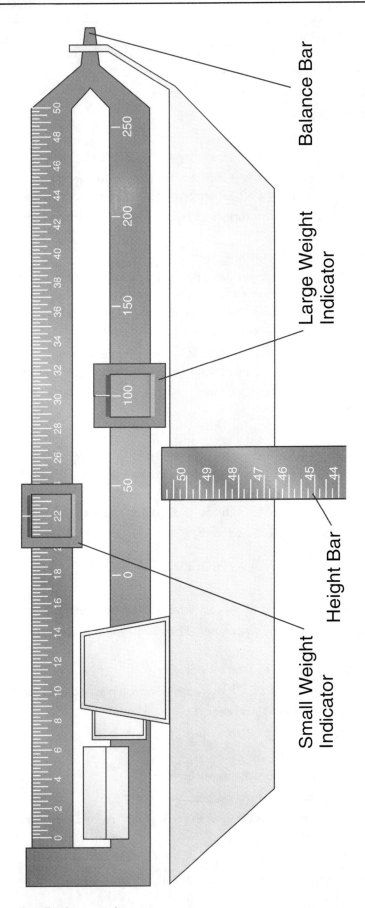

Balance Bar

Large Weight Indicator

Small Weight Indicator

Height Bar

TRANSPARENCY MASTER 50

**INITIAL PROCEDURE ACTIONS/
ENDING PROCEDURE ACTIONS**

INITIAL PROCEDURE ACTIONS

1. Wash your hands or use an alcohol-based hand cleaner.

2. Assemble supplies and equipment and bring to patient's room.

3. Knock on the door and identify yourself.

4. Identify the patient according to facility policy.

5. Ask visitors to leave the room and advise where they may wait (as desired by patient).

6. Explain what you are going to do and what is expected of the patient. Answer questions. (Maintain a dialogue with the patient during the procedure, and repeat explanations and instructions as needed.)

7. Provide privacy by closing the door, privacy curtain, and window curtain. (All three should be closed even if the patient is alone in the room.)

8. Wash your hands or use an alcohol-based hand cleaner.

9. Set up supplies and equipment at the bedside. (Use an overbed table, if possible, or other clean area. Cover with a clean underpad, according to nursing judgment, to provide a clean work surface.) Open packages. Position items for convenient reach. Position a container for soiled items so that you do not have to cross over clean items to access it.

10. Wash your hands or use an alcohol-based hand cleaner.

11. position the patient for the procedure. Support with pillows and props as needed. Place a clean underpad under the area, as needed. Make sure the patient is comfortable and able to maintain the position throughout the procedure.

12. Cover the patient with a bath blanket and drape for modesty. Fold the bath blanket back to expose only the area on which you will be working.

13. Raise the bed to a comfortable working height.

14. Apply gloves if contact with blood, moist body fluids (except sweat), secretions, excretions, or nonintact skin is likely.

15. Apply a gown if your uniform will have substantial contact with linen or other articles contaminated with blood, moist body fluid (except sweat), secretions, or excretions.

16. Apply a mask and eye protection if splashing of blood or moist body fluid is likely.

17. Lower the side rail on the side where you will be working.

ENDING PROCEDURE ACTIONS

1. Remove gloves.

2. Reposition the patient to ensure that he or she is comfortable and in good body alignment.

3. Replace the bed covers, then remove any drapes used. Place used drapes in plastic bag to discard in trash or soiled linen.

4. Elevate the side rails, if used, before leaving the bedside.

5. Remove other personal protective equipment, if worn, and discard in plastic bag or according to facility policy.

6. Wash your hands or use an alcohol-based hand cleaner.

7. Return the bed to the lowest horizontal position.

8. Open the privacy and window curtains.

9. Position the call signal and needed personal items within reach.

10. Wash your hands or use an alcohol-based hand cleaner.

11. Remove procedural trash and contaminated linen when you leave the room. Discard in appropriate container or location, according to facility policy.

12. Inform visitors that they may return to the room.

13. Document the procedure, your observations, and the patient's response.

TRANSPARENCY MASTER 51

FOOD GUIDE PYRAMID

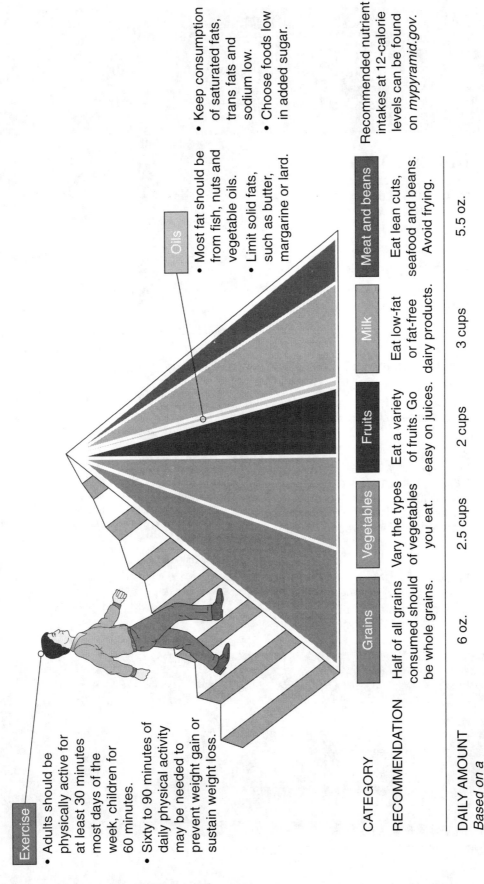

Exercise
- Adults should be physically active for at least 30 minutes most days of the week, children for 60 minutes.
- Sixty to 90 minutes of daily physical activity may be needed to prevent weight gain or sustain weight loss.

Oils
- Most fat should be from fish, nuts and vegetable oils.
- Limit solid fats, such as butter, margarine or lard.
- Keep consumption of saturated fats, trans fats and sodium low.
- Choose foods low in added sugar.

Recommended nutrient intakes at 12-calorie levels can be found on *mypyramid.gov*.

CATEGORY	Grains	Vegetables	Fruits	Milk	Meat and beans
RECOMMENDATION	Half of all grains consumed should be whole grains.	Vary the types of vegetables you eat.	Eat a variety of fruits. Go easy on juices.	Eat low-fat or fat-free dairy products.	Eat lean cuts, seafood and beans. Avoid frying.
DAILY AMOUNT *Based on a 2,000 calorie diet.*	6 oz.	2.5 cups	2 cups	3 cups	5.5 oz.

The USDA Food Guide Pyramid. The example food pyramid here was published in 2005. It is based on the average, 2,000-calorie-per-day diet. It contains 12 intake levels, ranging from 1,000 calories per day to 3,200 calories per day. The pyramid was designed to be individualized by each person to maintain a healthy weight. This can be easily done by visiting http://www.mypyramid.gov (Courtesy of United States Department of Agriculture)

TRANSPARENCY MASTER 52A   **DETERMINING MEAL INTAKE**

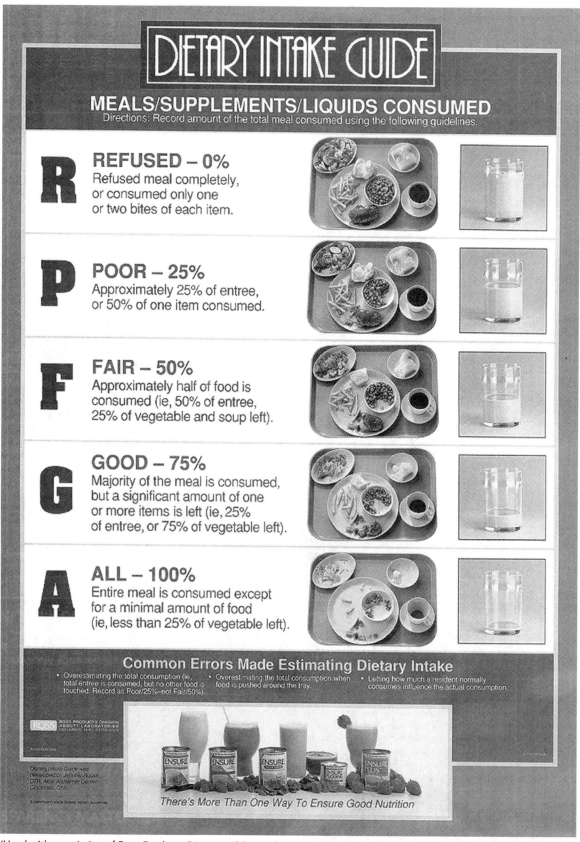

TRANSPARENCY MASTER 52B   **ALTERNATE METHOD OF DETERMINING MEAL INTAKE**

Alternate method of documenting meal intake

	Food Item	Percentage of Meal
Breakfast	eggs	35%
	eggs and bacon	40%
	eggs and sausage	45%
	toast *or* cereal	30%
	milk	20%
	fruit juice	15%
Dinner and Supper	meat group, including eggs, main dish, legumes	50%
	fruit group, including dessert items	15%
	bread or cereal group	10%
	vegetable group	15%
	fluids	10%

Alternate method of documenting meal intake

Breakfast

Egg, cheese or cottage cheese	50%
Hot or cold cereal	30%
Bread	10%
Bacon, ham or sausage	10%
Total	100%

Occasionally, a patient will request no protein foods (eggs, meat, cheese, cottage cheese) at breakfast. Please reassign the percentages to the other items on the tray and document accordingly.

Lunch and Supper

Meat, egg, cheese, or cottage cheese	40%
Starchy vegetable	20%
Vegetable or salad	20%
Bread	10%
Dessert	10%
Total	100%

The meat and starchy vegetables may be combined in some dishes, such as casseroles. If so, add the point values for these items together to total 60%. Sandwiches are also 60% because the two bread slices are the starchy vegetable. An additional bread item such as crackers may also be served at the meal.

TRANSPARENCY MASTER 53   **CALORIE/PROTEIN SUMMARY CHART**

Diet _____

CALORIE/PROTEIN SUMMARY

PATIENT _____   ROOM # _____

DAY 1					DAY 2					DAY 3				
DATE ___/___/___					DATE ___/___/___					DATE ___/___/___				
	% 0–25	% 25–50	% 50–75	% 75–100		% 0–25	% 25–50	% 50–75	% 75–100		% 0–25	% 25–50	% 50–75	% 75–100
Breakfast					**Breakfast**					**Breakfast**				
Meat					Meat					Meat				
Milk					Milk					Milk				
Fruit					Fruit					Fruit				
Starch					Starch					Starch				
Fat					Fat					Fat				
Other					Other					Other				
AM Supp.					AM Supp.					AM Supp.				
Noon Meal					**Noon Meal**					**Noon Meal**				
Meat					Meat					Meat				
Milk					Milk					Milk				
Juice					Juice					Juice				
Starch					Starch					Starch				
Vegetable					Vegetable					Vegetable				
Bread					Bread					Bread				
Fat					Fat					Fat				
Dessert					Dessert					Dessert				
Other					Other					Other				
PM Supp.					PM Supp.					PM Supp.				
Evening Meal					**Evening Meal**					**Evening Meal**				
Meat					Meat					Meat				
Milk					Milk					Milk				
Juice					Juice					Juice				
Starch					Starch					Starch				
Vegetable					Vegetable					Vegetable				
Bread					Bread					Bread				
Fat					Fat					Fat				
Dessert					Dessert					Dessert				
Other					Other					Other				
PM Supp.					PM Supp.					PM Supp.				
Total Kcal					**Total Kcal**					**Total Kcal**				
Total Pro					**Total Pro**					**Total Pro**				
Avg. for 3 days Kcal:						**Avg. Protein for 3 days:**								

PLEASE RETURN COMPLETED FORM TO NUTRITION CARE MANAGER

TRANSPARENCY MASTER 54   **INTAKE AND OUTPUT CHART**

INTAKE AND OUTPUT

Room:

Name:

Date:

Instructions:

Intake	Output	Intake	Output
Total		Total	

Drinking Glass........240 mL   Full Water Pitcher...950 mL   Milk Carton..............236 mL   Jello..............120 mL
Styrofoam Cup.......180 mL   Coffee or Teapot.....300 mL   Soup Bowl.............250 mL   Ice Cream Cup......90 mL
Juice Glass (small)..100 mL   Coffee Cup............150 mL   Soup Cup...............100 mL   Creamer............50 mL
Juice Glass (large)..240 mL

FOLEY CATHETER DRAINAGE: (Circle the following when applicable)

Color: Yellow   Amber   Brown   Red

Appearance: Cloudy   Clear   Sediment   Mucus   Bloody

Abdomen Distended   Catheter Irrigated   Catheter Changed

24 hour INTAKE _____

24 hour OUTPUT _____

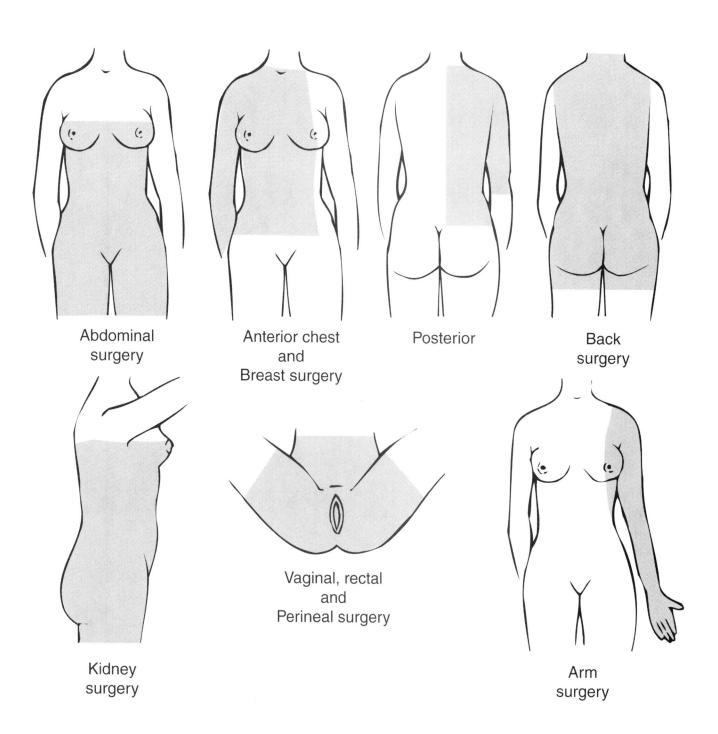

Abdominal
surgery

Anterior chest
and
Breast surgery

Posterior

Back
surgery

Kidney
surgery

Vaginal, rectal
and
Perineal surgery

Arm
surgery

SURGICAL CHECKLIST

- ■ Admission sheet

- ■ Surgical consent

- ■ Sterilization consent (if necessary)

- ■ Consultation sheet (if necessary)

- ■ History and physical

- ■ Lab reports (pregnancy test if necessary)

- ■ Surgery prep done and charted, if required

- ■ Latest TPR and blood pressure charted

- ■ Preoperative medication has been given and charted
  (if required)

- ■ Identification band on patient

- ■ Fingernail polish and makeup removed

- ■ Metallic objects removed (wedding band may be taped)

- ■ Valuables secured

- ■ Dentures removed

- ■ Other prostheses removed (glasses, contact lens, hearing aid,
  artificial limb, eye, wig, or hairpiece)

- ■ Bath blanket and head cap in place

- ■ Bed in high position and side rails up after pre-op medication
  is given

- ■ Patient has voided

- ■ Dentures removed

- ■ Catheter bag emptied and action documented

- Preoccupation with constipation
- Flatulence
- Bad taste in the mouth
- Burning tongue
- Vague oral discomforts associated with dentures
- Burning on urination
- Pain in lower abdomen
- Crying spells
- Trouble sleeping
- Loss of appetite
- Fatigue
- Headaches
- Backaches
- Stiff joints
- Apathy
- Inability to concentrate
- Lethargy
- Agitation
- Hallucinations
- Suicidal threats

EMOTIONAL RESPONSES TO DYING

Stages of Grief	Response of the Nursing Assistant
Denial	Reflect patient's statements, but try not to confirm or deny the fact that the patient is dying. **Example:** *"The lab tests can't be right—I don't have cancer."* *"It must have been difficult for you to learn the results of your tests."*
Anger	Understand the source of the patient's anger. Provide understanding and support. Listen. Try to meet reasonable needs and demands quickly. **Example:** *"This food is terrible—not fit to eat."* *"Let me see if I can find something that would appeal to you more."*
Bargaining	If it is possible to meet the patient's requests, do so. Listen attentively. **Example:** *"If only God will spare me this, I'll go to church every week."* *"Would you like a visit from your clergyperson?"*
Depression	Avoid clichés that dismiss the patient's depression ("It could be worse—you could be in more pain"). Be caring and supporting. Let the patient know that it is all right to be depressed. **Example:** *"There just isn't any sense in going on."* *"I understand you are feeling very depressed."*
Acceptance	Do not assume that, because the patient has accepted death, she or he is unafraid, or that she or he does not need emotional support. Listen attentively and be supportive and caring. **Example:** *"I feel so alone."* *"I am here with you. Would you like to talk?"*

TRANSPARENCY MASTER 59   **SIGNS AND SYMPTOMS OF DISORIENTATION**

- Inability to think clearly and quickly

- Bewilderment

- Faulty memory

- Drowsiness during the day and agitation during the night

- Alternating periods of excitability and drowsiness

- Inability to follow directions

- Misinterpretation of stimuli

- Lack of safety awareness

- Incoherent speech

- Illusions

- Delusions

- Hallucinations

TRANSPARENCY MASTER 60   **COMMON SITES FOR SKIN BREAKDOWN — PATIENT IN BED**

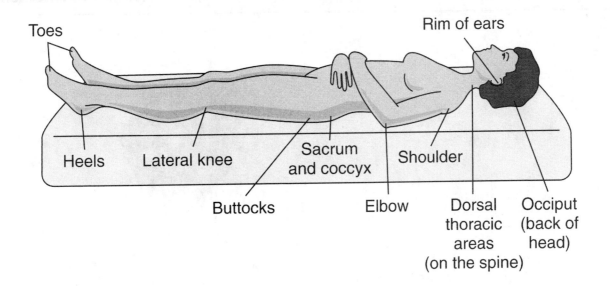

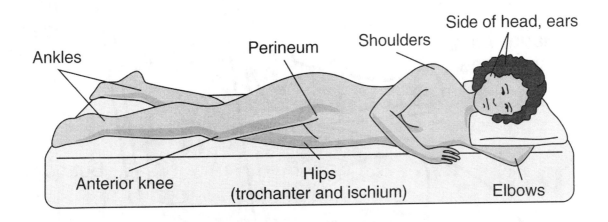

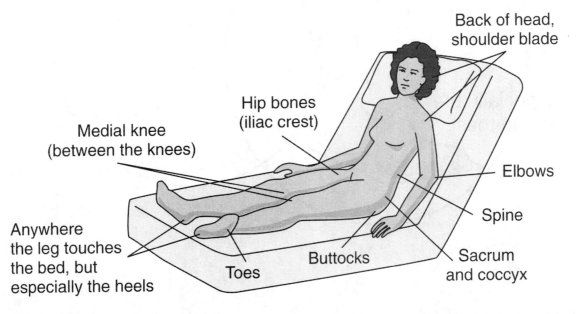

TRANSPARENCY MASTER 61

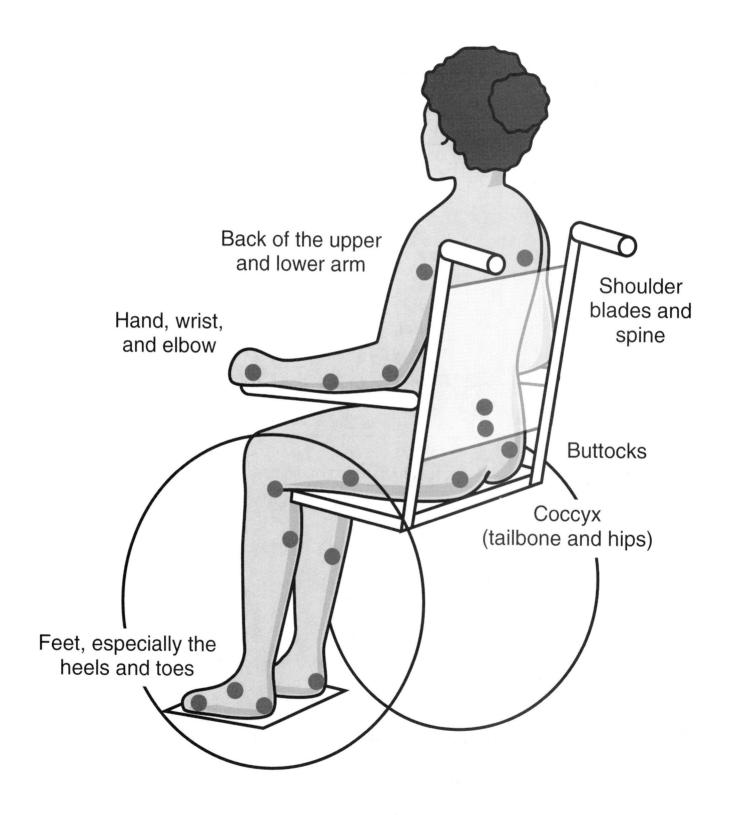

Back of the upper and lower arm

Hand, wrist, and elbow

Shoulder blades and spine

Buttocks

Coccyx (tailbone and hips)

Feet, especially the heels and toes

TRANSPARENCY MASTER 62   **SHEARING FORCES**

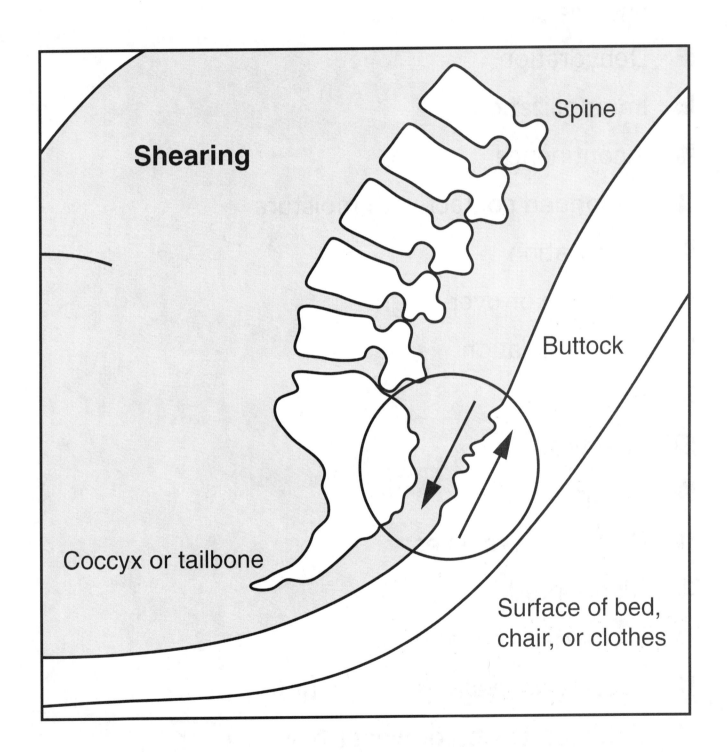

Shearing

Spine

Buttock

Coccyx or tailbone

Surface of bed, chair, or clothes

- Poor nutrition, eats less than half of meals and snacks
- Dehydration
- Immobilization
- Incontinence
- Prolonged contact with moisture
- Debilitation
- Very thin or overweight
- Poor circulation
- Edema
- Infection
- Aging
- Diminished reflexes
- Disoriented
- Prolonged pressure
- Subject to shearing and friction
- Confined to bed or wheelchair
- Discolored, thin, torn, or swollen skin

PRESSURE ULCER STAGES

Stage 1: Nonblanchable erythema of intact skin, the heralding lesion of skin ulceration. In individuals with darker skin, discoloration of the skin, warmth, edema, induration, or hardness may also be indicators. The lesion is not always round. Some pressure ulcers are irregular in shape.

Stage 2: Partial-thickness skin loss involving epidermis, dermis, or both. The ulcer is superficial and presents clinically as an abrasion, blister, or shallow crater. The skin surrounding this ulcer is tender and inflamed and at very high risk for further breakdown.

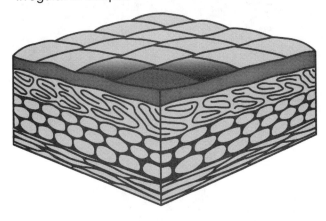

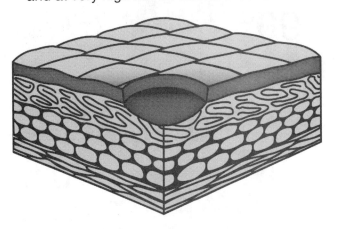

Stage 3: Full-thickness skin loss involving damage to or necrosis of subcutaneous tissue that may extend down to, but not through, underlying fascia. The ulcer presents clinically as a deep crater with or without undermining of adjacent tissue. Although the diameter of this pressure ulcer is not large, the patient has experienced full-thickness skin loss.

Stage 4: Full-thickness skin loss with extensive destruction, tissue necrosis, or damage to muscle, bone, or supporting structures (e.g., tendon, joint capsule). Undermining and sinus tracts also may be associated with Stage 4 pressure ulcers.

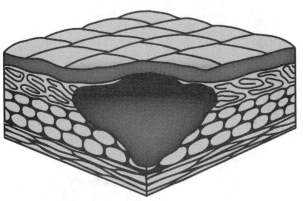

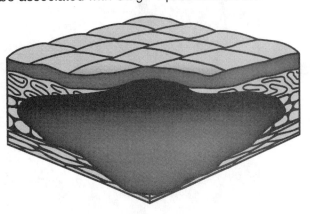

Avoidable and **Unavoidable** Pressure Ulcers [State Operations Manual. §483.25(c)]

- **Avoidable** means that the patient developed a pressure ulcer and that the facility did not do one or more of the following: evaluate the patient's clinical condition and pressure ulcer risk factors; define and implement interventions that are consistent with patient needs, patient goals, and recognized standards of practice; monitor and evaluate that impact of the interventions; or revise the interventions as appropriate.
- **Unavoidable** means that the patient developed a pressure ulcer even though the facility had evaluated the patient's clinical condition and pressure ulcer risk factors; defined and implemented interventions that are consistent with patient needs, goals, and recognized standards of practice; monitored and evaluated the impact of the interventions; and revised the approaches as appropriate.

The pressure ulcer stages reflect the amount of tissue destruction.

TRANSPARENCY MASTER 65A

DEGREES OF ELEVATION

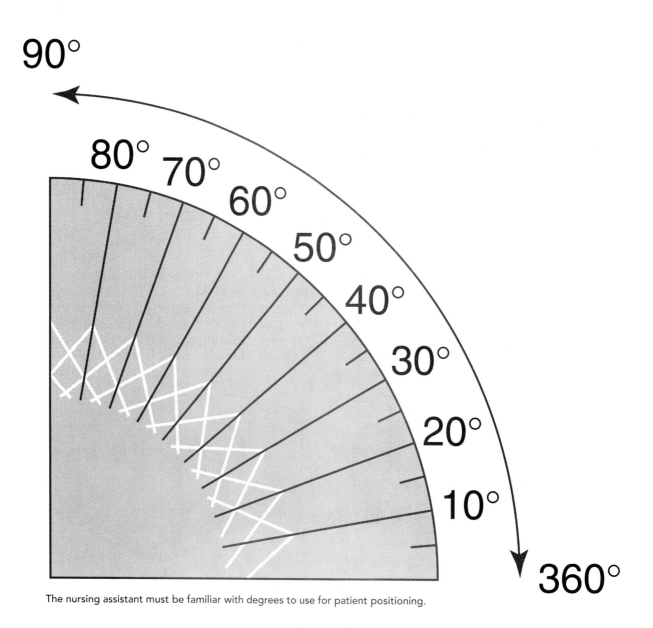

The nursing assistant must be familiar with degrees to use for patient positioning.

Range-of-Motion Terminology

- **Abduction** is moving an extremity *away from* the body.

- **Adduction** is moving an extremity *toward* the body.

- **Circumduction** is a circular movement of a joint, such as the thumb or wrist.

- **Dorsal flexion,** or **dorsiflexion,** is pulling the foot upward toward the head.

- **Eversion** is turning a joint outward.

- **Extension** is straightening a joint.

- **External rotation** is turning a joint outward *away from* the median line.

- **Flexion** is bending a joint.

- **Hyperextension** is gentle, excessive extension of a joint, slightly past the point of resistance.

- **Internal rotation** is turning a joint *inward toward* the median line.

- **Inversion** is turning a joint inward.

- **Medial** pertains to or is situated toward the midline of the body.

- **Median** means situated in the median plane or in the midline of the body.

- **Opposition** is touching each of the fingers against the thumb.

- **Palmar flexion** is the act of bending the hand down toward the palm.

- **Plantar flexion** is bending the foot downward, away from the body.

- **Pronation** is moving a joint to face downward.

- **Radial deviation** is turning the forearm toward the radius.

- **Retraction** is drawing back, away from the body.

- **Rotation** means moving a joint in, out, and around.

- **Supination** is moving a joint so it faces upward.

- **Ulnar deviation** is turning the forearm toward the ulna.

Terminology used for range-of-motion exercises

TRANSPARENCY MASTER 66   **IMPORTANT OBSERVATIONS OF PATIENTS WITH DIABETES**

Inadequate food intake

Eating food not allowed on diet

Refusal of meals, supplements, or snacks

Nausea, vomiting, or diarrhea

Inadequate fluid intake

Excessive activity

Complaints of dizziness, shakiness, racing heart

Blood sugar values outside of normal range

Signs and Symptoms of Hyperglycemia	**Signs and Symptoms of Hypoglycemia**
Gradual onset	*Rapid onset*
Nausea, vomiting	Complaints of hunger, weakness, dizziness, shakiness
Weakness	Skin cold, moist, clammy, pale
Headache	Rapid, shallow respirations
Full, bounding pulse	Nervousness and excitement
Fruity smell to breath	Rapid pulse
Hot, dry, flushed skin	Normal blood pressure
Labored respirations	Normal to rapid respirations
Low blood pressure	May complain of numb lips and tongue
Drowsiness	May act intoxicated, have tremors, convulse
Progressively worsening mental status or lethargy	Unconsciousness
Mental confusion	No sugar in the urine
Unconsciousness	Low blood sugar by fingerstick
Sugar in the urine	
High blood sugar by fingerstick	

TRANSPARENCY MASTER 67 PROGRESSION OF A FECAL IMPACTION

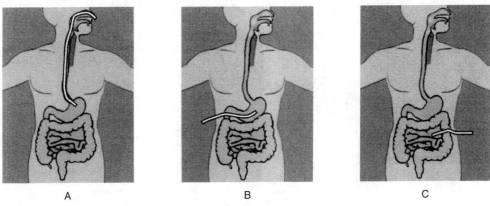

Enteral feeding methods. (A) Nasogastric (NG) feeding. (B) Gastrostomy (GT) feeding. (C) Jejunostomy (JT) feeding.

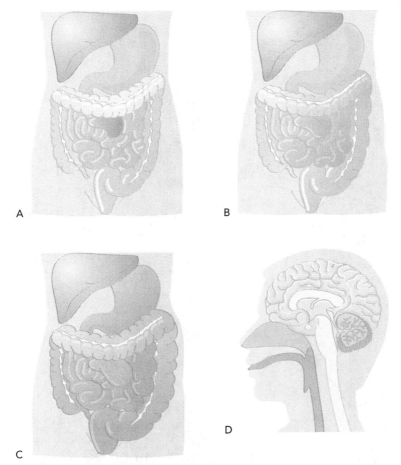

Progression of a fecal impaction, a life-threatening condition: (A) A fecal impaction blocks the rectum. The rectum and sigmoid colon become enlarged. (B) The colon continues to enlarge. (C) Fecal material gradually fills the colon. Digested and undigested food back up into the small intestines and stomach. The patient has signs and symptoms of acute illness, including lethargy, distention, constipation, and pain that is dull and cramping. (D) The entire system is full, and the patient vomits fecal material. The feces are commonly aspirated into the lungs.

TRANSPARENCY MASTER 68

SITES OF CONTAMINATION ON CLOSED URINARY DRAINAGE SYSTEM

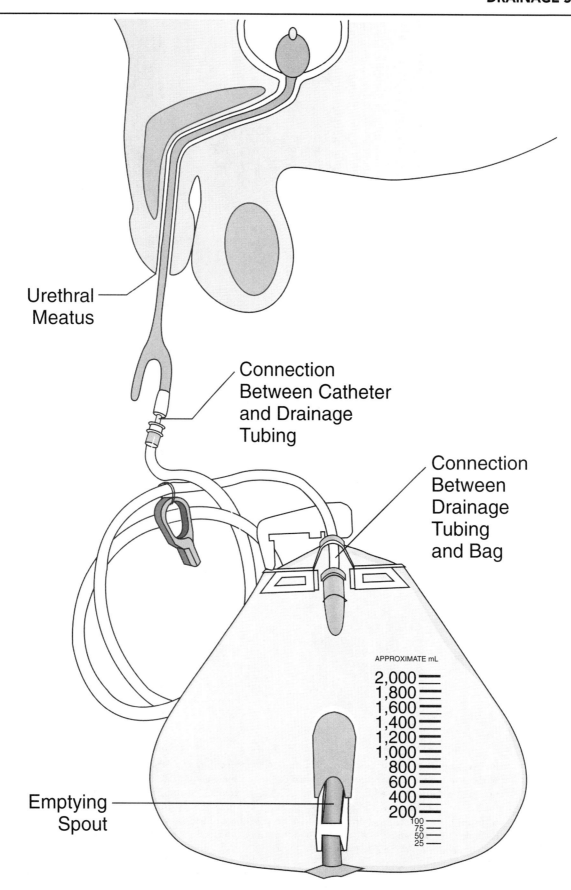

Urethral Meatus

Connection Between Catheter and Drainage Tubing

Connection Between Drainage Tubing and Bag

APPROXIMATE mL

2,000
1,800
1,600
1,400
1,200
1,000
800
600
400
200
100
75
50
25

Emptying Spout

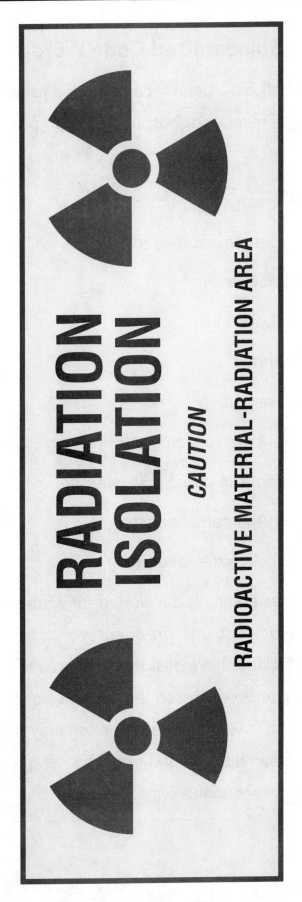

Standardized Code Words

The following code words have been recommended for standardization and have been adopted by a number of hospitals and long-term care facilities.

- Code Red: Fire

- Code Blue: Medical emergency—adult

- Code White: Medical emergency—pediatric

- Code Pink: Infant abduction

- Code Purple: Child abduction

- Code Yellow: Bomb threat

- Code Gray: Combative person

- Code Silver: Person with a weapon and/or hostage situation

- Code Orange: Hazardous material spill/release

- Code Triage Internal: An internal disaster

- Code Triage External: An external disaster

Please note: *This list was originally developed for acute care hospitals, and there is no code word for a patient or resident who elopes (wanders away). Some long-term care facilities have designated this as a "Code Brown." This omission was probably an oversight, so the code designation for an elopement may change in the future, or the color designation may be different in your facility. Facilities have been discouraged from changing the designation of the colors listed here, to prevent confusion.*

TRANSPARENCY MASTER 71A

POTENTIAL AREAS OF ENTRAPMENT

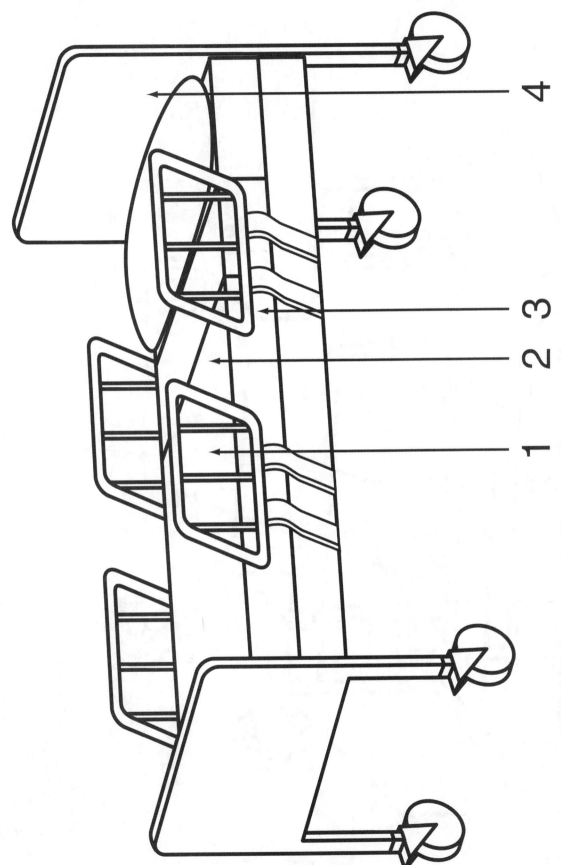

Entrapment between the mattress and side rails occurs in one of the following ways: (numbered 1 to 4 in the diagram):

1. through the bars of an individual side rail
2. through the space between split side rails
3. between the side rail and mattress
4. between the headboard or footboard, side rail, and mattress

TRANSPARENCY MASTER 71B   **ZONES OF ENTRAPMENT**

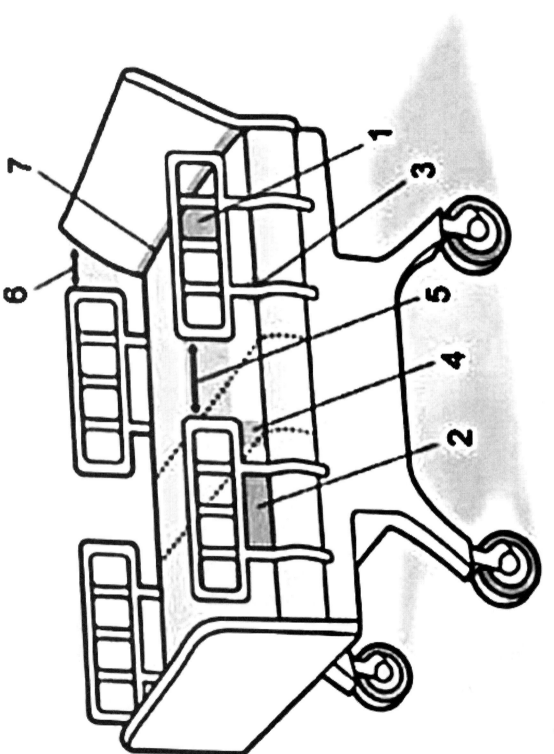

Potential areas of entrapment:

Zone 1—Within the rail

Zone 2—Between the top of the compressed mattress and the bottom of the rail, between rail supports

Zone 3—Between the rail and the mattress

Zone 4—Between the top of the compressed mattress and the bottom of the rail, at the end of the rail

Zone 5—Between the split bed rails

Zone 6—Between the end of the rail and the side edge of the headboard or footboard

Zone 7—Between the headboard or footboard and the end of the mattress

TRANSPARENCY MASTER 72   **IMPLANTED MEDICATION PUMP**

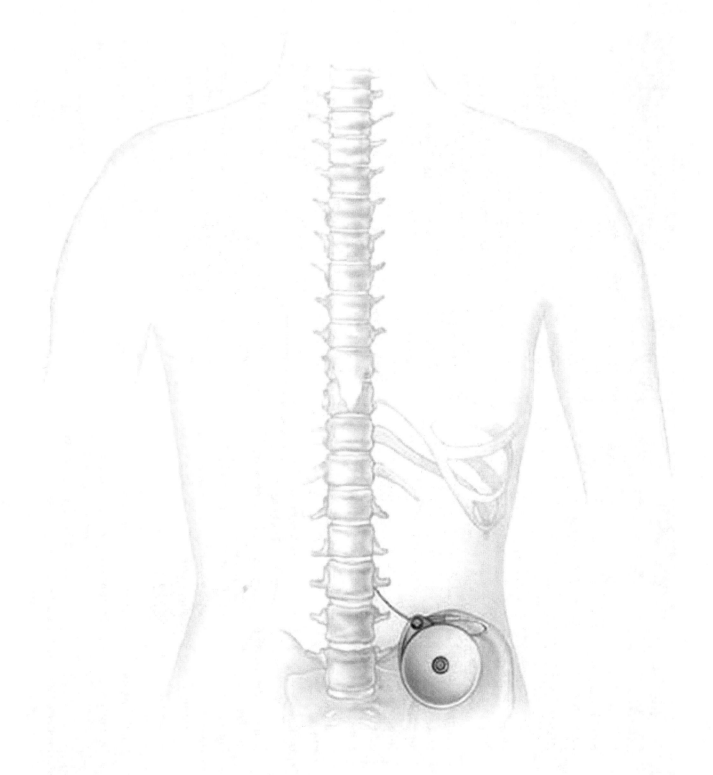

Guidelines for Documentation on the Computerized Medical Record

- Remember that audit trails track the computer, user, date, time, and exactly which medical records are accessed, based on your user identification data.

- The electronic record must note whether manual records are also being used. If this is the case (such as during a storm or electronic system failure), the records must cross-reference each other. Most hospitals have policies, such as reverting to paper documentation if the computer is down for a designated period of time.

- Make sure you enter the patient's correct identification code.

- Turn or position the monitor so it is not visible to others.

- Select a password that is not easily deciphered.

- Do not give your identification code or password to others.

- Do not allow others to find your password. Do not write it down or leave it where it is easily found, such as under the mouse pad, keyboard, or in an electronic file. Regularly change your password. Change it immediately if you suspect it has been compromised.

- Never let someone look over your shoulder when you are signing in or accessing patient data.

- Access only information that you are authorized to obtain.

- Document only in areas you are authorized to use.

- Do not print information unnecessarily. Destroy printed copies that are not part of the permanent record. Placing them in the wastebasket is prohibited in many facilities because of privacy laws.

- Never delete information from the electronic medical record.

- Many computer programs place expert reminders, messages, and/or error codes on the screen. These may be annoying, but they are important. Read them and follow the directions.

- The procedure for late-entry and addendum documentation will be different from a narrative system. Know and follow your facility policies for this type of charting.

- Electronic documentation must be signed by the person giving care. Your facility will have a procedure for doing electronic signatures. These are valid as long as they are accessible only to the person identified by that signature.

- Protect patient data transmitted electronically, such as by using an e-mail encryption service. Never transmit nonsecure, identifiable patient information.

- Always log off when you have finished using the computer.

- Wash your hands after using the computer. Many people use it, so the keyboard is a huge potential source of cross-contamination. If your facility uses plastic keyboard covers, routinely disinfect the cover with the recommended product. Avoid products containing alcohol when cleaning the computer and accessories. Use only products that are recommended for the surface being cleaned.

- Stay current. Attend continuing education programs to learn how to maximize your use of computerized charting and information systems.